HEALTH AND ILLNESS

A CROSS-CULTURAL ENCYCLOPEDIA

ENCYCLOPEDIAS OF THE HUMAN EXPERIENCE

David Levinson, Series Editor

HEALTH AND ILLNESS

A CROSS-CULTURAL ENCYCLOPEDIA

David Levinson
Laura Gaccione

ABC-CLIO

Santa Barbara, California
Denver, Colorado
Oxford, England

Library of Congress Cataloging-in-Publication Data

Levinson, David, 1947–
    Health and Illness: a cross-cultural encyclopedia / David
Levinson, Laura Gaccione.
      p. cm. — (Encyclopedias of the human experience)
    Includes bibliographical references and index.
    Summary: Offers information on a variety of health-related topics,
from acupuncture and faith healing to reflexology and yoga,
emphasizing traditional and alternative approaches.
    1. Alternative medicine—Encyclopedias, Juvenile. 2. Traditional
medicine—Encyclopedias, Juvenile. [Alternative medicine—
Encyclopedias. Traditional medicine—Encyclopedias.]
I. Gaccione, Laura. II. Title. III. Series.
R733.L477   1997   610'.3—DC21   97-29638

ISBN 0-87436-876-6 (alk. paper)

03 02 01 00 99 98   10 9 8 7 6 5 4 3 2 (cloth)

ABC-CLIO, Inc.
130 Cremona Drive, P.O. Box 1911
Santa Barbara, California 93116-1911

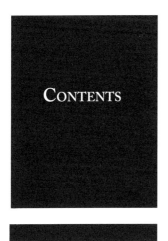

Contents

CONTENTS

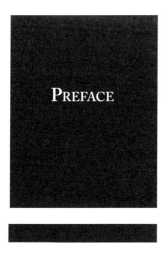

PREFACE

This volume provides information about three different though interrelated types of health care systems—biomedicine, alternative and complementary, and traditional. Biomedicine, meaning scientific (or "conventional") health care or medicine is what most people mean when they talk about *medicine.* It is the dominant approach to health care in the United States and other Western nations and with varying degrees of success is being transferred to non-Western nations and cultures around the world. Alternative and complementary health care refers to approaches that are used in Western and some non-Western nations in place of or as adjuncts to biomedicine. Some of these, such as homeopathy and natural medicine, are *alternatives* to biomedicine in that practitioners argue that they can prevent or cure the same, or at least many of the same, ailments attended to by biomedicine. Other approaches in this category are more accurately described as *complementary,* as they are not seen as replacements to biomedicine but as approaches or techniques that will make scientific ones more effective. For example, visual imagery and relaxation techniques might help speed the recovery of a person who has undergone major surgery.

The third category of health care systems covered here is what we call *traditional,* although it is called by other labels, including non-Western, indigenous, folk, and primitive. This category includes medical systems that developed mainly in non-Western cultures and that continue to be used in many cultures, often alongside biomedicine. There is, of course, some overlap between the three categories. Some traditional systems or techniques have been incorporated into both biomedicine and alternative medicine. For example, many drugs used in biomedicine are derived from plants that were first identified as medically useful by indigenous peoples. Similarly, the Ayurvedic medical system of Hindu India is an indigenous system, although aspects of it have now been adapted for use in Western cultures. In addition to these three approaches, we also cover specific health care issues and disorders in non-Western cultures. Examination of these points to the often close relationship between disease and culture.

The major reason we have chosen to cover these three major approaches to health and healing in this one volume is because in the modern world they do coexist and in many societies people seeking health care often have a choice among approaches and techniques based on all three. Despite predictions by some health care planners that biomedicine would eventually replace alternative and traditional approaches all around the world, by the 1990s that has not happened. Nor does it seem likely to happen in the near future. In most cultures—including the United States—people often pick and choose among these different approaches until they find the one that works best for them. A decision on which approach works best is based on criteria that involve a number of considerations for most people—effectiveness of the treatment, their beliefs about what causes illness, the seriousness of the illness, and the cost of treatment. For most people in most cultures, health care is a complicated matter.

An interesting issue concerning health care across cultures is the role of Western medicine, which is now available, although sometimes in very limited and primitive form, all around the world. Rather than replacing other approaches to treatment, an argument can be made that the spread of biomedicine has instead actually stimulated the development of alternative approaches, as the number of these available has mushroomed in the last several decades. Perhaps a more reasoned argument would suggest that it is not biomedicine itself that has encouraged people to look elsewhere but rather the effectiveness of biomedicine in treating some types of illness such as infectious disease and its lack of attention to diseases or discomforts that are not life-threatening. It is for these types of illnesses that people often seek alternative cures and for which they look to other cultures for effective treatments.

While there are numerous differences among these three approaches, many of which are documented throughout this volume, perhaps the major difference is how each views the basic cause of disease. In biomedicine, disease is viewed as the result of either external agents, such as viruses or bacteria, or internal forces, such as genetic factors or aging, that disrupt the normal functioning of the body. Treatment centers on identifying the specific cause, eliminating it, and relieving symptoms. In alternative approaches the causal agent is often seen as any factor—internal or external—that upsets the normal balance within the body. Although all alternative approaches are based on theories about disease causation, diagnosis does not focus on pinpointing a specific virus or bacteria. Treatment focuses instead on restoring the proper balance so that the body can heal itself. In most traditional systems, the causal agent is usually believed to be some supernatural force that seeks to cause injury, illness, or death, and treatment focuses on identifying the agent and ending its influence. A second major difference among the three approaches is

the means that are used to determine what causes illness and what treatments are effective. In biomedicine, the scientific approach is used to develop and test theories about the cause of illness and illnesses and to test the effectiveness of possible treatments. Thus, the treatments that are used are the ones that have been shown through experimentation to be the most effective ones for that illness and that patient. In alternative healing, there is far less reliance on the scientific method. Instead, choice of treatment is often based on a combination of the healer's experience and the patient's preferences. In traditional systems, ideas about the cause and treatment of illness are not developed in isolation from other ideas about the world. Rather, beliefs about disease causation and treatment are typically enmeshed in a religious belief system and reflect broad and deep beliefs about the natural and supernatural worlds and the place of humans in them.

Although we cover all three major health care approaches in this volume, our emphasis is on the alternative and traditional approaches. This is because, unlike biomedicine, both are clearly cross-cultural. Traditional approaches are by definition cross-cultural, and most alternative approaches are cross-cultural in the sense that key elements are borrowed from non-Western cultures. That many of these key elements have been redefined to appeal to a Western audience does not mean that they are now Western, although in their Westernized form they would probably not be meaningful to people in the cultures where they first developed.

In gathering the information for this volume, we have relied mainly on four sources of information. First, for the alternative approaches, we have reviewed the very large and ever-expanding literature on these topics. There are thousands of books devoted to all the different alternative approaches, a dozen or so general alternative health encyclopedias, many magazines, and much information made available by advocacy organizations.

While we have not looked at everything available, we have reviewed a great deal of material, a process made easier by our living in a community that has emerged as a major international center for alternative health care. With some key exceptions, it is important to note that this alternative literature is advocacy literature in that it is written by practitioners, patients, or others who strongly believe in the approach or technique they write about. It works for the writer's patients or worked for the writer and they want to share that with other people. In using this information, we have tried not to be advocates and instead have tried simply to describe the approaches and review claims for their effectiveness. Regardless of what their advocates say, we do not recommend any treatments to readers of this book. To round out the information provided in these publications we have also tried some treatments ourselves and have interviewed providers of various alternative approaches.

Our two other major sources of information cover traditional health and healing. The first is the ethnographic record—books, articles, doctoral dissertations, reports, etc., whose purpose is to describe the way of life of a particular culture. Most general ethnography contains information about health care in the culture being described. To some extent, we have relied on the older ethnography because it describes the culture before it was influenced by Western culture and thus gives a clearer picture of the indigenous health care system. Second, we have consulted the more recent literature of medical anthropology, which focuses specifically on health care in non-Western cultures.

As noted above, our goal is to describe health and illness around the world, with an emphasis on health care in non-Western cultures and the use of non-Western health care approaches in Western cultures. This book is descriptive. It is about what people know and do around the world about their health. It is not a health care manual and we offer no advice about health care in general or for any specific illness or treatment.

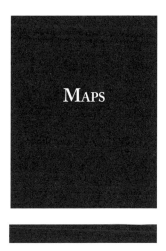

MAPS

The following maps show approximate locations
of the cultures mentioned in the text.

Africa and the Middle East

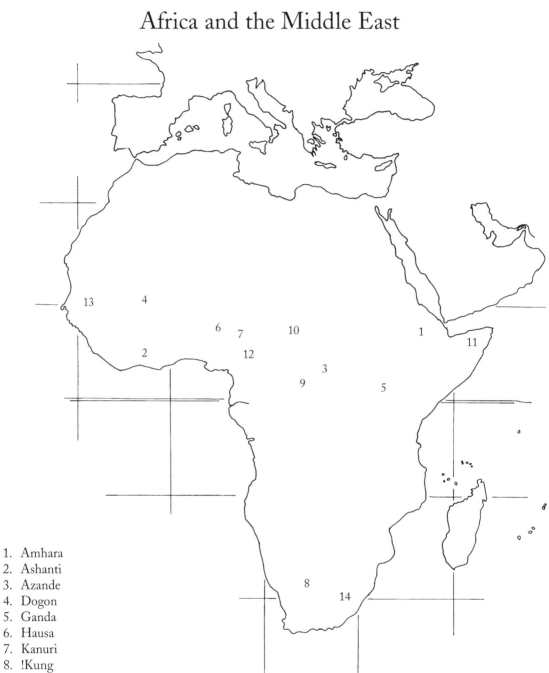

1. Amhara
2. Ashanti
3. Azande
4. Dogon
5. Ganda
6. Hausa
7. Kanuri
8. !Kung
9. Mbuti
10. Sara
11. Somali
12. Tiv
13. Wolof
14. Zulu

Central and South America

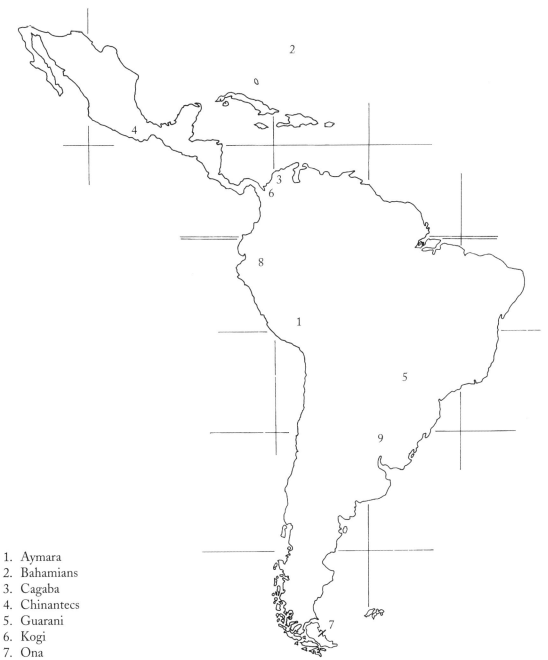

1. Aymara
2. Bahamians
3. Cagaba
4. Chinantecs
5. Guarani
6. Kogi
7. Ona
8. Quichua
9. Toba

Europe and Asia

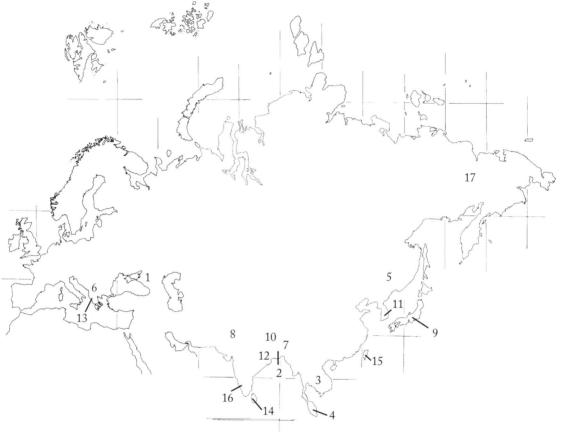

1. Abkhazians
2. Bengali
3. Central Thai
4. Chewong
5. Chinese
6. Gypsies
7. Garo
8. Hunza
9. Japanese
10. Khasi
11. Koreans
12. Santal
13. Serbs
14. Sinhalese
15. Taiwanese
16. Tamil
17. Yakut

North America

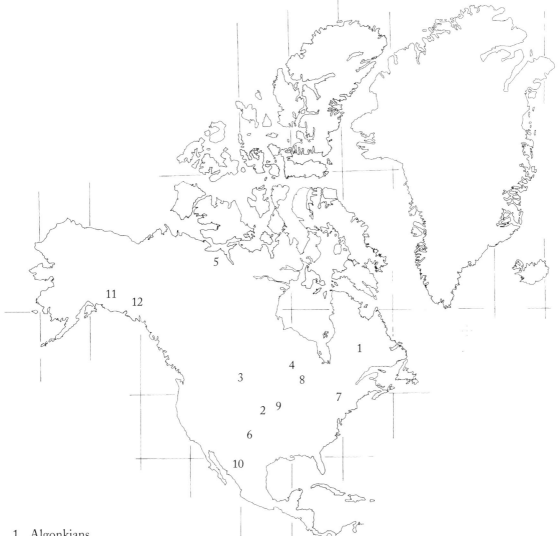

1. Algonkians
2. Arapaho
3. Blackfoot
4. Chippewa
5. Copper Inuit
6. Hopi
7. Iroquois
8. Ojibwa
9. Pawnee
10. Tarahumara
11. Tenino
12. Tlingit

Oceania

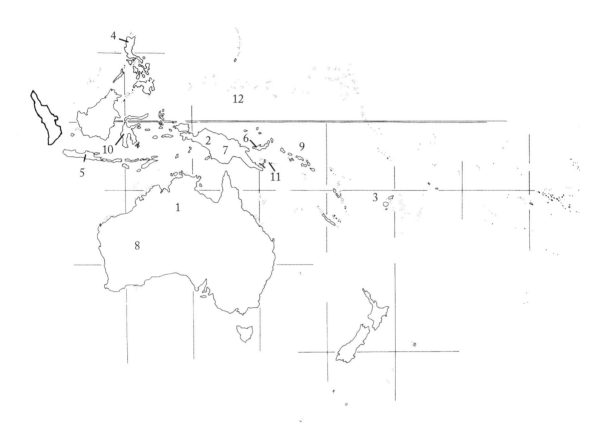

1. Aranda
2. Dani
3. Fijians
4. Ifugao
5. Javanese
6. Lusi-Kaliai
7. Maenga
8. Mardudjara
9. Tikopia
10. Toradja
11. Trobriand Islanders
12. Truk

HEALTH AND ILLNESS
A CROSS-CULTURAL ENCYCLOPEDIA

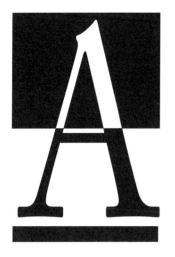

Acupuncture is recorded in the Yellow Emperor's classic textbook of medicine in the third century B.C. The word is derived from the Latin words *acus* (needles) and *punctura* (pricking). Its original application was for arthritis, gout, and gastrointestinal distress. The earliest needles were made of flint until metals such as bronze, silver, and gold were discovered. Most needles today are made of stainless steel. The needles are much thinner than needles used for vaccinations and injections in the West and generally do not hurt when inserted. They often have a copper or aluminum handle and range from one-half inch in length for head and facial points to three to four inches for insertion into deep tissue or thick muscle. Three types of needles with varying lengths are used: one for insertion, one for light tapping (especially used with children), and a triangular needle for bloodletting. They are twirled to produce the desired effect, the building of energy, or chi, at the spot of insertion. The acupuncturist usually combines one central point with sensitive spots near the source of the illness. Each point has a particular effect alone and in combination.

There are three approaches, which may be used alone or in combination:

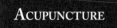

ACUPUNCTURE

Acupuncture is an ancient Chinese art and science of healing. It is based on a belief in an energy system within the body by which energy flows between its various organs. The healing of illness occurs when the flow of energy in the body is balanced. This energy is called chi and is comprised of two opposing forces called yin and yang. The Chinese work with the concept of balancing opposites in food, healing herbs, and massage. Acupuncture is more invasive, involving the insertion of needles into the body at specific points that are believed to control or regulate the flow of chi. The points are configured along invisible lines in the body called meridians. Each organ is connected to a meridian and along each lies a series of points that produce different effects when stimulated. The meridians end and begin at the fingers and toes. Maps of these meridians, which can be found in the offices of acupuncturists, depict long lines, some running the length of the body. In keeping with the original philosophical scheme of traditional Chinese medicine, there are 365 points, one corresponding to each day of the year.

1. **Distant point.** Though the diseased organ may be in the center of the body, distant points in the arms and legs may be stimulated. There is an aphorism that states that for ailments of the upper body, use points on the lower body, and for ailments of the lower body, use points on the upper body. Hand points might be stimulated for head and neck problems and points on the feet or legs for stomach problems. A point on the head might be used for diseases of the lower colon.

2. **Local point.** An acupuncture point near a sensitive spot that has been located by touch is chosen and stimulated with a needle.

3. **Adjacent or neighboring point.** The acupuncture points nearest the diseased organ or the trouble are stimulated. These points may be used together with the local point or in place of it.

In addition, specific points known to have a beneficial effect for a particular area may be added, and points in the ears may be used.

For anesthesia, points along the meridian of the sick organ or body part are used. The amount of time the needle is twirled and the point is stimulated is critical to allow the chi to gain force. Experiments with acupuncture anesthesia have

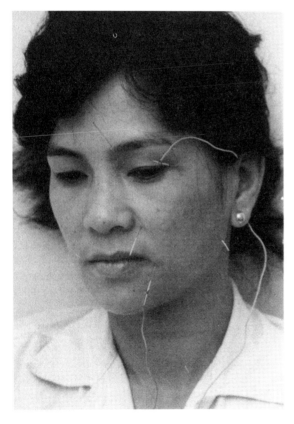

Acupuncture, treatment with needles placed at carefully selected sites on the body, was developed in China and is based on balancing the flow of energy within the body.

been going on in the People's Republic of China since the 1950s. One of the differences between acupuncture for healing and for anesthesia is that, for anesthesia, the needles must be constantly stimulated for the analgesic effect to continue. This has prompted experiments with electrical hookups to continue the stimulation. The mental condition of the patient is considered when contemplating the use of acupuncture anesthesia. Breathing techniques are often employed as the person remains completely conscious during surgery. The body must be "quiet" enough and the skin healthy enough to take the needles. While backup of traditional anesthesia is usually still used, acupuncture has proven to be inexpensive and safe in most cases.

Another form of stimulation is called moxibustion. Dried plant leaves called moxa are burned at the site of the selected acupuncture points. They are usually in the form of cones or rolled up in tissue paper like a cigarette and are held at a short distance above the point. Moxibustion is considered effective for relieving abdominal pain.

Possible complications of acupuncture include infection and hepatitis. Bleeding resulting from the inadvertent needling of internal organs or major blood vessels may occur. Strong stimulation of the central nervous system may result in temporary paralysis.

A number of legends have arisen to explain the origins of acupuncture. One is that ancient Chinese warriors who had been wounded by arrows noticed that other aches and pains had disappeared, and they deduced a cause-and-effect relationship between the wound and their healing. Another is that they noticed the soothing effect of massage.

Acupuncture's popularity has grown since its arrival in the United States in the early 1970s. It is practiced in many urban areas of the United States by both Chinese immigrants and American students of the technique. Word of acupuncture first appeared in the report of the distinguished journalist James Reston of the *New York Times,* who had been on location in China covering diplomatic events. He was taken ill and had to undergo surgery for appendicitis, and acupuncture anesthesia was used. He subsequently wrote about his experience, and Americans have been interested ever since.

There are schools of acupuncture in the United States, and a national commission exists to oversee certification. Students who have completed the required number of hours of study are given a diploma of acupuncture and, depending on the laws of each state, may obtain a license to practice. This includes but is not limited to medical doctors. Since January 1996, students have been required to complete a significant number of hours in the study of Chinese herbs in addition to acupuncture to become a certified acupuncturist. Some states do not allow the licensing of acupuncture.

Acupuncturists in the United States have had most success treating myofascial conditions—inflammations of the soft tissue. These include muscle injuries, tendonitis, and arthritis. Musculoskeletal, gastrointestinal, respiratory, and gynecological problems are said to respond well to acupuncture. Migraine headaches are also treatable, but, as one acupuncturist reminds us, the technique is aimed at correcting energetic imbalance, not curing the illness per se. According to Peter Goldberg, a licensed acupuncturist, "If we are working with your migraine, what we are doing is working with the energy system so the energy can flow properly." The energy or force of chi that is released through acupuncture can often be felt by the patient. Some report feelings of energetic well-being and balance. One person described the feeling of being four years old again—open to life and full of youthful energy.

See also CHINESE MEDICINE.

Risse, Gunther, ed. (1973) *Modern China and Traditional Chinese Medicine.*

Tan, Leong T., Margaret Y. C. Tan, and Veith Ilza. (1973) *Acupuncture Therapy: Current Chinese Practice.*

Weil, Andrew. (1983) *Health and Healing: Understanding Conventional and Alternative Medicine.*

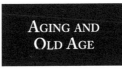

AGING AND OLD AGE

Aging is a universal. In all cultures all people change biologically as they get older and in all cultures all people experience the same types of biological changes. In addition to being a biological universal, aging is also a cultural universal, as in all cultures the process of aging is recognized, the status of old age is marked by special words, and there are norms that govern the treatment afforded the aged. Variation across cultures concerns mainly the issues of when a person is considered to be old and how they are treated. In the United States and many other modern nations, old age is defined in economic and political terms. One reaches old age when one retires from regular work and is eligible to begin collecting retirement, Social Security, and other societal benefits to which old people are entitled. In most cultures, however, chronological age is not so clearly a marker of aging and old age. Although old people are clearly older in years than younger people, other factors such as physical appearance and the ability to continue working are far more important markers of aging.

Across cultures and nations there is considerable variation in how long people live. In the absence of reliable birth records, it is difficult to accurately measure the average life expectancy in many cultures. However, the information has become much more reliable and standardized in many nations of the world. Two sets of information are

Sample Average Life Expectancies

Over 75 Years	Over 70 Years	Over 65 Years	Over 60 Years	Over 50 Years	Under 50 Years
Australia	Albania	China	Brazil	Bolivia	Afghanistan
Canada	Argentina	Ecuador	Egypt	Botswana	Bangladesh
Iceland	Bahrain	Guyana	Iraq	Cameroon	Burkina Faso
Israel	Belgium	Lebanon	Mongolia	India	Cambodia
Italy	Chile	Mexico	Morocco	Iran	Chad
Japan	Cuba	Qatar	Nicaragua	Liberia	Congo
Spain	Germany	Syria	Peru	Oman	Ethiopia
Sweden	Great Britain		Philippines	Sudan	Gambia
United States	Greece		Thailand	Togo	Mali
	Hungary		Tunisia	Uganda	Nepal
	Kuwait			Zambia	Niger
	New Zealand				
	Portugal				

of most interest in regard to aging. First, the percentage of the population over sixty-five years of age and, second, average life expectancy. As regards the percentage of the population over age sixty-five, the nations of the world can be divided into four categories:

1. Those with aged populations in which more than 10 percent of the population is older than age sixty-five, such as Australia, Austria, Belgium, Canada, Denmark, France, Japan, the Netherlands, Norway, Portugal, Sweden, and the United States
2. Those with mature populations in which between 7 percent and 9 percent of the population is older than age sixty-five, such as Cuba, Grenada, Israel, Martinique, Puerto Rico, and Romania
3. Those with youthful populations in which between 4 percent and 6 percent of the population is older than age sixty-five, such as Albania, Algeria, the Bahamas, Brazil, Chad, Chile, China, Egypt, Gabon, Jamaica, Lebanon, Malaysia, Mexico, Myanmar, Panama, Taiwan, Turkey, and Vietnam
4. Those with young populations in which 4 percent or less of the population is older

than age sixty-five, such as Angola, Congo, Guatemala, Indonesia, Iran, Kuwait, Mali, Nigeria, Tanzania, and Togo

Average life expectancy also varies across nations, with a sample of nations shown above. The most striking pattern in this information is the disparity between economically developed and economically less developed nations. People in developed nations live longer and those nations have more aged people than do less developed nations. This is due to a combination of conditions in developed nations, including better sanitation, more extensive health care, a better diet, better living conditions, and less dangerous work. One of the more intriguing issues raised by the study of aging across cultures is finding that there are a few cultures where people live to exceptionally old ages. These include the Hunza in Pakistan, Aegean islanders, the Yakut in Siberia, the Azerbaijani Turks, people in some villages in the Andes in South America, and the Abkhazians in the nation of Georgia in the Caucasus region of Eurasia. The Abkhazians have drawn the most attention, spurred by reports from journalists in the 1970s that they regularly lived to ninety years or more, looked decades younger than their actual ages, and continued to lead full and active lives. More careful research suggests that the claims about looking young and living active lives are exaggerations and experts disagree about the claims of unusual longevity. Assuming that a larger number of Abkhazians than most other peoples live into their nineties and even over 100 years of age, a number of explanations have been suggested. First, there may be some genetic factor at work that allows the Abkhazians to live longer. Some support for this comes from the fact that the Abkhazians marry relatively late in life and have children later, women continue to menstruate into the mid-fifties, and men are sexually potent well into their seventies. Thus, the entire life-course may be longer—for genetic or cultural reasons—for Abkhazians than for other people. Another explanation is that their diet, which is rich in unprocessed fruits and vegetables and low in fat and calories, may prevent diseases of old age, including cardiovascular disease and cancers. A third possible cause is psychological in that the Abkhazians tend to take responsibility for their own lives and rarely blame others for their problems, suggesting that they experience less

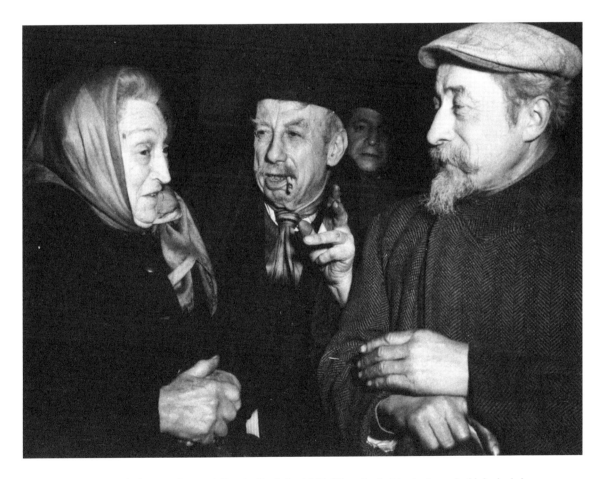

Apartment building workers socialize in Paris in 1949. These individuals show the biological changes associated with aging, a process recognized with special treatment by cultures around the world.

conflict and stress. A fourth and final factor is the role and treatment afforded elderly Abkhazians. The old are honored and are cared for by family and friends—two factors associated across cultures with a more comfortable aging experience.

BIOLOGICAL AGING

Whether or not there are cultures where people live an especially long time, in all cultures aging is a biological process and the body tends to change in similar ways in most people in most cultures. Predictable biological changes associated with aging across cultures include changes in body composition, bone structure, metabolism, and neurological functioning. With regard to body composition there is greater accumulation of fat in the body as one ages, and especially in the upper body. For women, there is marked change in body shape, with the middle and upper body increasing in size. There is also a reduction in the amount of muscle, which is one reason elderly people have less energy than younger people. The most dramatic change in bone structure as one ages is progressive bone loss, a process that effects women to a far greater extent than men and is associated with a high rate of broken bones in elderly women. The problem is so severe and widespread in women that it is categorized as a medical condition called osteoporosis, which is caused by an estrogen deficiency following menopause that leads to loss of calcium from the bones. The bones then become weak and break easily. In the United States, many medical experts now recommend that postmenopausal women undergo hormone replacement therapy to prevent osteoporosis as well as other estrogen deficiency–related disorders such as cardiovascular disease. The major metabolic changes associated with aging that occur across cultures are an increase in the blood sugar level and a reduced capacity for the immune system to fight disease. The final category of biological change is a change in neurological functioning, which is reflected in memory lapses and loss, confusion, and serious neurological disorders such as Alzheimer's disease.

SOCIAL AGING

Across cultures there are a number of indicators that tell an individual and his or her family and friends that he or she is aging. One marker is chronological age, as even in cultures where age is not measured in chronological terms both the biological changes associated with aging and the expectations people have about realistic behavior at different ages or life stages tend to mark people as aging or aged. Another important marker is physical appearance. Again, changes in physical appearance are largely biologically determined, but the meanings assigned them vary across cultures. For example, the Aymara of Bolivia distinguish between loss of sight and hearing in someone who is old and the same losses in someone who is young. Such losses are considered a natural part of aging (the Aymara say that "the eyes [or ears] of the person have gone on ahead") but are considered unnatural for younger people and are believed to be caused by evil forces. Loss of hair is a major marker of aging for men in the United States, but not so in many Native American cultures. Hair turning gray is an important marker in many cultures, and Taiwanese women mark themselves as old when they stop dying their hair black and let it go gray.

In addition to physical appearance, across cultures a major indicator of aging or of a shift in one's status from being an adult to being aged is a diminished capacity to perform the routine activities of adulthood. For people in rural Taiwan, there is a clear reduction in regular activity:

> Men begin to retire for reasons other than wealth or sickness, and women begin to leave the management of the household, not just

the routine chores, to their daughters-in-law. Parents of brothers who have set up separate households show their age by their inability to control the previously joint family. (Harrell 1981: 194)

Among the Truk of Oceania, men point to their diminished capacity as a sign of aging: "I don't think I will live much longer, for I am an old man and I am a little weak. I am still able to work, but in the past I was very strong; now I cannot lift heavy things." (Gladwin and Sarason 1953: 142)

While diminished capacity is often associated with old age, it is not always perceived as a negative development and in some cultures the aged might be assigned new, less difficult, but equally important responsibilities. For example, old Kogi men in South America define their new status as "seated":

> The state of this phase of life, that of the mature man, of the father of a family, is represented by a word which the men use all the time in their conversations: "seated." "What are you doing?" one is asked. "I am seated," he will answer with pride.
>
> To grow old is thus pleasant for the Kogi. As the years pass, his knowledge and his status increase. Children and young people respect him and ask his advice. Society esteems him. And so long as he lives thus, now with grandsons and great-grandsons to whom he teaches his knowledge, he is sure of being near the Mother who will soon receive him into her arms. (Reichel-Dolmatoff 1951: 258)

Similarly, for the rural Taiwanese, while their work and responsibilities are reduced, the quality of their life may actually improve:

> In general, however, old age is a time of great freedom and leisure for men and women. Since they have few pressing responsibilities, they are free to wander about the village and visit each other. At most, old people

of either sex may help watch their young grandchildren during the day. Some of the older people, especially one or two grandmothers in Hsin Hsing, are known for their ability to tell wonderful stories based on Taiwan opera or puppet shows which they have seen in the surrounding villages or in Lukang. (Gallin 1966: 215)

AGING IN THE LIFE CYCLE

In many cultures, aging is seen a natural stage in the course of one's life. In the United States, for example, most people see an individual's life as progressing through a number of stages, with each stage marked by certain age, role, and behavioral expectations. A fairly detailed stage scheme for the United States is as follows:

Birth
Infancy
Early Childhood
Late Childhood
Adolescence
Early Adulthood
Adulthood
Middle Age
Old Age
Death

In other cultures, the life course is conceptualized in the same linear pattern, although the stages may differ. The Dogon of West Africa, for example, mark only four life stages—adolescent, adult, mature man, and old man, with each stage lasting for about nine to twelve years in an individual's life. The Trobriand Islanders of New Guinea have a more precise scheme, which also differentiates among men and women at various stages, as on page 10. (Malinowski 1929: 60)

The Trobrianders also simplify their system into three stages:

> There are, besides these more specific subdivisions, the three main distinctions of age,

Life Stages in the Trobriand Islands

Stage	Male Name	Female Name
infant until age of crawling	Waywaya	Waywaya
infant until the age of walking	Pwapwawa	Pwapwawa
child until puberty	Gwadi	Gwadi
child	Monagwadi	Inagwadi
youth from puberty	To'ulatile	Nakapugula
mature man/ripe women	Tobubowa'u	Nabubowa'u
married man/woman	Tovavaygile	Navavaygile
old man/woman	Tomwaya	Numwaya

between ripe man and woman in the full vigour of life and the two stages—those of childhood and of old age—which limit manhood and womanhood on either side. The second main stage is divided into two parts, mainly by the fact of marriage. Thus, the words under [youth from puberty to marriage] primarily designate unmarried people and to that extent are opposed to [married man/woman], but they also imply youthfulness or unripeness, and in that respect are opposed to [mature man/ripe woman]. (Malinowski 1929: 61)

The Trobriand system points to a common organizing principle of life-stage schemes in many cultures—the importance of biological changes associated with sexual activity and reproduction. Individuals are classified in a pre-adult stage before they are to reproduce, as adults when they can reproduce, and as aged after their reproductive ability ends or is diminished. The importance of the ability to reproduce as an organizing principle in the notion of the life stages is indicated by the life-stage scheme of the Pawnee of the central United States. The Pawnee classify individuals into five life stages, with sexual function an important organizing principle:

The Skidi recognized five distinct periods or epochs in the life history of an individual of either sex. For the male these periods were as follows:

1. Pirau. This means "child," or more properly, "baby," carried no distinction of sex, and was applicable only to a child during the nursing period.
2. Piruski, "boy." This term covered the period from the termination of childhood to the age of puberty. The word, pisiks, "covered up" (closed foreskin), was also used as a nickname for a boy of this period, referring to the fact that he had not yet had connection with women.
3. Pitisutki. The term was applied to a boy after he had reached the age of puberty but had not yet married, and means "grown or straight up."
4. Pita. This referred to the period after marriage until old age, and is the general term for "man."
5. Kurahus, meaning "old man," was applicable to that period of a man's life when he no longer took active part in the hunt or went out with the warriors.

The corresponding names for the female were:

1. Pirau.
2. Tcoraki, "girl."
3. Tcoras. This corresponded to the third period of the man; that is, the

period after reaching puberty and extending up to marriage.

4. Tcapat, "woman" (blood-from-delivery), especially referred to the fact that she had given birth.

5. Tcostit applied to all women after menopause. (Dorsey 1940: 87)

This linear conceptualization of the life cycle is not found in all cultures, because in some cultures the life cycle is seen as circular. For example, Hindus in India, who believe in reincarnation, see life as a never-ending circle of births, deaths, and rebirths. Similarly, the Hopi of Arizona see life as existing both above and below the ground, with those who die physically moving to the underground world, where they continue to "live."

Treatment of the Aged

Despite tales of old Eskimos sent off to die on ice floats, in most cultures the elderly are well cared for. Similarly, the belief that aged Americans were better cared for by their families in the past than today is not supported by any research. The cultures where abandoning or killing the elderly is an acceptable practice are mostly ones that are nomadic and it is only the aged who are no longer able to travel on their own and thus become a burden to the group who experience such treatment. Most aged people die before they reach this point. Still, the aged are not always well-treated. In about 15 percent of societies, some aged people might be persecuted as witches, some might have to give their property away, some might have to live apart from the group, and some are killed when they are old.

In cultures where the elderly are abused, abuse begins only when an old person reaches decrepitude, that is, when he or she is no longer able to care for him- or herself and becomes a burden to the group. The treatment that might be afforded

someone who has reached decrepitude is indicated by this example from the Dogon of Mali:

> In proportion as these intellectual qualities diminish, as the man grows old, as his mind becomes dim, a vacuum is made around him. When the old man weakened by age drags himself to the men's shelter in order to rest sunk against a post in a senile reverie, his neighbors move away. Undoubtedly, one comes across adults who show filial affection toward their parents; but often, too, an old man in his second childhood, a helpless old woman, are left to themselves; the boy of ten or twelve years whom one sends to carry a meal to the grandfather may eat the millet porridge, announcing afterwards that he fulfilled his task. The ones who complain most among these old people are those who, no longer having children, fall into the care of more distant kinsmen, nephews or cousins; even now the latter scarcely feed the old men; in the old days they used to let them die of hunger. (Paulme 1940: 466)

In some cultures there is much variation in the responsibilities and status of old men in comparison to old women. For example, among the Taiwanese old men give up authority in the household readily while old women seek to maintain authority over their daughters-in-law and continue to perform the religious rituals required of the senior woman in the family. This variation may be a result of the different experience Taiwanese men and women have with responsibility over their life-course. Boys are indulged and are not expected to be very responsible. As a young adult the man often continues to live with his family and the responsibilities of being the head of the household, a husband, and a father come as a shock. Thus, they are not eager to keep these responsibilities as they get old. Girls, on the other hand, carry numerous child care and household responsibilities from an early age. These responsibilities multiply for a woman when she marries and goes to live with her husband and his family. Thus, being responsible in the household is a lifelong woman's role and one she is not eager to give up. Additionally, a Taiwanese woman has considerable control over her daughter-in-law, and this power may be difficult to give up as well.

See also DEATH.

Albert, Steven M., and Maria G. Cattell. (1994) *Old Age in Global Perspective.*

Benet, Sula. (1974) *Abkhasians: The Long-Living People of the Caucasus.*

Dorsey, George A. (1940) *Notes on Skidi Pawnee Society.*

Gallin, Bernard. (1966) *Hsin Hsing, Taiwan: A Chinese Village in Change.*

Garb, Paula. (1987) *Where the Old Are Young: Long Life in the Soviet Caucasus.*

Gladwin, Thomas, and Seymour B. Sarason. (1953) *Truk: Man in Paradise.*

Glascock, Anthony P., and Richard A. Wagner. (1986) *HRAF Research Series in Quantitative Cross-Cultural Data. Vol. II. Life Cycle Data.*

Harrell, Clyde S. (1981) "Growing Old in Rural Taiwan." In *Other Ways of Growing Old: Anthropological Perspectives,* edited by Pamela T. Amos and Stevan Harrell, 193–210, 259–260.

LaBarre, Weston. (1948) *The Aymara Indians of the Lake Titicaca Plateau, Bolivia.*

Malinowski, Bronislaw. (1929) *The Sexual Life of Savages in Northwestern Melanesia.*

Paulme, Denise. (1940) *Social Organization of the Dogon of French Sudan.* Translated from the French by Frieda Schutze.

Reichel-Dolmatoff, Gerardo. (1951) *The Kogi: A Tribe of the Sierra Nevada de Santa Marta, Colombia.* Vol. 2. Translated from the Spanish by Sydney Muirden.

Rosenow, Hill Gates. (1970) *Prosperity Settlement: The Politics of Paipai in Taipei, Taiwan.*

Rubenstein, R., ed. (1990) *Anthropology and Aging: Comprehensive Reviews.*

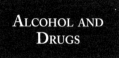

ALCOHOL AND DRUGS

The use of chemicals that can alter one's mood or behavior is a cultural universal. This does not mean that every individual in every culture uses drugs but only that some people in every culture use drugs, at least on some occasions. Although the pharmaceuticals used most commonly around the world today are mass produced in economically developed nations and exported around the world, throughout human history thousands of drugs—in the form of raw or processed plant material—have been discovered or developed for human use. These drugs may be raw plant materials that are eaten, chewed, smoked, rubbed on the skin, or snorted, or plant materials that are processed and then eaten, drunk, smoked, chewed, or injected. Across cultures, the most common drug throughout human history has been the alcoholic beverage, consumed in thousands of forms. There are few cultures lacking indigenous methods of producing alcoholic beers, wines, or spirits from fermented plant material, although in some cultures such as the Mormon and Islamic cultures the use of alcohol is forbidden. Although not usually thought of as drugs, coffee and tobacco have now replaced alcoholic beverages around the world as the most commonly consumed drugs. As discussed below, both coffee and tobacco contain mood-altering substances (caffeine and nicotine), both are addictive, and both are consumed regularly by hundreds of millions of people because of their psychoactive effects. The list at the end of the article contains a short list of only a few drugs used in cultures around the world.

One of the more interesting topics in the history of alcohol use across cultures is how indigenous patterns of use were influenced by the arrival of European colonists. European colonization influenced indigenous drug use in two major ways. First, the colonists often introduced or promoted the use of drugs not previously used or not used as frequently. Second, colonists introduced new alcoholic beverages such as rum and whiskey that had much higher alcohol contents than indigenous beverages and much stronger physiological and behavioral effects.

Europeans promoted the use of drugs either to induce indigenous peoples to supply the colonists with items of economic value or to enhance their work performance. Use of inducements seems to have been confined to the early years of colonization when alcohol and tobacco were often sold or traded for furs, minerals, or other items desired by the colonists. Drugs as enhancers were used in situations where indigenous people were used as laborers. The drugs used in this situation were usually ones that contain stimulants such as caffeine and nicotine that would increase worker productivity by allowing them to work longer, harder, or faster. While native peoples themselves used both narcotic and hallucinogenic drugs for religious and social purposes, colonists discouraged the use of these drugs because they interfered with productivity.

The introduction of strong alcohol beverages to native peoples, and especially to American Indians, has proven to be one of the major disasters of colonization. Along with the new beverages such as rum and whiskey, Indians adopted the drinking style of the European traders who brought the beverages to them. Thus, Indian drinking, contrary to traditional patterns of drug use, became solitary and angry, accompanied by violence and abuse, and often associated with addiction. The role of whites in encouraging native drinking and its effects are documented in these two accounts concerning the Tlingit of the Northwest Coast and the Ojibwa of the Great Lakes region:

> "There are plenty of irresponsible whites," writes Ballou, "ready to make money out of the aborigines. Rum is the native's bane, its effect upon him being singularly fatal; it maddens him; even slight intoxication means to him delirium and all its consequences, wild brutality and utter demoralization."
>
> More crimes, cruelty, brutality and misery among the natives are due to drink than to any other one thing—yea, than to all other things put together. Many have died directly from overdrink and poisonous drinks. Many have been killed in drunken brawls or crippled for life. Children are abused, neglected and made to suffer by drunken parents. (Jones 1914: 217)

The situation among the Ojibwa is described in much the same way and the change from traditional use of drugs is noted:

> Consumption of liquor was undoubtedly the greatest evil on the reservation. It was illegal to sell liquor to an Indian, yet whites in every community sold liquor to persons who were easily distinguishable as Indians. (Hilger 1939: 35–36)
>
> . . . The Chippewa in their traditional culture had no intoxicating liquor. Smoking, chewing, and drinking decoctions of steeped herbs and roots gave them some exhilaration, but none of these caused loss of judgment, of consciousness, or of control of faculties. Today, intoxication is one of the evils on the White Earth Reservation. (122)

The following sections survey the use of seven substances—alcohol, coffee, tea, coca, khat, kava, and betel—that are commonly used either across cultures or by a number of cultures in a particular region.

ALCOHOL

Of all the drugs regularly used by humans, alcohol is the one used most often for "health" reasons. In many cultures people believe that drinking alcoholic beverages promotes good health, as suggested by toasts in many languages: "To your health," "*L'chaim,*" "*Salud,*" "*Viva,*" "*Kan pei,*" and "*Na zdrowie.*" In addition, in many cultures, alcoholic beverages have been used as a pain killer, as a disinfectant, to induce sleep, to reduce anxiety, and to relive boredom and unhappiness. In fact, some experts believe that alcoholics use alcohol to "self-medicate." Medical research, of course, provides a different perspective on alcohol consumption and indicates that most alcohol use and especially heavy, regular use lead to worse rather than better health. It is also clear that for many people regular use can lead to addiction to alcohol, which is related to many other life problems including accidents, family problems, and poor work performance. The only known health benefit of alcohol consumption is a slightly reduced risk of cardiovascular disease in some moderate drinkers.

The regular use of alcohol for social and religious purposes in many cultures raises the question of why people drink. This is really two questions. First, the question of why certain individuals drink or drink to excess, which is an issue beyond the scope of this work. The second question of why cultures vary in the degree to which their members drink alcoholic beverages requires first that we note some patterns in alcohol consumption across cultures:

1. In most traditional, non-Western cultures drinking is a group activity with clear rules about who, what, where, when, and how drinking may take place and what behaviors are considered appropriate during or following drinking.
2. In addition to social rules about alcohol use, in many cultures alcohol and alcohol use also have clear and important social roles. An example of the many social roles filled by alcoholic beverages is provided by the Bemba of Zimbabwe:

> Beer is the present of honour between kinsmen. It is carried to chiefs as tribute, used to reward labour, or given as an offering to spirits. Nowadays, it may be one of the few ways by which a woman, left deserted by her husband, can make money for clothes. Men cultivate extra ground in order to have enough millet for brewing. Abundance of beer is the glory of a commoner's hospitality, or a chief's court. Without it tribal councils cannot be held, and marriage or initiation ceremonies do not take place. For all these reasons it is impossible to describe the physical effects of native beer-drinking without knowing the part it plays in the Bemba's whole social life. (Richards 1939: 77)

3. In most traditional, non-Western cultures solitary drinking is unusual and alcohol addiction is equally rare.
4. How an individual behaves while drinking is not related to the amount of alcohol consumed. While consuming large enough quantities of alcohol will induce sleep in all individuals, how people behave when drinking is determined more by the social context of the drinking and the expectations the drinker has about what effects the alcohol will have on him or her. Across cultures, the most common expected effect of alcohol consumption is that it is a social facilitator. Bemba drinking is typical of many cultures:

> But it is probably the fact that beer-drinking is such a social event that accounts for the people's quick sense of exhilaration and even intoxication. Natives gather together from surrounding villages to drink at their relatives' huts and exchange gossip. . . . Further, beer

is drunk by the maximum number of people who can crowd into one hut. At an average brewing three or four calabashes might be available for distribution, and of these one would be given to the headman to share with the leaders of the village, another might be given to the son-in-law of the brewer to drink with the younger men of the village, and a third kept in the owner's hut for his near family or special friends. But in each case, after the formal drinking has begun, the original guests are joined by others who enter with a polite salutation, take a short pull at the beer, and stay for a short talk. When there is only one calabash to be divided in the village, each inhabitant will probably join the crowd in the hut at one time or another in the evening. Thus there is a constant coming and going of men and women, and the children who are too small to be left at home. (Richards 1939: 78–79)

5. In all cultures the rules that govern drinking behavior allow for behaviors that are not permitted in other contexts. These rules usually allow for the public expression of anger, aggression, and sexual desires that other times are kept private. For the Bemba:

> Beer is recognized as making a man more talkative, liable to quarrel, or indulge in illicit love-making, and men whose hearts get hot quickly, to repeat the native phrase, are avoided at beer drinks, if possible, because they may involve their friends in legal liabilities. (Richards 1939: 77)

6. In most cultures alcohol is used for ceremonial and religious purposes. While alcohol plays a ritual role in world religions such as Roman Catholicism and Judaism, it is also important in many traditional religions, as for the Tarahumara of northern Mexico:

> Tesguino [corn beer] has a sacred character somewhat analogous to that of the

ubiquitous kava of the Pacific. It was said that tesguino was given to the Indians by onoruame or tata diosi (god) so that they could get their work done and that they might enjoy themselves. Whenever a jar of the beer is drunk, it must be first dedicated to tata diosi by symbolically tossing three small gourdfuls dipped from a larger gourd towards each of the four directions. This is done in front of a wooden cross and is for the purpose of allowing God to drink first so that he will not get angry.

The ritual significance of the beer is further shown by the fact that it is included as an integral part of most ceremonies. For example, in the "curing" ceremonies for assurance of good crops, protection of animals, killing of worms, petition for rain, or protection from lightning, a jar of tesguino is placed at the foot of a wooden cross throughout the ritual. It is drunk by the ritual specialist and important men as part of the ceremony and later serves as one of the "medicines" that is sprinkled on the new corn and animals.

The only ceremonial act that resembles a rite of passage besides child curing rituals and funerals, is the time a boy about the age of fourteen is allowed to drink tesguino for the first time.

Besides the importance of the beer as a sacred part of ceremonies themselves, each religious fiesta is followed by a large tesguinada which may last as long as forty-eight hours. (Kennedy 1963: 623)

In addition to these patterns in alcohol use, there are also some clear differences across cultures in how much people customarily drink, whether drinking is mainly recreational or for religious purposes, and what types of beverages are consumed. When we look at information about how much alcohol people in different nations consume, it is clear that there is considerable variation across cultures. One survey of drinking in nations indicates that France has the highest rate, with the average person consuming 16.8 liters of absolute alcohol per year, and Egypt and Syria the lowest with only 0.1 liters per year. The following rates of the liters of absolute alcohol consumed per person in a year give some idea of the breadth of alcohol consumption across cultures:

Nation	Liters of Absolute Alcohol Consumed
France	16.8
Italy	13.6
Spain	11.4
Argentina	10.6
Canada	7.6
Great Britain	6.9
United States	6.8
Poland	6.0
Japan	5.5
Greece	5.4
Panama	3.6
Mexico	2.5
Congo	0.7
Senegal	0.3
Algeria	0.3
Egypt	0.1

This sample of rates across nations indicates that there is some patterning to this wide range of alcohol use. First, alcohol use is heaviest in European nations or nations outside Europe with large European populations. Second, alcohol use is highest in southern Europe—four of the six nations at the top of the full list (France, Italy, Portugal, and Spain) are in southern Europe. Third, within Europe there is a clear declining gradient of use from the south to the north. And, fourth, alcohol use is the lowest in the Middle East and North Africa. Many cultures in these regions are Islamic, and Muslims abstain from alcohol use in accord with the Koran.

Social and behavioral scientists have set forth a wide range of biological, psychological, sociocultural, psychosocial, ecological, demographic, and economic explanations for alcohol addiction in individuals and for the variation in alcohol use across cultures. The explanation that seems to answer best the variation across cultures is that alcohol is consumed by people to reduce stress and anxiety. Thus, alcohol use is greater in cultures where there is more stress. Stress, in this sense, may take any number of forms, including anxiety over food shortages, feelings of weakness or powerlessness, and unresolved conflicts from childhood.

TOBACCO

Tobacco is a plant indigenous to South America. When Europeans arrived in the Americas in 1492 tobacco was used both recreationally and medicinally by native peoples in South America, Central America, the Caribbean islands, and parts of North America. As cigarettes were not mass-produced until the twentieth century, indigenous use of tobacco included smoking it in pipes or rolled in leaves, chewing it, or inhaling it in the form of snuff. The variety of tobacco used was probably *Nicotiana rustica*. The following description of tobacco use by a Miskito healer of Central America indicates its medicinal use:

> Through the use of narcotics, especially the excessive use of tobacco, the sukya throws himself in a condition of wild ecstasy, and goes into trances and hypnotic states. During such an abnormal condition he is supposed to be in relation with friendly spirits whom he had invoked previously, and who reveal to him the source of the illness and the mode of cure.
>
> The cure proper consists in whistling over the sick person, blowing tobacco smoke over him, and massaging and sucking the afflicted body parts. The sukya purifies the drinking water, or any other beverage intended for the patient, by exposing it to the dew for some time, and then blowing into it with a bamboo rod or tobacco pipe so as to produce bubbles. . . . (Conzemius 1932: 123–124)

Tobacco was quickly adopted by the European settlers who desired what they took to be its qualities as a sedative, an aphrodisiac, and a cure for various ailments, as indicated by this entry in a French dictionary from 1573:

> Nicotaine: a herb of marvellous virtue against all wounds, ulcers, face ulcers and similar things, which M. Jean Nicot, Ambassador to the King of Portugal, sent to France and from whom it has derived its name.

Europeans distinguished between *Nicotiana rustica* and *Nicotiana tabacum.* The latter is indigenous to Brazil and is the variety adopted by the British for cultivation in North America and eventually became the basis for tobacco growing and smoking around the world. Although there was some early interest in tobacco as a medicine, use of *Nicotiana tabacum* has been mainly for recreational purposes around the world for several centuries. Although the Roman Catholic, Russian Orthodox, and Islamic religions have at times tried to ban tobacco smoking, these efforts failed, and regular smoking of tobacco is a daily activity for hundreds of millions of people around the world.

The most important active component of tobacco is nicotine, an oily substance concentrated in the large leaves of tobacco plants. Nicotine is both a stimulant and sedative. It acts initially as a stimulant by causing the release of epinephrine, which in turn stimulates a sudden rise in the blood sugar level. This stimulation of the nervous and muscle systems is then followed by a depression of the central nervous system. In order to control the depression and associated feeling of fatigue, many smokers then smoke

The AMERICAN COLONIES.

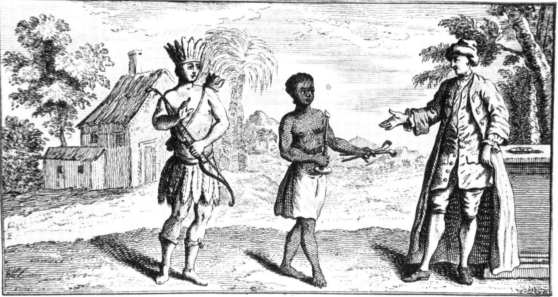

A Native American offers an Englishman tobacco pipes in a mid–eighteenth-century engraving. Along with coffee, tobacco, unknown to Europeans prior to exploration of North and South America, has replaced alcohol as the most commonly consumed drug worldwide.

another cigarette and the process continues. Nicotine is both psychologically and physiologically addictive and persons who attempt to stop smoking experience withdrawal symptoms such as cravings for tobacco, headaches, nervousness, and insomnia. Despite the early health claims for tobacco, it is now clear from years of scientific research that there are no health benefits from the use of tobacco and, to the contrary, the ingestion of nicotine, tar, carbon monoxide, and other components of tobacco through smoking or chewing is associated with numerous major health problems. It is a major cause of lung cancer and emphysema and a large contributor to other diseases, such as congestive heart disease, coronary disease, and cancers of the stomach, esophagus, throat, and mouth. It also makes the symptoms of other illnesses, such as colds, allergies, and bronchitis, considerably more severe. There is considerable evidence that smoking causes harm to the health of others in the smoker's vicinity through their breathing "secondary smoke" and that smoking leads to more stillborn births and babies with health problems. Although tobacco use has been declining in some nations, such as the United States, tobacco is produced and consumed around the world, and China is now both the leading producer and consumer.

COFFEE AND TEA

Coffee and tea are consumed by adults and sometimes children in many cultures, and both may be consumed by individuals drinking alone, at meals, or in social settings. Although not often thought of as drugs, coffee and tea contain caffeine, which is a stimulant that increases the heart rate, raises blood sugar levels, interferes with sleep, and may make an individual more alert and talkative. Regular use (four cups of coffee per day) can lead to physical dependence and side effects such as severe headaches when caffeine is

not consumed. Because of its presence in coffee, tea, chocolate, and numerous brands of mass-produced soft drinks, caffeine is the most commonly used drug in the world. It is also one that provides relatively few serious side effects, although long-term, heavy use can lead to addiction and problems such as insomnia, shortness of breath, anxiety, and possibly other health problems.

Coffee has been consumed by humans for more than 1,000 years. Its earliest use has been traced to northeastern Africa in the area of present-day Ethiopia, where berries and perhaps leaves from the *Coffea arabica* tree were mixed with other foods and eaten to prevent drowsiness. The first widespread use of coffee was evidently for medicinal purposes, as Islamic physicians recommended what is believed to be coffee to improve the general state of one's health. At some point people—in Ethiopia or across the Red Sea in Arabia—discovered that the berries and leaves or the berries alone could be boiled to produce a drink with the same effects as the eaten berries. Subsequently, the process was refined still further and the coffee beans were separated from the plant and ground before boiling to produce a beverage. Coffee spread from northeast Africa along with Islam across North Africa, throughout the Middle East and Asia, and into southern Europe. In all these regions, wherever people started drinking coffee they soon began to meet in establishments called coffeehouses, where they drank together and talked. Coffeehouses developed in Islamic nations in place of the inns, taverns, and pubs of Europe because alcohol was forbidden by Islam. While drinking did occur in private, it was forcibly controlled in public places. Governments routinely looked upon coffeehouses with suspicion, as places where a revolution might begin, and sought to control or shut them down, usually with little or limited success. Religious leaders saw them as encouraging sinful behavior, especially gambling. Today, in nations such as Turkey, the coffeehouse remains a central institution in community life.

Coffee entered Western Europe through Venice in 1615 and regular use quickly spread across the continent, despite efforts by church officials to control its consumption. As elsewhere, in a number of nations coffeehouses (called the *caffè* in Italy) sprung up in towns and cities. From Europe coffee spread to the Americas. Not only did coffee as a drink spread, but also cultivation of the coffee plant, with Brazil, Colombia, Indonesia, Guatemala, and Mexico all becoming major locales for coffee plantations, in addition to African nations such as the Ivory Coast. These nations have the hot, wet climates ideal for coffee cultivation and both the more desirable *Coffea arabica* and the less desirable *Coffea robusta* are grown for export. The major consumer nations today are the United States and Germany, although coffee is a daily drink in most nations.

Tea, according to Chinese folklore, was first cultivated and used in China in 2737 B.C. Although that date is probably too early an estimate, tea was discovered and first cultivated and consumed in China. Its earliest use, which dates to about 1000 B.C., was for medicinal purposes, and tea is mentioned in the pharmacopeia of early Chinese medical manuals. By about 350 B.C. the boiling of green tea leaves in water to produce a tonic for treating headache, indigestion, ulcers, lethargy and other ills was a common medical practice. Up until the fifth century A.D. tea in China was made by boiling green tea leaves. In the fifth century the process began to change and leaves were dried before boiling. The use of dry leaves that could be crushed into bales for storage and shipping led to the use of different varieties of tea leaves and to tea trade across China. In A.D. 780 the *Ch'a Ching* (Classic of tea) was published. It included detailed instructions for all phases of tea growing, processing, prepara-

tion, and consumption within a Taoist framework, placing tea clearly within the framework of Chinese culture. Tea use was transferred to Japan by Buddhists, where it, like Buddhism itself, was transformed and absorbed into Japanese culture. The distinctive Japanese tea ceremony remains in use in the 1990s.

After 1644 in China, black, oolong, and green tea became the major types of teas used, and eventually these types were traded around the world. Tea came to the Western world through traders in the Netherlands, who brought it from Japan, and in Russia, where it had been obtained from Mongolia. At first, it was seen as a medicine and used for much the same ills as in China, although throughout the seventeenth and eighteenth centuries there were debates about whether it was actually curative or harmful. Tea consumption is typically associated with England and it arrived there in the 1600s from the Netherlands. Although there was resistance by religious leaders and concern among the ruling classes about its use by the masses, by the early eighteenth century tea was being used as a medicine, served at coffeehouses and public tea gardens, and consumed in homes. It also played a role in the American Revolution (the Boston Tea Party protest against British taxation) and the Opium Wars in China in the 1800s. The medicinal claims made for tea are indicated by the following public notice posted at Garway's Coffee House in London in 1657:

> The Drink is declared to be most wholesome, preserving perfect health until extreme Old Age. . . .
> It maketh the body active and lusty.
> It helpeth the Headache, giddiness and headyness thereof.
> It removeth the obstructions of the Spleen.
> It is very good against the Stone and Gravel, cleaning the kidneys and Uriters,

being drank with Virgins Honey instead of Sugar.

It taketh away the difficulty of breathing, opening Obstructions.

It is good against Lipitude Distillations and cleareth the sight.

It removeth Lassitude and cleaneth and purifyeth adult Humors and hot Liver.

It is good against Crudities, strengthening the weakness of the Ventricle and Stomack, causing good Appetite and Digestion, and particularly for Men of a corpulent Body, and such as are great eaters of Flech.

It vanquisheth heavy dreams, easeth the Brain, and strengtheneth the Memory.

It overcometh superfluous Sleep, and prevents Sleepiness in general, a draught of the Infusion being taken, so that without trouble whole nights may be spent in study without hurt to the Body, in that it moderately heateth and bindeth the mouth of the Stomack.

It prevents and cures agues, Surfeits, and Feavers, by infusing a fit quantity of the Leaf, thereby provoking a most gentle Vomit and breathing of the Pores, and hath been given with wonderful success.

It (being prepared with Milk and Water) strengtheneth the inward parts, and prevents Consumptions, and powerfully assuageth the pains of the Bowels, or gripping of the Guts and Looseness.

It is for Colds, Dropsies, and Scurveys, if properly infused, purging the Blood by sweat and Urine, and expelleth infection.

It drives away all pains in the Collick proceeding from Wind, and purgeth safely the Gall.

And that the Vertues and excellencies of this Leaf and Drink are many and great is evident and manifest by the high esteem and use of it (especially of the late years) among Physicians and knowing men in France, Italy, Holland and other parts of Christendom. (McCoy and Walker 1976: 141–142)

In order to end their reliance on tea from China, the British East India Company transplanted trees to India and Sri Lanka in the 1700s and also used the tea plant indigenous to north-eastern India to develop a tea industry. These two nations along with China are now the major producers of tea around the world. The tea plant, *Camellia sinensis,* is indigenous to China and northeastern India. Today, the two major varieties of tea plant are the Chinese and Assam varieties, with a number of types of each used to produce the different teas available in the marketplacc. In addition, the definition of tea has now broadened and, especially in holistic and herbal healing, it is used to mean any vegetable matter that is boiled in water and then drunk. These teas play a major role in herbal medicine.

COCA AND COCAINE

Coca and cocaine are derived from the *Erythroxylon coca* shrub, which is native to the highlands of Ecuador, Bolivia, Peru, and Chile and which, through contact among Indian groups, spread to other areas of South and Central America. Coca is the name given to the drug used by Indians in South America, who mix dry leaves with lime and then chew or suck on them to withdraw the cocaine that "alleviates the pangs of hunger and fatigue, gives an apparent increase in energy, and produces a pleasurable 'lift'" (Tschopik 1951: 157). It is estimated that some 90 percent of adults in some Indian groups such as the Aymara chew coca daily. The practice was spread through the region by the Inca, whose rulers used coca for religious purposes and who encouraged its use by the general population—and especially miners—as a means of increasing productivity. Cocaine is the common name for the psychoactive agents of the coca shrub, whose chemical name is benzoylmethylecognine. It was first extracted in pure form from coca leaves by German chemists in the 1850s and was used medicinally and for other purposes (such as in Coca-Cola) into the early twentieth century. Concerns about addiction then led many countries to restrict its sale and use. Since the

1960s it has emerged in North America and Europe as a major illegal drug and is called "leaf," "coke," "snow," "blow," and other names by users. It is used in crystal form and is inhaled through the nose, injected, or smoked in a form called crack. The drug is desirable because of the feeling of euphoria it creates. It is highly addictive psychologically as users seek a continuation of the euphoria they experience, which, over time, requires greater and greater doses.

KAVA

Kava is used ceremonially in many Polynesian societies and is an important symbolic component of the social stratification systems of traditional Polynesian cultures such as the Marquesans, Tongans, and Samoans. It is consumed on various occasions such as the installation of a chief, greeting visitors from other societies, and welcoming higher status people into one's home. In addition, the rules that govern the actual drinking also indicate one's rank, as in some cultures only high ranking people can drink kava, while in other cultures drinking proceeds in the order of the social rank of those present, with those of highest rank drinking first. The social rules governing kava use in Polynesian societies are indicated in this description of a meeting of village chiefs in one district of Fiji:

> Nabadua entered bearing a great stalk of kava which he presented to the visiting elders, on behalf of Nakoroka. Ratu Kitioni of Lekutu, who had been sitting with the chiefs, slid quietly down into the rank of commoners; his strong Wesleyanism and weak digestion prohibited his enjoying the quiet intoxication that kava brings. Young Nakoroka men entered to mix kava in Nakoroka's largest bowl. As they poured water into the bowl, guests clapped out lusty songs which he who mixes must follow in the rhythm of his movements; the clapping with supped palms resounded pleasantly through the village. Ratu Luke

> came to sit before the bowl with Vatili as presiding chief while the kava was served to the visitors. Peni came to serve the cup. . . . There was a sudden flurry of confusion; Peni had forgotten that the church comes before the state. The Buli refused the cup and indicated the missionary. . . . Peni rose again gracefully, refilled the cup and knelt before the missionary, who drank as the assembled guests clapped out the song that always accompanies the first cup of kava and the drinking of the highest chief. Then a commoner drank as "messenger" for the missionary. Then the Buli drank to the song that indicates the second highest chief. A hereditary chief from Tavua followed the Buli's "messenger." When all visiting elders in the upper part of the house had drunk, Vatili and Ratu Luke took their turn; Vatili's status as "village chief" permitted him to drink on this occasion as a true chief at Nakoroka. The cup went the round of "chiefs" again before the kava bowl was twisted on its base as a signal that the more formal part of the ceremony was complete and that now the commoners could drink in their turn. (Quain 1948: 75)

The long history of kava use, its supernatural origins, and its ties to royalty are indicated by these verses from the festival song "The Kava of Miru Grows in Avaiki," performed at the installation of a chief in New Zealand in 1790:

Solo: Go on !
Chorus: The finest and most pleasing drink.
Solo: Ay! E!
Chorus: Tane', god with the yellow teeth,
                was once expelled from Tahiti,
                Yellow, with devouring mankind.
Solo: Let the red kava carefully be plucked,
                As a draught for dancers in the upperworld.
                Let the drink be prepared for the priests.
Chorus: The sacred bowl of the priests is ready,
                To be quaffed by yon sacred men.
Solo: Is there not yet another sort?

Chorus: 'Tis too sacred for mortal use.
Solo: Two shoots may we only strip; the parent stem
    Belongs to Miru only, is reserved for the destruction of souls.

In addition to its social role, kava also plays a role in religion and is used ceremoniously. For example, the Tikopia use kava as an offering to the gods:

> There was a big hurricane at Tikopia not long ago in which so many coconut trees were blown down or damaged that there was a great scarcity of food. Many houses were also destroyed and the inhabitants had to sleep in the open. The people thought that the atua had sent the storm, being angry because they had not been giving him enough kava, and in their turn the people were angry with the atua. To make matters worse there followed a drought; the sun shone continuously and dried up the earth and starvation was staring the people in the face. Offerings of kava were made daily to bring rain without result. At last the brother of the chief of the Taumako asked John if he could do anything and John prayed for rain which fell three days later so that the taro and yams grew again.
>
> The apparent success of John led to a division among the people, some believing that the rain was due to his intervention while others believed that it had been sent by the atua to whom at last the long continued offerings of kava had become acceptable. (Rivers 1914: 317)

KHAT

Khat is the common name for the *Catha edulis* plant, which is native to northeast Africa. It is also called kat or qat. The leaves and buds are brewed into a tea or are chewed for the mild hallucinogenic effect and euphoria caused by a number of psychoactive agents in the plant. Khat is drunk or chewed by some men in northeast Africa and the neighboring Middle East.

BETEL

Betel is the name of the seed of the *Areca catechu,* a variety of palm tree widely distributed through mainland and insular South and Southeast Asia. Indigenous peoples in these regions routinely chew betel. The chew consists of a slice of the seed mixed with lime and a piece of leaf from the *Piper betel* vine. Betel is a mild stimulant and thus has an effect much like the caffeine in coffee. It also increases salivation and thus the regular spitting of large quantities of the red betel juice is a required component of chewing. The chew also turns the teeth black, and black teeth are a common indicator of regular betel use in Southeast Asia.

Although betel chewing has declined somewhat under Western influence, it remains common in rural areas. Its ubiquitous use in the past is indicated by this description of betel chewing by the Ifugao of the northern Philippines:

> The Ifugao have the two great luxury-dissipations of the world: smoking and drinking together with a third which they share with the Malayo-Polynesian area: betel-chewing. The last named ranks second in religious importance and first in social and economic importance.
>
> Everybody, even the poorest, chews betel. The common salutation is "Give me a betel nut," and the answer is "All right, where is your lime box?" "your betel leaf," as the case may be. Betels are offered the deities in feasts; betels are ceremoniously chewed in the arrangement of marriages.
>
> The areca palm, which produces the betel-nut, grows sometimes fifty feet high. To obtain the nuts a woman will, in the case of a tall tree, tie her ankles so as to leave a space between the feet about the size of the palm trunk. Then by a series of bodily convolutions resembling the locomotion of a "measuring worm" she ascends the tree. . . . The trees are valued at fifty centavos. Between the divisions of the Ifugao tribe betel

A Partial List of Commonly Used Psychoactive Agents

Hallucinogens

Common Name	Region
Agara	New Guinea
Bolek-hena	Venezuela
Canary Island Broom	Canary Islands
Coral Tree	United States, Mexico, Guatemala
Deadly Nightshade	Europe, Asia
Ergot	Europe
Fly Agaric	World
Hemp, Pot, Grass	India
Henbane	Europe
Iboga	Central Africa
Jimson Weed	United States
Khana	South Africa
Kwashi	West Africa
Lion's Ear, Lion's Tail	South Africa
Madagascar Periwinkle	Madagascar
Magic Mushrooms	Mexico
Mandrake, Satan's Apple	Europe
Marula	South Africa
Mescal Bean	United States, Mexico
Niando	West and Central Africa
Nutmeg	Southeast Asia
Peyote	Mexico, United States
Piule	Mexico, Guatemala
Puffball	Mexico
Quiebra Plata	Mexico
Rape dos Indios	Brazil
San Pedro	Ecuador
Shansi	Ecuador
Silver Morning Glory	Southeast Asia
S'Keng-keng	South Africa
Soma	India
Sweet Calomel	United States, Canada
Syrian Rue	Middle East
Taique, Chapico	Chile
Thle-pela-kano	Mexico, Guatemala
Thorn Apple	Mexico, United States
Tupa	Chile
Vilca	Peru, Bolivia, Argentina

Tranquilizers and Sedatives

Common Name	Region
American Ginseng	United States
Asiatic Ginseng	Korea
Cabeza de Ángel	Mexico, Guatemala
Chinese Cat Powder	Japan
Hop	Europe, Asia, North America
Intoxicating Mint	Russia, Central Asia
Kava-kava	Oceania
Opium Poppy	Europe, Asia
Palo copal	Mexico
Pinque-pinque	Central America, Caribbean
Sarpaganda	South Asia

Stimulants

Common Name	Region
Arabian Coffee	Middle East, Africa
Betel, Areca Nut	South Asia, Southeast Asia, Oceania
Coca	Peru, Ecuador, Bolivia
Coffee	South America, United States
Cola (Kola) Nut	West Africa
Khat	Middle East, Africa
Mate	Brazil, Argentina, Paraguay
Pituri	Australia
Tea	China, South Asia

nuts are one of the most important export crops. (Barton 1922: 407)

The religious and magical role given to betel in some cultures is found among the Toradja of Indonesia:

> Some use this means of enjoyment in moderation, others are addicted to it and declare that they would die if they had to do without the sirih quid. With the inflicting of imprisonment, many declare that absence from sirih-pinang is harder to bear than the confinement.
>
> The Toradja carries the sirih-pinang with him in an unfastened bag, which can be pulled closed with a cord. . . . A sirih bag is the most common gift that a girl makes for a boy. In addition to what he needs for his

betel quid, the Toradja keeps in it his flint and steel, means of divining, home remedies, money, and other trifles. It is regarded as great rudeness to take anything from someone's sirih bag without permission, for through this harm is easily done to the magic power of the magic remedies kept in it. For this reason too, one does not step over a sirih bag: it might be that the genitals would be affected by the remedies mentioned. (Adriani and Kruyt 1951: 353)

See also DIET AND NUTRITION; HERBAL MEDICINE.

Adriani, N., and Albert C. Kruyt. (1951) *The Bare'e-Speaking Toradja of Central Celebes (the East Toradja).* Translated from the Dutch by Jenni K. Moulton.

Andersen, Johannes C. (1995) *Myths and Legends of the Polynesians.* First published in 1928.

Babor, Thomas. (1986) *Alcohol: Customs and Rituals.*

Barton, Roy F. (1922) *Ifugao Economics.*

Conzemius, Eduard. (1932) *Ethnographical Survey of the Miskito and Sumu Indians of Honduras and Nicaragua.*

Emboden, William A., Jr. (1972) *Narcotic Plants.*

Heath, Dwight B., ed. (1995) *International Handbook on Alcohol and Culture.*

Hilger, M. Inez. (1939) *A Social Study of One Hundred Fifty Chippewa Indian Families of the White Earth Reservation of Minnesota.*

Jankowiak, William, and Dan Bradburd. (1996) "Using Drug Foods to Capture and Enhance Labor Performance: A Cross-Cultural Perspective." *Current Anthropology* 37: 717–720.

Jones, Livingston F. (1914) *A Study of the Tlinghets of Alaska.*

Kennedy, John G. (1963) "Tesguino: The Role of Beer in Tarahumara Culture." *American Anthropologist* 65: 620–640.

Levinson, David, and Martin J. Malone. (1980) *Toward Explaining Human Culture.*

Lewis, Bernard. (1995) *The Middle East: A Brief History of the Last 2,000 Years.*

McCoy, Elin, and Frederick Walker. (1976) *Coffee and Tea.* 3d ed., revised.

Marshall, Mac, ed. (1979) *Beliefs, Behaviors, & Alcoholic Beverages: A Cross-Cultural Survey.*

Quain, Buell. (1948) *Fijian Village.*

Richards, Audrey I. (1939) *Land, Labour, and Diet in Northern Rhodesia: An Economic Study of the Bemba Tribe.*

Rivers, W. H. R. (1914) *The History of Melanesian Society.*

Sahlins, Marshall D. (1958) *Social Stratification in Polynesia.*

Tschopik, Harry, Jr. (1951) *The Aymara of the Chucuito, Peru: 1. Magic.* Anthropological Papers of the American Museum of Natural History 44: 133–308.

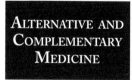

ALTERNATIVE AND COMPLEMENTARY MEDICINE

Alternative and complementary medicine is a general label applied to some healing approaches that do not fall within the framework of scientific medicine. That is, the approaches used are either an alternative to or complementary to biomedicine. Alternative approaches are ones that are promoted as equally or more effective approaches, at least for some purposes, than are those of biomedicine. Homeopathy and Ayurvedic medicine are general alternative health systems. Chiropractic adjustment for back pain, on the other hand, is a specific alternative treatment to such scientific approaches as anti-inflammatory drugs or surgery. Alternative approaches are used in place of scientific approaches. Complementary approaches, on the other hand, are used in conjunction with scientific approaches. For example, chiropractic adjustment for back pain becomes a complementary approach when it is used alongside anti-inflammatory drugs prescribed by a medical doctor. Alternative and complementary is a fairly recent label for this broad category of approaches. Other labels that have been and continue to be used include primitive, ethnic, marginal, unorthodox, unofficial, folk, popular, and vernacular healing. These labels reflect the belief among many health experts that biomedicine would eventually replace these alternative approaches, which were believed to be popular because (1) the users were ignorant of biomedicine, (2) biomedicine was unavailable, or (3) biomedicine was of little value—as in advanced cases of cancer—and people were desperate for anything that might work. A survey published in the January 1993 issue of the *New England Journal of Medicine* did much to destroy these beliefs and showed that at least 30 percent of Americans use alternative forms of healing. And compared to other nations, the United States is at the low end of the scale of alternative medicine. In European nations, 50 percent of people routinely use alternative approaches. In Germany, for example, 20 percent of physicians are homeopaths, anthroposophical physicians, or routine prescribers of herbal remedies. The Germans do not require that treatments be shown to be effective to be used, only that they are not harmful. Similarly, homeopathy and chiropractic are popular in Great Britain, along with other alternative approaches. Queen Elizabeth II employs a homeopath as one of her personal physicians and Princess Diana makes use of a half-dozen alternative methods for health maintenance purposes.

The hundreds of systems, approaches, and techniques that fall within the alternative and complementary rubric can be classified into six general categories:

1. Alternative medical systems such as homeopathy and Ayurvedic medicine
2. Mind/body interventions such as meditation and yoga
3. Diet and nutritional approaches that seek to prevent disease
4. Manual healing or bodywork such as chiropractic and massage
5. Herbal healing
6. Pharmacological and biological healing such as chelation therapy or the use of shark cartilage to prevent cancer

Of these six general categories, only the last remains truly controversial, as many health experts believe that these treatments are ineffective and that their use for life-threatening disorders such as cancer creates a situation where some people may use them and ignore effective treatments.

Although alternative approaches use a wide range of techniques, most share a number of common features. These include:

1. A focus on disease prevention and health maintenance
2. A holistic approach in which the whole person—mind, emotions, and spirit are considered
3. The use of natural processes and materials in healing
4. A focus on the cause of the disease rather than symptoms
5. A consideration of lifestyle and emotional issues
6. A belief that the body has an innate ability to heal itself when it is brought into balance or harmony

At the same time, however, different alternative approaches do reflect different beliefs about health and healing. Two popular though somewhat different approaches are found in the ideas of two leading proponents of alternative healing, Deepak Chopra and Andrew Weil. Both are medical doctors who have incorporated alternative approaches into their healing philosophy.

Deepak Chopra has combined his Western medical experience with Indian Ayurveda and posits the existence of an inner world where intelligence, thoughts, beliefs, and feelings are formed, and *can be changed,* directly impacting health. This inner world is called the quantum body, and Chopra believes that we experience it as a level of awareness. In it, perfect health resides. The more we access this quantum body, the more our body will begin to restore itself to health. Chopra's techniques, which include transcendental meditation, a purification regime called panchakarma to rid the body of toxins (or ama),

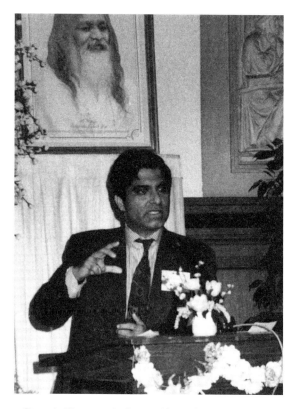

Deepak Chopra, who has combined his Western medical training with principles of Indian Ayurvedic medicine, speaks at the International Law and Peace Conference.

pulse diagnosis, a massage technique called marma therapy, music therapy, and aromatherapy, ultimately encourage a healthy lifestyle, but also provide contact with this quantum body: "In a serious or life-threatening illness, there can be many layers of imbalance concealing the depths where healing exists. Each layer is like a mask hiding the self from itself—one could spend a lifetime never suspecting that the quantum mechanical body exists. Perfect health is a reality at this deepest level, and it waits to be brought to the surface of life." (Chopra 1991: 111)

Andrew Weil leads a small number of conventionally trained physicians who are combining alternative approaches with orthodox methods. Weil is a proponent of "integrative medicine," combining the holistic philosophies and strategies of traditional medicine with the life-saving scientific methods of emergency and surgical care. He prescribes herbal remedies far more often than pharmaceutical drugs, which he finds overwhelming to the human body in many cases. He approximates that, after more than twenty-five years of personal research, he would recommend a conventional cure in only about 20 per cent of the cases he treats. He, and others, not only feel that this approach is more effective, but it would also drastically cut the cost of medical care and solve many of the nation's health care problems.

Alternative approaches became more mainstream in the United States in 1991 when Congress appropriated funds for the creation of an Office of Alternative Medicine (OAM) and placed it under the auspices of the National Institutes of Health (NIH) in 1993. The mission of the office is to facilitate the "evaluation of alternative medical treatments, including acupuncture and Oriental medicine, homeopathic medicine and physical manipulation therapies . . . establish an information clearinghouse to exchange information with the public about alternative medicine and support research training in this field." The office is supporting research on the effectiveness of acupuncture, massage therapy, hypnosis, music therapy, homeopathy, traditional Chinese medicine and herbs, and Qi gong. There is also a grant to create a center for alternative treatment of HIV/AIDS.

In addition to effectiveness, proponents of alternative treatments point to the lower costs for treating some ailments, as suggested by the examples below.

RECURRENT EAR INFECTIONS

Conventional Therapy: Antibiotics, with tubes surgically implanted in the ear canal(s) if condition persists. Estimated annual cost of conventional therapy: $650 million (10 million ear infections annually at a cost of $50 for office visit and medication and 100,000 children with tubes put in ears at $1,500 per procedure).

Alternative Therapy: Allergy elimination diet with individual food challenges to identify allergenic foods. This approach eliminates recurrent ear infections and eliminates the need for tubes in the ears at least 75 percent of the time. Estimated annual cost savings with alternative treatment: $487.5 million.

ACUTE MYOCARDIAL INFARCTION (HEART ATTACK)

Conventional Therapy: Fibrinolytic ("clot-busting") drugs such as tissue plasminogen activator (TPA) or streptokinase. Estimated annual cost of conventional therapy: TPA costs $2,300 per dose, streptokinase $280 per dose. Approximately $500 million to $1 billion spent annually on these drugs.

Alternative Therapy: Intravenous magnesium. Controlled studies show that magnesium reduces the death rate from acute myocardial infarction as much as or more than the fibrinolytic drugs and has fewer side effects. Magnesium costs about $5 per dose. Estimated annual cost savings with alternative treatment: the cost of magnesium is negligible, so approximately $500 million to $1 billion would be saved annually if doctors used magnesium instead of fibrinolytic drugs.

ALTERNATIVE AND COMPLEMENTARY APPROACHES

The following list provides a brief overview of the major approaches and techniques classified as alternative. The approaches that are covered in detail in separate articles in this volume are in ALL CAPITAL LETTERS.

Alternative Medical Systems

Acupressure
ACUPUNCTURE
AYURVEDIC MEDICINE
CHINESE MEDICINE
FAITH HEALING
HERBAL MEDICINE
HOMEOPATHY
NATUROPATHIC MEDICINE
Shamanism

Mind/Body Interventions

Bioenergetics
Biofeedback
Biorhythms
Body-Oriented Psychotherapy
Breathing Techniques
Color Therapy
Growth Astrology
Hypnosis
Hypnotherapy
Human Aura
Martial Arts

MEDITATION
Music Therapy
Past Life Therapy
Relaxation Techniques
Spiritual Healing
Therapeutic Touch
YOGA

Diet and Nutritional Approaches

Macrobiotics
Nutritional Therapy
Veganism
Vegetarianism

Manual Healing or Bodywork

Alexander Technique
Applied Kinesiology
Belly Dancing
CHIROPRACTIC
Massage
Myotherapy
Osteopathy
Polarity Therapy
REFLEXOLOGY
REIKI
Rolfing
Shiatsu
Trager Work

Herbal Healing

AROMATHERAPY
Bach Flower Remedies
Flower Healing

Pharmacological and Biological Healing

Bee Venom
Chelation Therapy
Colonics
Copper
Ginseng
Shark Cartilage

General

ASTROLOGY
Iridology

ALTERNATIVE HEALERS

While medical doctors and allied medical personnel sometimes employ what are classified as alternative methods in their practices, most alternative modalities are employed by healers who are not medical doctors. The training, licensing, and supervision required of these healers varies widely from individual to individual, although there has been a movement over the last two decades toward more training and state licensing. Regardless of whether they are licensed or not, no alternative healers are allowed to practice medicine in the United States. That is, they are not allowed to prescribe drugs, to conduct invasive tests, or to perform surgery. Some, however, are trained and permitted to use the results of medical procedures such as X rays. At least twenty-six medical schools in thirteen states, including Columbia and Harvard universities, offer course work in alternative medicine. Dr. Marc. S. Micozi (1996), author of the first American medical textbook on alternative and complementary medicines, states that

medical education must expand to include discussion of alternative medicine—why patients seek it, what forms may help certain illnesses, and what types are potentially useless or harmful. We also must fundamentally alter the manner in which students are trained. Medical students should study and observe the practitioners of alternative medicine. They should take fewer courses in the subspecialties of conventional medicine and spend more time working directly with patients, learning to appreciate their different cultures and attitudes toward health and disease. And adding to the curriculum more information about nutrition and other practices of good health should be seen as an important part of instructing students in the "art" and science of medicine. (Micozi 1996: 48)

While medical doctors earn the M.D. degree, alternative practitioners may earn any number of other degrees. The most common ones include:

B.A.M.S.	Bachelor of Ayurvedic Medicine and Surgery
C.A.	Certified Acupuncturist
C.A.T.	Certified Acupressure Therapist
D.Ac.	Diplomate of Acupuncture
D.C.	Doctor of Chiropractic
D.H.A.N.P.	Diplomate of Homeopathic Academy of Naturopathic Physicians
D.O.M.	Doctor of Oriental Medicine
L.Ac.	Licensed Acupuncturist
L.M.T.	Licensed Massage Therapist
M.Ac.	Master of Acupuncture
M.A.Sc.	Master of Ayurvedic Science
N.D.	Doctor of Naturopathy
O.M.D.	Oriental Medical Doctor

Experts who believe that biomedicine and alternative healing should coexist suggest that when searching for a practitioner of one of the alternative medicines, the following questions seem wise:

1. Are they willing to work with your physician in a complementary way?
2. Have they completed a proven course of study appropriate for their mode of treatment? Is the specialty licensed by the state or a regulating body, and if so, are they licensed?
3. Have they treated your condition, and do they have any way of demonstrating this?
4. Is it covered by health insurance?

Health insurance companies in the United States are slowly beginning to fund alternative medicine treatments. Massage, acupuncture, and chiropractic are covered more than most other alternatives. The cost effectiveness and the preventative aspects of these techniques may help to defray the rising costs of technological medicine.

See also BIOMEDICINE.

Chopra, Deepak. (1991) *Perfect Health: The Complete Mind/Body Guide.*

Dunkin, Amy. (1995) " 'Complementary' Medicine: Is It Good for What Ails You?" *Business Week* (November 27): 134.

Eisenberg, D. M., et. al. (1993) "Unconventional Medicine in the United States: Prevalence, Costs, and Patterns of Use." *New England Journal of Medicine* 328: 246–252.

Gottlieb, Bill, ed. (1995) *New Choices in Natural Healing.*

Hill, Ann, ed. (1979) *A Visual Encyclopedia of Unconventional Medicine: A Health Manual for the Whole Person.*

Hulke, Malcolm, ed. (1979) *The Encyclopedia of Alternative Medicine and Self-Help.*

Kastner, Mark, and Hugh Burroughs. (1993) *Alternative Healing: The Complete A–Z Guide to over 160 Different Therapies.*

Micozi, Marc S. (1996) "The Need to Teach Alternative Medicine." *The Chronicle of Higher Education* (August 16): 48.

O'Connor, Bonnie B. (1995) *Healing Traditions: Alternative Medicine and the Health Professions.*

Olsen, Kristin G. (1989) *The Encyclopedia of Alternative Health Care.*

Payer, Lynn. (1988) *Medicine and Culture.*

Weil, Andrew. (1983) *Health and Healing: Understanding Conventional and Alternative Medicine.*

Woodham, Anne. (1994) *HEA Guide to Complementary Medicine and Therapies.*

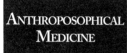

ANTHROPOSOPHICAL MEDICINE Dating back to the early 1900s, anthroposophical medicine is based on the philosophy of the German philosopher Rudolph Steiner and consists of an integrated body of knowledge and belief for healing the body, soul, and spirit. All anthroposophical physicians are licensed medical doctors, but they also embrace the Steiner philosophy that illness can be a powerful tool for spiritual growth.

Anthroposophical medicine rests on two core beliefs. First, illness represents a deviation from wholeness, and in this regard anthroposophical medicine is similar to many holistic approaches, including Ayurvedic and Chinese medicine. Second, the anthroposophical approach holds that illness serves the purpose of aiding the soul's learning and evolution, with the goal of realigning a person with the design of their higher self or Ego.

This transformative process of healing can only be accomplished with the conscious and willful participation of the patient. Though trained as medical doctors, anthroposophical physicians prescribe mostly homeopathic remedies, using their intuition to both diagnose and prescribe. Their key task, however, is to intuit the condition of the person's soul and spirit and to be a sort of midwife to the patient's personal unfoldment in the healing of the illness.

An example of this approach is found in the following description of the anthroposophical approach to treating back pain and why, after chiropractic and traditional medical treatment, problems can persist:

> In a lot of back problems it's difficult for a human to stand upright—not just in a physical sense. In our medicines we help strengthen the uprightness, which is a function of the Ego. You can wriggle a person's spinal column, but if you don't help a person feel stronger inwardly about their life, they keep succumbing to the enormous pressures. (Leviton 1988: 15)

Thus, the physical problem is seen as a reflection of a weakness in an emotional or spiritual sense.

The Ego is defined as "the individual spark of spiritual creative energy" (Leviton 1988: 9). It is what makes a person an individual and unique. The Ego is believed to be a part of a four-part model of the human being, which, in turn, is an integral part of the natural and metaphysical worlds. The first "body" incorporates the earth and mineral spheres and is the physical body. The etheric body is the second and is composed of life forces that facilitate growth and healing. It is aligned with the plant world. The astral component contains the emotions, feeling, and thinking and makes consciousness possible. It relates to the animal realm. The Ego is the fourth "body" and is related to the heart. It holds the blueprint for an individual's spiritual evolution. These bodies interpenetrate to create the physical, mental, emotional, and spiritual life that we experience.

Steiner called anthroposophical medicine a broadening of mainstream medicine. In its examination of the parts of the human being excluded from the experiments of biomedicine, he sought to treat the whole person, including their spiritual dimension. Since biomedicine focuses on the more easily observed physical realm, anthroposophical medicine can be viewed as the "art" of medicine that complements the science. In his writings, Steiner set forth ideas about the emergence of each of the four bodies, with a timetable corresponding to age. He identified possible illnesses that can develop when there is conflict or barrier to the proper development of each. Each of the bodies is the seat of aspects of being that enhance healing, that is, imagination is believed to be a function of the etheric realm, inspiration of the astral realm, and intuition of the Ego.

The astral body is felt to be the place where illness begins. The concept of karma plays a part in understanding how illness comes into a person's life and the place it plays in one's overall spiritual evolution. Karma is the energetic consequence of thought and action and includes the idea of reincarnation. Anthroposophists believe that the Ego (spirit) carries the past "record" of a person's thought and action from lifetime to lifetime. The evolutionary plan includes the patient's responsibility for addressing any negative influences from the past and for developing strategies for personal improvement. It is in this context that illness is seen as more than an accident or a negative twist of fate, rather it is seen as a catalyst for personal growth.

An anthroposophical doctor speaks at length with the patient, trying to first determine a nonphysical basis for the illness. It may be that the patient is involved in an emotional or spiritual crisis, in which the illness is an opportunity for healing a wound from the past. A good example is of a very aggressive man who developed eczema. With continued caring and concerned listening, he finally became very emotional as he expressed the great suffering he had witnessed during World War II. It eventually emerged that he had been burned with napalm in the very place on his skin where he was now developing eczema.

Through art therapy and healing conversations, he eventually had a powerful dream of healing, after which physical healing came about. But he had also become respectful of his own

and others' feelings, in the process becoming a more compassionate individual. This is an example of the type of spiritual growth that can accompany the experience of illness in the context of anthroposophy.

In addition to the spiritual overview, Steiner developed theories about the function of the human system. He believed that there is an energetic polarity process that includes a building-up pole, a breaking-down pole, and a balancing pole. One pole, the nerve-sense, is located in the head and is cool, draws inward, and serves the functions of conscious thinking. On the opposite end is the metabolic-limb system, which is warm and active and involves will and instinct. It is connected to the digestive organs and motor system. The rhythmic system of circulation and respiration harmonizes these two poles. It provides the physical basis for feelings and is believed to unite thought and will.

Illness can be viewed as too much activity in one or the other pole. If it is at the cold pole, the result is sclerosis, or degenerative disease; if it is at the warm pole, inflammation or fever is the result. The effect of inflammation or fever is actually believed to be a purgative to the system and is found most often in the first stage of development (birth to age seven). This process of reaction and healing is believed to clear the body of foreign materials. At this stage, the Ego is believed to be in conflict with forces of parental heredity. The astral body becomes active between seven and fourteen, and from fourteen to twenty-one the struggle between the Ego and independent rational thinking comes into play. It culminates at age twenty-one, when the Ego truly comes into its own.

Again, the goal of treatment is to work out the personal development of the client. "Healing occurs when the Ego's intentionality is liberated, when the patient experiences herself as a creative being, as much the creator of the illness as the facilitator of the healing." (Leviton 1988: 13)

At the same time, however, medicines may be given and there are some specialized diagnostic tools. One method of diagnosis is called the sensitive blood crystallization process and works by analysis of the patterns created when blood droplets are mixed with copper chloride. The patterns indicate the effects of etheric forces in particular organs of the body.

The oneness of man and nature is the philosophy that underlies the prescription of the remedies. Most medicines are homeopathic, but prescribed intuitively, taking into account the "nature" of the medicine as well as the symptoms that the remedies cure. Steiner believed that plant and mineral substances, as well as animal ones, have essential natures that correlate with different organs.

As in homeopathy, the remedies are believed to have captured the vital force of the material through the process of "potentization." In this process, the substance is placed in water and alcohol, shaken vigorously, and then diluted many times, with shaking at each dilution. This shaking and dilution is believed to transform the substance into a spiritual and medicinal force. Controversy exists over the remedies, as the successive dilutions often continue until there is no detectable trace of the original material.

Anthroposophical societies exist around the world from Argentina to Switzerland. Professional associations of anthroposophical doctors exist in sixteen countries. There are several anthroposophical hospitals and clinics in Germany, and clinics in Austria, Brazil, Italy, the Netherlands, Sweden, and the United Kingdom. A worldwide center of the Anthroposophical Medical Movement exists in Switzerland. Anthroposophical medical education is offered in Germany, the United Kingdom, Switzerland and the Netherlands. In the United States, the Physician's Association for Anthroposophical Medicine offers courses for physicians.

See also HOMEOPATHIC MEDICINE.

Bott, Victor. (1982) *Anthroposophical Medicine: An Extension of the Art of Healing.*

Evans, Michael, and Iain Rodger. (1992) *Anthroposophical Medicine: Healing for Body, Mind and Spirit.*

Hill, Ann, ed. (1979) *A Visual Encyclopedia of Unconventional Medicine: A Health Manual for the Whole Person.*

Leviton, Richard. (1988) *Anthroposophical Medicine Today.*

AROMATHERAPY

It is still something of a mystery how fragrance affects our well-being, but since the time of ancient Egypt and Persia, aromatic oils have been used to soothe physical and mental complaints, attract sexual partners, and embalm the dead. Cleopatra strewed her boudoir with rose petals during her seduction of Mark Anthony, massage using aromatic oils for health and healing has been around since ancient times, and the mummies of ancient Egypt are proof of the power of aroma.

Initially discovered as a by-product of herbalism, the use of essential oils in healing and cosmetics has its own lexicon. The oils are distilled from plant sources and stored in dark, air-tight containers because of their high volatility. The knowledge of the healing effects of various oils has been passed down through the ages to those who study aromatherapy. Oils are applied singly, or mixed with others that have similar properties.

The term aromatherapy is only about seventy years old. A French cosmetic chemist named Rene Maurice Gattefosse found a link between the use of essential oils and improvement in skin conditions. He had burned his hand and found that lavender oil sped its healing. He began research into the healing properties of many oils and discovered antibacterial properties in some of the oils. A colleague opened a clinic in the United States, where treatments for skin cancer, gangrene, and facial ulcers were developed.

Interest, though limited, continued in the research of Dr. Jean Valnet, an army surgeon, who used antiseptic essential oils to treat war wounds during World War II. In France today, medical doctors may study aromatherapy and include it in their spectrum of healing arts, as herbalists have done for centuries.

Aromatherapy's use as a rejuvenator was popularized by Marguerite Maury, a contemporary of Dr. Valnet, whose book *The Secret of Life and Youth* was published in France in the 1960s. Maury conceived the idea of treating the whole person by blending oils to meet the needs of each individual. Her idea was that the proper combination of oils could restore balance to an unbalanced body, mind, and spirit. She resurrected the ancient idea of skin application of the oil, which was the forerunner of the most popular form of aromatherapy used today, holistic aromatherapy.

Holistic aromatherapy is widely practiced in the United States and the United Kingdom and is generally used to promote relaxation and as preventative health care. Stress-related illnesses are also a focus. Depression, anger, anxiety, insomnia, acne, eczema, minor digestive complaints, menstrual cramps, and arthritic pain are some of the conditions that aromatherapists treat.

Oils may be diluted in hot water and inhaled, massaged into the body, added to baths, used as a compress, or (occasionally) swallowed. Creative uses include adding oils to a humidifier, placing drops of oil on wood to be burned in the fireplace, pouring diluted oil onto coals in a sauna, and using oils in potpourri, scented candles, perfumes. Massage is the most common usage.

The oils are distilled from plants as follows: plant materials are heated until vapor rises, then through the use of a cooling system the vapor is condensed. The liquid that condenses is a mixture of water and the essential oil. The two are easily separated, as the oil floats on the water. The oil is quickly bottled or it will evaporate. It takes five tons of rose blossoms to create just two pounds of rose oil. But only a few drops of oil are used in a typical treatment. Various parts of plants are used to obtain the oil, including leaves, roots, and flowers.

Like many holistic practitioners, an aromatherapist will interview clients about diet, lifestyle, general health and medical history, as well as the specific complaint. She will then consult the wealth of traditional remedies and choose oils to apply through one of the methods of application.

Aromatherapists combine oils with similar or complementary properties to meet the needs of the individual. Intuition plays a part in the healer's choices, in addition to knowledge of the oil's properties. The norm is to combine between two and five oils. They are said to work synergistically, with the result being greater than the individual properties of each. When applied through body massage, the essential oils are diluted in a carrier oil, a less-expensive and less volatile oil such as sesame oil, sweet almond oil, or a vegetable oil.

Some practitioners use the technique of dowsing to choose a healing oil: this technique is also used in herbal medicine. A pendulum is swung over the array of oils that are selected as possibilities; it is believed that the pendulum will gravitate toward an effective remedy. Sometimes the client chooses between several oils on the basis of the pleasantness of the smell.

Aromatherapists who use massage may use a number of techniques, including shiatsu, Swedish massage, and reflexology. The experience is relaxing and revitalizing and clients sometimes fall asleep. Massage has been proven to stimulate circulation, strengthen the immune system, reduce tension, and relieve pain. Some believe that it removes dangerous buildups of toxic waste that become stored in muscles when tension prevents natural elimination. The nurturing effect of touch has proven to be life-giving in the case of infants and those suffering from illness. The general effect of the aromas plus massage gives a deep feeling of well-being.

Occasionally, repressed feelings will surface and be released through talking or tears. Practitioners must be empathetic listeners when this occurs. For those suffering from mental illness, the effect of positive touch and the relaxing effect of the proper oils can aid healing.

The properties of the oils are categorized as stimulating, relaxing, or uplifting. Some, like garlic and hyssop, have what is referred to as a "normalizing" effect; both may be used to treat either high or low blood pressure, with good results. Short-term reactions to treatment include a slight worsening of symptoms for some. This effect is also seen in homeopathy, as the body reestablishes homeostasis.

Some common remedies for essential oils include: peppermint for irritable bowel syndrome, lavender for post-operative stress in heart patients and for burns and infections, eucalyptus for influenza, neroli for shock and stress-related conditions like indigestion and insomnia, marjoram for asthma, and rose for depression. Aromatherapy is a complementary therapy: it is not meant as a substitute for conventional medical care but as an adjunct that will stimulate the body's natural systems of healing.

The healing properties of the oils work in three ways: they reach the blood stream through the digestive system when taken orally, through the skin into the blood stream when massaged, and through vapors into the brain when inhaled. Odors dissolve in nasal tissue and then pass on to the hypothalamus through the olfactory nerves. The hypothalamus regulates body functions like temperature, blood sugar level, sexual arousal, and emotions. The "message of an odor" then travels to the limbic system, which handles emotions, and to the hippocampus, the part of the brain that has to do with memories. This explains why odors can so easily evoke nostalgia for other times and places.

An ancient form of aromatherapy, called marma therapy, is still used in India today. It is part of a healing system called Ayurveda, which means science of healthy living or longevity. Marmas are pressure points similar to acupuncture points, invisible to the eye but part of an energetic healing system within the body. Oils are used to massage the marma points.

Ayurveda is a healing system that seeks to balance body, mind, and spirit. Sensations to the body, including fragrances, are believed to consist of energy vibrations. Certain fragrances vibrate in a way that is more beneficial to one person than another. A system of types of people—called doshas—describes people based on their physical and mental and emotional characteristics. The make-up of certain types of foods or smells affects each dosha type differently. For example:

> Vata is balanced with a mixture of warm, sweet, sour aromas like basil, orange, rose, geranium, clove, and other spice.
> Pitta is balanced by a mixture of sweet, cool aromas like sandalwood, rose mint, cinnamon, jasmine and Kapha, similar to Vata, is balanced by a mixture of warm aromas, but with spicier overtones like juniper, eucalyptus, camphor, clove and marjoram. (Chopra 1991: 152)

The rejuvenating quality of essential oils led to many cosmetic uses, and the first perfumes were mixtures of essential oils. In ancient Egypt, female royalty were massaged by slaves with aromatic oils, conditioning the skin as well as making it fragrant. Most perfumes today are chemically based and lack the natural energy believed to be a part of the rejuvenating effect of the oils themselves. The art of embalming the dead with oils came from the belief that a person's physical body would be needed in the next life. Certain oils retarded the decomposition of the body. Oils were also used during times of plague and drought as a way of disguising offensive body odor.

See also AYURVEDIC MEDICINE; BODYWORK.

Chopra, Deepak. (1991) *Perfect Health: The Complete Mind/Body Guide.*

Davis, Patricia. (1995) *Aromatherapy A–Z.*

McGilvery, Carole, and Jimi Reed. (1994) *Essential Aromatherapy.*

Tisserand, Robert. (1988) *Aromatherapy: To Heal and Tend the Body.*

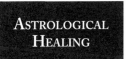

ASTROLOGICAL HEALING

A holistic view of the universe postulates that there are interrelationships among and parallels between all aspects of the natural and supernatural world. In many ancient systems of healing and philosophy, the idea that synchronous events are continually happening and reflect cycles of nature and similarities of properties was a guiding principle.

In the world view presented in modern astrology, the psyche of a person is believed to be a microcosm of the entire universe. It contains all qualities of experience, all talents, all predilections of behavior and feeling. The sun, moon, and planets represent *specific qualities.* What makes a personality and what life experiences are played out within this personality are defined by the particular alignment of planets within the zodiacal circle of star constellations that encircles the earth. This information is then mapped over a circle of twelve "houses,"

or aspects of experience, at the time of a person's birth.

Astrology means "star knowledge" in Greek. Its Western roots are in Mesopotamia and Sumer. Originally, the use of knowledge of the qualities and placements of the sun, moon, and planets in the star system was used as a tool for predicting events for royalty—who represented the divine on earth. Court astrologers would advise on the wisdom of taking particular courses of action and the most advantageous time to do so. This was called horary astrology.

Philosophical, humanistic, or growth astrology, which deals with aspects of personality for individuals and groups of people, came later, as individual human rights grew and as humans began to see themselves as the center of their own universe. Today many astrologers practice growth-oriented astrology, which uses astrological analysis as a tool for facilitating the spiritual growth of individuals, couples, families, and organizations. Closely related to this idea of spiritual growth is a desire for physical health; for some people, astrology is part of that process.

BASICS OF ASTROLOGY

Astrology is based on the observations of ancient times that the sun, moon, and planets move in our field of vision through the stars. Stars themselves move only incrementally. But as the earth rotates, twelve constellations, or star groups, appear to be circling overhead in a band around the earth. These constellations were discerned by ancient astrologers as the twelve signs of the zodiac, each having a different meaning, and together representing all of human experience. This band is called the ecliptic or zodiacal circle.

At different times during the day, month, and year, and depending on where on the earth you are looking out from, the planets, sun, and moon are seen against a backdrop of a particular star group, or constellation. A planet is then said to be in a particular zodiacal sign, for example, Venus is in Cancer. Due to the movement of the stars, called the precession of the ages, the correspondence is *not* exact, but that is the principle.

Using a reference work called an ephemeris, which contains the positions of the sun, moon, and planets as they move through the zodiac, and computer programs to perform mathematical calculations, modern astrologers plot these planets on a paper chart that includes the zodiacal circle of twelve 30-degree segments, overlaid by twelve houses (arranged like twelve pie slices of varying widths in 360 degrees of pie). When referencing the date and place of someone's birth, the resulting chart is called a birth chart, natal chart, or horoscope.

The qualities ascribed to the planets (it is an astrological convention to refer to the sun and moon as planets as well) are modified by those of signs of the zodiac they appear in. They function within the realm of life experience presented by the house in which they appear, forming the basis for describing the life experience of an individual. Another way of understanding this is to make a theatrical comparison: the houses are the stage set, the signs determine what the set looks like, and the planets are the actors.

The completed chart then contains planets and signs in each of the twelve houses. The interpretation of the interrelationship of all of these qualities, energies, and life dramas will identify talents; potential character strengths and defects; hobbies; career choice; quality of relationships with family, friends, and mate; and a host of other possibilities. The goal of humanistic astrology is to obtain information about these life patterns and innate tendencies from birth to death so that one can be active in life's events and turning points in pursuit of spiritual evolution.

The placement of the sun at the time of one's birth determines one's astrological sign. The signs of the zodiac are:

- Aries, the ram
  (March 21–April 20)
- Taurus, the bull
  (April 21–May 21)
- Gemini, the twins
  (May 22–June 21)
- Cancer, the crab
  (June 22–July 23)
- Leo, the lion
  (July 24–August 23)
- Virgo, the virgin
  (August 24–September 23)
- Libra, the scales of balance
  (September 24–October 23)
- Scorpio, the scorpion
  (October 24–November 22)
- Sagittarius, the archer
  (November 23–December 21)
- Capricorn, the goat
  (December 22–January 20)
- Aquarius, the water carrier
  (January 21–February 19)
- Pisces, the fish
  (February 20–March 20)

Aries starts the first day of spring and the signs always follow each other in the same order in 30-degree increments around the circle. They are represented on the chart with a symbolic letter, or glyph. The signs' element will be of earth, water, fire, or air; their mode will be cardinal, fixed, or mutable; and they can be expressed as masculine or feminine. Cardinal signs initiate, fixed signs stabilize, and mutable signs are receptive to change.

Aries is the ram, the life force, the will to exist. Its element is fire, and its mode is cardinal. It represents unyielding force in the face of life's challenges. Its lesson is courage, but its shadow side is a daredevil mentality and getting caught in the very crises that are meant to teach that lesson. Aries needs a force to push up against. Other Aries qualities are honesty, intensity, and directness.

Taurus, the bull, is the most physical sign, preferring the communication of music to that of words. Its element is earth and its mode is fixed. Taureans love silence, nature, simplicity, solidity. Its shadow side is the proverbial stubbornness of the bull, possessiveness, predictability, and a security bred from fear rather than choice.

Gemini represents the twins. Its element is air, its mode is mutable. Geminis are quick-thinking, intelligent collectors of information who strive to see clearly and who straddle unconventional and seemingly irreconcilable ideas regardless of how unorthodox their position may be. They revel in making sense of confusion. Their shadow side is the flip side of their quick minds—they never lose an argument and can reconstruct the elements of the truth to fit a less-than-true outcome. Geminis embody curiosity, vitality, and wonder in life.

Unlike Gemini, Cancer's exploration of the universe is an internal affair: Cancer leads with his or her feelings. Cancer's element is water, its mode is cardinal, and its archetype is the mother. Cancers develop an armor to protect their soft insides. The challenge for Cancer is to develop and evolve to the point where he or she outgrows his or her shell. Its shadow side is a tendency to hide from life, to hide beyond a nurturing persona instead of confronting the crises and challenges that are needed to grow.

Leo the Lion's strength is brash self-aggrandizement. Leo's element is fire, its mode is fixed. Leo trusts in life and knows how to be happy. Leo is the sign of the actor, the politician, the creative personality. You always know that Leo is in the room. Leo's shadow side is the tendency to alienate others by displaying a seemingly huge ego. Pride is another pitfall.

Virgo is the sign of wholeness, of the purity of mind embodied in Eastern philosophies like Buddhism and Taoism. Virgo's element is earth, its mode mutable. Perfection, unfettered

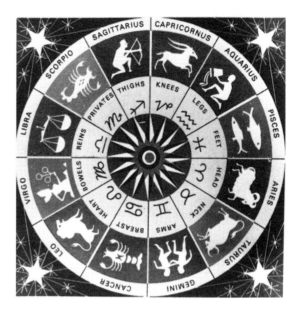

Astrology became popular in the United States in the 1930s. Today growth astrology is practiced to facilitate physical health, an aspect of spiritual growth.

freedom of the mind, is the goal of Virgo. Virgo loves order and may tend to seriousness and self-absorption, but service is the key to happiness. Self-criticism and self-abnegation are pitfalls for Virgo.

Libra's symbol is the scales of harmony and balance, the reconciliation of opposites. Libra's element is air, its mode is cardinal. Libra both appreciates and creates beauty in the search for a harmonious mental and spiritual structure within which to live or a harmonious relationship where he or she can dare to be his or her most vulnerable self. Libras are always able to see both sides of an issue, but this ability often makes decision making agony. Indecisiveness and dalliance are the shadow side of Libra.

Scorpio is intensely focused on the present, using feelings rather than reason to move forward in life. Scorpio's element is water and its mode fixed. Actions based on feelings lead to satisfaction; Scorpio wants his. Emotional encounters must be lived at a fever pitch. Repression is not a part of

Scorpio's makeup, but introspection is intense. Self-absorption and despair, a lack of balance in the consciousness, are the shadow sides of Scorpio.

Sagittarius is the wanderer, the student, the thinker. The search for meaning through travel and intellectual stimulation is paramount. Sagittarius's element is fire, its mode is mutable. Enthusiasm, free-spiritedness, and resilience mark the Sagittarian. There is not much from which Sagittarius cannot recover. In Sagittarius's search for wholeness, he or she seeks to discover his or her true place in life. Naiveté and placing too much faith in others may lead to tragedy.

Capricorn's vision is to have self and public personality become one. Capricorn's power, cunning, and ambition must be tempered with introspection and solitude to achieve balance. Capricorn's element is earth, its mode is cardinal. Patience, practicality, and self-discipline are hallmarks of Capricorn's success. Its shadow side is difficulty in forming close interpersonal relationships; feelings are a challenge.

Aquarius is the sign of human freedom, the rebellion against social conformity. Aquarius's element is air and its mode is fixed. Single-mindedness may lead to loneliness as Aquarians search for truth. Alienation is the shadow for this sign.

Pisces, the fish, lives in the mother ocean of emotions. Its element is water and its mode is mutable. An easy awareness of higher consciousness is central to the Piscean personality—formless, structureless, and creative. Subjectivity and madness may be a shadow side of Pisces, as well as escaping into addiction.

Next we will examine the qualities of the planets. Planets activate a particular energy in an area of life experience determined by the house and colored by the sign or signs in the house. Qualities of the "planets" are as follows:

1. The sun represents the essential self
2. The moon represents the expressed self or personality
3. The rising sign, which is the astrological sign and degree of the zodiac that was rising on the eastern horizon at the time and place of birth, represents the body through which this self and personality are anchored
4. Mercury is the trickster, the messenger, and represents mind, daily experience, and communication
5. Venus represents beauty and love, the emotional realm
6. Mars represents the ability to be aggressive and effective in the world
7. Jupiter represents hospitality, faith, and trust and expansion into the benefit in community
8. Saturn represents patience, limitation, and structure
9. Uranus represents the higher mind, the warrior
10. Neptune helps discern what is illusion and challenges us to go with what is real
11. Pluto rules transmutation and transformation, death and birth at a cellular level

Every planet rules a sign of the zodiac or has a natural affinity with one. Mercury rules Gemini, for example. Mercury is the planet of communication, and Gemini the sign of connections. Planets can rule more than one sign.

When a planet appears in the corresponding sign, its qualities are amplified and said to be "exalted." They may be said to be "in detriment" if the qualities of the planet are in conflict with those of the sign. In this case, the ruling planet of a sign appears in its opposite sign—180 degrees around the chart. Worse yet is if a planet is in its "fall."

The positions of the planets in relation to each other are significant and are called aspects. At 120 degrees, the aspect is called a trine and represents major harmony aspects of the chart. At 60 degrees is the sextile, which it not as strong and exerts minor benefit. At 90 degrees, the planets are square, which represents a challenging opportunity for growth. At 180 degrees, they are in opposition, and determining how to embrace both natures of the planets must be explored. When planets are said to be conjunct, they appear within a few degrees of each other.

Planets may be clustered in various ways, which are referred to as the bowl, the bucket, the seesaw, the scatter, the cluster, the splay, and the locomotive.

The houses of the zodiac are a function of the angles created by the division of the horizon line into unequal pie-like pieces. There is more than one house system: the most commonly used house system in the United States is called Placidus; the most commonly used house system in Europe is called Koch. There is also an equal-house system. The boundary line that separates one piece of "pie" from another is called a cusp.

The first house begins in the east and represents the way we put ourselves out in the world, the expression of our physical, genetic heritage and clothing styles. It includes the rising sign and begins the east to west movement. The second house has to do with possessions, valuables, and income. The third house rules communication, humor, community, siblings, the elementary school years, and short-distance travel or commuting. The fourth house is the psychic ground we stand on, the unquestioned assumptions about the world and one's family of origin. It represents the home that we create.

The fifth house rules gambling, love affairs, and children, as well as all aspects of creativity. The sixth house represents health, community service, and more mundane life activities. Traditional relationships are the basis of the seventh house—major commitments like marriage and business partnerships.

In the eighth house, power issues come to the foreground. Death, taxes, other people's money, and legacies are also at issue, as are natural ways of accessing healing energy and connection with inner divinity. In the ninth house, higher education and consciousness are played out, as well as long-distance travel, expansion of the mind, and goals and planning. The tenth house is the place of career or vocation and how we are seen in the world. In the eleventh house, larger groups of people, organizations, friendship groups, and manifesting one's dreams are key. The twelfth house is the house of karma—meaning the inter- and intrapersonal issues that are part of our life's work to solve. The challenge it holds out is growth on a soul level.

Growth Astrology

Astrology became popular in Western cultures in the early 1930s when Paul Clancy published *American Astrology* magazine. Evangeline Adams had introduced it to a smaller audience a few years earlier with a book called *Sun Sign Astrology*. After the success of *American Astrology*, newspapers began to print daily horoscopes (to the chagrin of serious astrologers).

Rather than take the view that these calculations set our lives in stone, most growth-centered astrologers take the view that the birth chart represents a spectrum of possibilities and that the individual knows best which aspects can be applied. What is not written is how the soul responds to the set-up; how these life patterns are played out depends on the person's own evolution. Particular energetic situations can warn of times of upheaval or trouble and can make the person mindful during that time. They need not portend disaster. Creative analysis of the chart can result in a picture of the best possible reality for the person being charted.

Astrologer Steven Forrest sets forth seven principles of growth-oriented astrology:

1. Astrological symbols are neutral. There are no good ones, no bad ones.
2. Individuals are responsible for the way they embody their birth charts.

3. No astrologer can determine a person's level of response to his or her birth chart from that birth chart alone.

4. The birth chart is a blueprint for the happiest, most fulfilling, most spiritually creative path of growth available to the individual.

5. All deviations from the ideal growth pattern symbolized by the birth chart are unstable states, usually accompanied by a sense of aimlessness, emptiness, and anxiety.

6. Astrology recognizes only two absolutes: the irreducible mystery of life and the uniqueness of each individual viewpoint on that mystery. (1984: 8–9)

7. Astrology suffers when wedded too closely to any philosophy or religion. Nothing in the system matters except the intensification of a person's self-awareness.

Each of these seven principles is basic. Subtract or distort even one of them and the whole edifice crumbles into a ruin of fortune-telling.

We are free. Celestial forces and the human will function together in an open, synergistic relationship.

Avery, Jeanne. (1982) *The Rising Sign: Your Astrological Mask.*

Forrest, Steven. (1984) *The Inner Sky: The Dynamic New Astrology for Everyone.*

Jones, Marc Edmund. (1972) *Astrology: How and Why It Works.*

Lofthus, Myrna. (1980) *A Spiritual Approach to Astrology.*

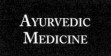

AYURVEDIC MEDICINE

Ayurveda, a 5,000-year-old system of healing from India, means "knowledge of the life span" in Sanskrit. "Ayur" is "the contact of our body with the soul that results in the state of living." (Thakkur 1974: 3) Ayurveda rests on the belief that by using techniques that treat the body, mind, and spirit equally a person will be restored to his or her natural balance. Health is seen to be the product of balance and the absence of disease. Unhappiness in work or family life, incompatibility with a particular climate or season of the year, and a diet of foods not compatible with one's body type are believed to cause disease in much the same way that in Western medicine germs are seen as causing disease.

The system relies on the belief in three organizing principles of nature called doshas. The Vata, Pitta, and Kapha doshas exist in all people, but vary in degree in each person. They are interdependent and work together. They are believed to be various combinations of any two of the five elements of the natural world: earth, water, fire, air, and space (ether).

Ayurveda also operates from the belief that by harnessing the power of the mind we can contact a center of awareness, where the mind and body are one, and that by bringing this awareness into balance, the body's balance will follow and healing will occur. It is believed that balance, even more than our Western medicine concept of immunity, keeps the body in a state of health.

Ayurvedic treatment involves identifying a patient as having one of the three doshas, or some combination of two, as predominant. Once the type is determined, and the imbalance identified, a particular diet, specific exercises, and certain routines are prescribed. Lifestyle changes are often recommended. The goal is to bring the patient into balance with his or her own nature or constitution. It is believed that this strengthens the mind-body connection.

Each of the dosha types has particular physical and psychological characteristics and differences in metabolism and dietary preferences. The person with a predominant Vata, for example, is said to be thin, enthusiastic, and vivacious by nature, with an active and imaginative mind.

They often have trouble falling asleep. The Pitta type is precise and orderly, quick to anger, fond of cold food and drink, and irritable if a meal is missed. They have sharp intellects and are articulate. The Kapha gains weight easily, needs lots of sleep, and has a calm personality. Kaphas have good physical stamina and are bothered by cool weather.

To understand the philosophy of Ayurveda, the following quote from the Indian writer Chandrashekhar G. Thakkur is helpful:

> To understand the patient as a whole is the physician's foremost task, but how and in what terms? Not merely as a victim of certain adventitious factors like germs, etc., but as a complex of certain basic factors which are liable to derangement and disorder through various causes such as age, diet, climate, season and the rest; and, having done this, to go on to prescribe matching modes of treatment, to restore him not only to a state where his particular complaint has disappeared, but to a condition of happiness wherein the mind and body are completely involved. (1974: xx)

According to ancient teachings, a person's predominant dosha is determined at the time of their conception in the womb. The two other doshas exist in a particular proportion. This proportional relationship between the three doshas remains constant throughout one's life, determining one's constitution or nature. An Ayurvedic doctor will not prescribe the same drug to two people with the same disease, but takes into account the person's dosha type and prescribes accordingly.

It is believed that balancing these doshas provides health without creating an imbalance in the form of the side effects or suppression of symptoms that may arise from using synthetic drugs. It is often felt by Ayurvedic physicians that drugs are more dangerous than the disease because of their sometimes debilitating side effects, which further push the doshas out of balance.

In Ayurvedic medicine the body is seen as perpetually changing, rather than solid. Our bodies are constantly creating new cells and replacing old ones. It is often said that the body completely replaces itself every seven years. Individual organs of the body replicate themselves even more quickly. Thus, the body is viewed as in process all the time.

The early exponents of Ayurveda had two different concerns: (1) to determine what is normal and (2) to determine what is pathological. The first would be described today as preventative medicine—to focus on and promote what keeps us healthy. Knowledge of this is considered as important as how to treat a disease or illness.

Important to their understanding of health is the Ayurvedic belief that the universe consists of five elements or factors in the natural world. These elements—earth, water, fire, air, and space—are the same elements found in the rest of the universe—in our food, water, and air. Humans are believed to be comprised of the same "stuff" as the world outside of us. It is the balance of these elements in ourselves that creates harmony between ourselves and our outer world, resulting in optimal health.

The five elements are said to have the following properties:

> **Earth.** Smell, density, heaviness, and solidity; its taste is slightly astringent, mostly sweet
> **Water.** Density, softness, moistness, flowing, cold; its tastes are slightly astringent, sour, and salty, but mostly sweet
> **Fire.** Light, active, rough, dry, hot, clear; its tastes are slightly sour and salty, mostly pungent
> **Air.** Light, rough, dry, cold, transparent; its tastes are slightly bitter, mostly astringent
> **Space (ether).** Light, soft, smooth, transparent; its taste is not manifested

From these five factors come the three doshas. Vata is believed to be composed of space and air energies, Pitta of fire and earth, and Kapha of earth and water. These doshas together constitute a dynamic that links the body and mind. Within the three doshas are twenty-five gunas, or fundamental qualities.

Vata is dry, moving, cold, light, changeable, subtle, rough, and quick. If your skin is too dry, your Vata is becoming unbalanced. Vata controls movement and its seat is in the heart. Its season bridges late autumn and winter.

Pitta is hot, sharp, light, moist, slightly oily, fluid, and sour smelling. Pitta relates to heat: burning sensations in the body indicate unbalanced Pitta. Its season is summer and early autumn and its seat is in the digestive system.

Kapha is heavy, cold, oily sweet, steady, slow, soft, sticky, dull and smooth. Gaining weight and depression make Kapha rise. Kapha controls the structure of the body and is expressed by the mucous membranes. Its season is in spring.

When one dosha grows in prominence by a particular diet or climate or disruptive influence, the others shift as well. The term Vyadhi refers to that which causes unhappiness, and Roga to that which causes discomfort. Stress and poor diet might fall under these categories, which unseat the balance of the doshas and cause disease.

One component of Ayurvedic medicine are myths regarding the imparting of the knowledge of Ayurveda to humans. One, described in the ancient Charaka Samhita, tells of a time when the earth was full of disease and the sages (wise and compassionate people) gathered near the Himalayas. They selected one of themselves, Bharadwaja, to go to the goddess Indra to learn the science of life. On his return he taught another sage, Atreya. Atreya had six pupils and each wrote a separate text. Two have been preserved, Charaka Samhita and Bhlea Samhita. This course of events is believed to have occurred between the sixth and seventh centuries B.C. An-

other story says that Indra sent the physician of the gods to earth to teach medicine with an emphasis on surgery. Sushruta was the most skilled and wrote the Sushruta Samhita.

AYURVEDIC MEDICAL PRACTICE

There are eight branches of Ayurveda:

1. Kaya (general medicine)
2. Shalya (major surgery)
3. Shalakya (ear, nose, throat, mouth, and eye diseases)
4. Bhuta Vidhya (psychiatry)
5. Kumara Bhritya (pediatrics)
6. Agada (toxicology)
7. Rasayana (rejuvenation or tonics)
8. Vajiarana (aphrodisiacs)

The Charaka Samhita describes six virtues of a skillful physician: knowledge, logic, science, remembrance, adaptability, and practical demonstration. He or she must be constantly learning. Thakkur says, "For a fool this whole world is full of enemies, but for an intelligent man, this whole Universe is full of experts and tutors." (1974: 7) Diagnosis by an Ayurvedic physician differs from that of a Western medical doctor, although in the West today, some doctors may use Ayurvedic techniques in combination with Western medicine. The pulse is felt, and a trained Ayurvedic physician "reads" the state of the patient's doshas from it.

This ancient skill of diagnosing from the pulse, called Nadi Vigyan, is also present in Chinese medicine. What the doctor is feeling for is the "quality" of the pulse. According to the Charaka Samhita, "The characteristic of earth is roughness, that of water is liquidity, of air expansion, of fire, heat and that of ether (space) non-resistance. All of these qualities are perceived through the sense of touch." (Thakkur 1974: 17)

If the doshas are in normal proportion and activity, the person will be healthy and happy. Therefore, the diagnosis consists of identifying which dosha is out of balance. Treatment consists of reducing the dosha that is in excess and increasing the dosha that is in deficit. The patient is questioned about his or her symptoms, but also about his or her mental state, family life, and overall strength. The season of the year is considered as well as the state of the "appetites" of the patient.

The disease process consists of six stages:

1. Accumulation: the buildup of one or more doshas
2. Aggravation: the dosha spreading outside its normal boundaries
3. Dissemination: the doshas moving throughout the body
4. Localization: the dosha settling where it should not
5. Manifestation: the physical symptoms arising at that point of localization
6. Disruption: full-blown illness

Vata is considered to be "king" of the doshas and, after a person's primary dosha, the most likely to go out of balance and cause stress-related problems. In Vata imbalance headaches, backaches, insomnia, and menstrual cramps are typical manifestations. Grief and depression are signs of Vata imbalance since Vata controls the nervous system. The physical indications would be constipation, dry skin, low stamina, high blood pressure, irritable bowel syndrome, intolerance to cold, and weight loss, among others. It is the energetic Vata that is likely to eat on the run while pursuing many interests and activities that cause overstimulation.

To balance Vata a doctor might prescribe regular habits of eating and sleeping, quiet, warmth, a steady supply of nourishment, attention to fluids, and a decreased sensitivity to stress.

A Vata-pacifying diet would include warm foods with added butter and fat, salt, sour, and sweet tastes, and satisfying foods such as stews and soups, casseroles, and fresh bread. Although sweet snacks may be eaten, too much sugar adds to Vata's restless nature. It is recommended that some fruits, such as apples and pears, be cooked before eating. Certain vegetables are to be eaten, and others avoided.

Pitta imbalance manifests itself as heartburn, ulcers, heart disease, and other stress-related problems. Pittas often drive themselves to extremes, becoming perfectionists. Anger, resentment, self-criticism, and irritability are out-of-balance Pitta qualities. To balance Pitta, moderation is called for. Coolness, attention to leisure, exposure to natural beauty, decreased stimulants, and a balance of rest and activity are advised.

A Pitta-pacifying diet would include cool or warm, but not hot, foods, bittersweet and astringent tastes, and less butter or fat. A Pitta is advised to avoid pickles, yogurt, sour cream, and cheese.

Kapha imbalance reflects excessive heaviness, whether it be obesity, heavy digestion, or depression. Diabetes or allergies reflect Kapha imbalance. Procrastination, greed, oversleeping, and possessiveness are some of the mental or psychological indications. To restore balance, stimulation is called for. Exercise, weight control, warmth and dryness, and reduced consumption of sweets are also ordered. Dry toast, apples, crackers, and raw vegetables are recommended.

MODERN AYURVEDIC MEDICINE

A modern system of Ayurveda was developed by Maharishi Mahesh Yogi, the founder of Transcendental Meditation, also called TM. This method of meditation became popular in the United States in the 1970s. His Ayurvedic system was brought to the United States in

1985. An American doctor of Indian descent named Deepak Chopra studied with him and has combined and extended his Western practice to include Ayurveda. He has also trained many other American physicians.

In the reemergence of Ayurveda by the Maharishi there is an emphasis on the power of the patient to heal himself or herself. A patient's attitude toward illness is considered to be a strong factor in this new approach. Chopra believes that freedom from sickness can be achieved by contacting the level of awareness where the mind and body are one, and bringing balance to that area. The body is then believed to heal itself.

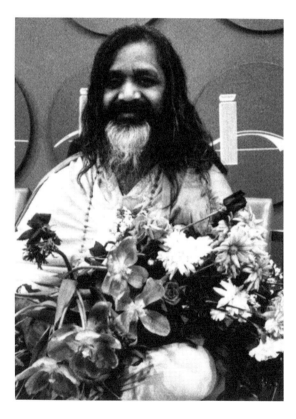

Maharishi Mahesh Yogi, in New York in 1968, developed transcendental meditation, which enables a practitioner to balance mind and body through meditation.

In addition to dosha diagnosis and diet and lifestyle change, some of the techniques used in Maharishi Ayurveda include TM and Primordial Sound. To transcend is to go beyond—in this case it means to go beyond the activity of the mind. TM seeks to reach a place of relaxation beyond even thought.

TM is practiced by repeating a mantra (a special syllable or word) over and over silently. Eventually an inner balance or repose is achieved. It is hoped that old thought patterns and mental blocks will fall away, and the mind will begin to heal itself.

In Primordial Sound, sound is believed to be a form of energy that "glues" the body together in balance. In illness, one is literally viewed as being out of tune. A daily technique is taught to reintroduce "lost" sounds.

Practicing the asanas (postures) of yoga is part of the treatment, as is the use of medicinal herbs, in the form of teas, tinctures, and massage oils. There are herbs that are believed to balance different doshas, as well as various smells. Aromatherapy may be part of a treatment, during which aromatic oils are placed in hot water and inhaled by patients.

Marma therapy is a form of massage that has as its starting point a series of 107 points on the body. These points, similar to acupuncture points in Chinese medicine, are believed to be very potent points of connection for the mind and body. When stimulated, a person's energy is believed to increase and balance is reached in the body.

A purification practice called panchakarma is often prescribed to clean out toxins and ama, the impurities deposited in the cells as a result of poor digestion. This practice takes about a week and includes the cleansing of the digestive tract.

Part of the philosophy of Ayurveda involves making correct choices. It believes that, at the center of being, everyone has healthy desires that will further their personal spiritual evolution. This quality is called sattva. The impulse to regress or stay the same is called tamas. Between the two is rajas, the impulse that tells a person when a choice must be made.

Everyone consists of a mixture of all these impulses. Sattva is said to combat mental ama—impure or negative thoughts that can build up and cause the doshas to go out of balance. Avoiding mental ama, which can be created through psychological stress, negative emotions, and witnessing acts of violence, is critical for health. Routines for increasing Sattva include

1. a pleasant, generous temperament;
2. acting from reason instead of impulse;
3. refraining from anger or criticism;
4. taking time for fun and play every day;
5. rising with the sun, watching the sunset, and occasionally strolling in the moonlight; and
6. eating light, natural foods.

While these may seem like common sense recommendations for living a happier life, in Ayurveda a happier life is a healthier life.

See also AROMATHERAPY; BODYWORK; DIET AND NUTRITION; YOGA.

Chopra, Deepak. (1989) *Quantum Healing: Exploring the Frontiers of Mind/Body Medicine.*

———. (1991) *Perfect Health: The Complete Mind/Body Guide.*

Maharishi Mahesh Yogi. (1968) *Science of Being and Art of Living.*

Thakkur, Chandrashekhar. (1974) *Ayurveda: The Indian Art and Science of Medicine.*

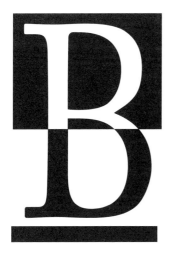

Biomedicine is the dominant type of medicine around the world. It is also called scientific, conventional, or allopathic medicine to distinguish it from alternative medicine, and Western medicine to distinguish it from traditional non-Western medicine. Biomedicine began and developed in Europe, with influences from the Middle East, spread to the United States, where it has also developed, and then spread to all areas of the world. As improving local health care, which usually means more biomedical care, has been a goal of nearly all governments and all international health organizations, biomedicine is now available in some form to all people around the world.

Three key features of biomedicine are (1) use of the scientific method to explain disease and develop and use treatment, (2) reliance on technology, and (3) specialization in treatment.

SCIENCE IN MEDICINE

Science and scientific medicine constitute the primary belief system of biomedicine. Science is based on objectivity, experimentation, rationality, facts, and truth. The basic assumption is that through careful and unbiased observation and experimentation, humans can discover and understand the true nature of the world. In biomedicine, this assumption is reflected in the use of observation and experimentation to study the human body and its interactions with the environment, to identify and explain the causes of disease—in general and in specific illnesses—and to develop and use treatments.

In the Western world, magic preceded science as the basis of medicine until about the sixth century B.C., when the scientific approach began to slowly emerge in ancient Greece. The Greek form of humoral medicine in which the body is composed on the four humors—blood, phlegm, yellow bile, and black bile—was perhaps the first attempt to explain human health in natural terms. In the fifth century B.C., disease came to be viewed as a natural rather than a supernatural phenomenon and physicians were trained to look for physical causes such as diet, occupation, and climate. The promulgation of the Hippocratic Oath in about 460 B.C. marked the beginning of scientific medicine, as opposed to magical medicine, in the West.

Throughout the Greek era and into the Roman era, medicine continued to develop as a science, with detailed studies of human anatomy and physiology and the founding of medical schools. Scientific medicine made little progress during the Middle Ages, but during the Renaissance began to develop again. The interest in the human form in art spurred the development of anatomy, physiology, and surgery. With the emergence of modern science during the Enlightenment in the seventeenth century, scientific medicine took major strides with the use of the experimental method and the microscope. In the eighteenth century, advances continued with the introduction of effective vaccinations, the further refinement of surgery, and, most importantly, the emergence of the body as a machine

THE OATH OF HIPPOCRATES
∴

I SWEAR BY APOLLO THE PHYSICIAN· AND AESCULAPIUS· AND HEALTH·AND ALL·HEAL· AND ALL THE GODS AND GODDESSES · THAT · ACCORDING TO MY ABILITY AND JUDGMENT · I WILL KEEP THIS OATH AND THIS STIPULATION— TO RECKON HIM WHO TAUGHT ME THIS ART EQUALLY DEAR TO ME AS MY PARENTS · TO SHARE MY SUBSTANCE WITH HIM · & RELIEVE HIS NECESSITIES IF REQUIRED · TO LOOK UPON HIS OFFSPRING IN THE SAME FOOTING AS MY OWN BROTHERS · AND TO TEACH THEM THIS ART · IF THEY SHALL WISH TO LEARN IT · WITHOUT FEE OR STIPULATION · AND THAT BY PRECEPT · LECTURE · & EVERY OTHER MODE OF INSTRUCTION · I WILL IMPART A KNOWLEDGE OF THE ART TO MY OWN SONS · AND THOSE OF MY TEACHERS · AND TO DISCIPLES BOUND BY A STIPULATION AND OATH ACCORDING TO THE LAW OF MEDICINE · BUT TO NONE OTHERS· I WILL FOLLOW THAT SYSTEM OF REGIMEN WHICH · ACCORDING TO MY ABILITY AND JUDGMENT · I CONSIDER FOR THE BENEFIT OF MY PATIENTS · AND ABSTAIN FROM WHATEVER IS DELETERIOUS AND MISCHIEVOUS · I WILL GIVE NO DEADLY MEDICINE TO ANYONE IF ASKED · NOR SUGGEST ANY SUCH COUNSEL · AND IN LIKE MANNER I WILL NOT GIVE TO A WOMAN A PESSARY TO PRODUCE ABORTION • WITH PURITY & WITH HOLINESS I WILL PASS MY LIFE & PRACTICE MY ART• I WILL NOT CUT PERSONS LABORING UNDER THE STONE · BUT WILL LEAVE THIS TO BE DONE BY MEN WHO ARE PRACTITIONERS OF THIS WORK • INTO WHAT· EVER HOUSES I ENTER · I WILL GO INTO THEM FOR THE BENEFIT OF THE SICK · AND WILL ABSTAIN FROM EVERY VOLUNTARY ACT OF MISCHIEF & CORRUPTION · AND FURTHER · FROM THE SEDUCTION OF FEMALES OR MALES · OF FREEMEN AND SLAVES • WHATEVER · IN CONNECTION WITH MY PROFESSIONAL PRACTICE · OR NOT IN CON· NECTION WITH IT · I SEE OR HEAR · IN THE LIFE OF MEN · WHICH OUGHT NOT TO BE SPOKEN OF ABROAD · I WILL NOT DIVULGE · AS RECKONING THAT ALL SUCH SHOULD BE KEPT SECRET • WHILE I CONTINUE TO KEEP THIS OATH UNVIOLATED · MAY IT BE GRANTED TO ME TO ENJOY LIFE AND THE PRACTICE OF THE ART · RESPECTED BY ALL MEN · IN ALL TIMES · BUT SHOULD I TRESPASS AND VIOLATE THIS OATH · MAY THE REVERSE BE MY LOT

The beginnings of biomedicine are traditionally attributed to the Greeks of the sixth century B.C. Hippocrates (c. 460–c. 377 B.C.) is known as the father of medicine. An oath attributed to him states that a physician will "follow that system of regimen which according to my ability and judgment I consider for the benefit of my patients and abstain from whatever is deleterious and mischievous. . . ."

model. In the 1880s, scientific medicine came into full bloom with a nearly complete knowledge of human anatomy and physiology, the proving of the germ theory of disease, the development of general anesthesia, and the recognition of insects as carriers of disease. In the twentieth century, scientific medicine has been closely linked with biomedical research and with basic science, which have produced antibiotics, chemotherapy, immunizations for many diseases,

organ transplants, and gene splicing, among many such advances.

As an applied science, clinical medicine (which is often described as both an art and science) is closely dependent on research in molecular biology, biochemistry, and genetics. The following concepts are central to biomedicine:

Homeostasis. All organisms seek to maintain a stable internal environment
Unity. All organisms have certain similarities, most importantly cells and the genetic material (DNA) within them
Evolution. All organisms have developed into their current forms through a process of random variation and selective retention
Diversity. In all populations there is variation caused by changes in DNA in some organisms
Ecology. All living organisms interact with their environment
Continuity. All living organisms reproduce

TECHNOLOGY

Modern biomedicine is based on the use of technology in research, diagnosis, and treatment. Some technology remains low level, such as the stethoscope to listen to chest sounds, scales to record a person's weight, and the inflatable sleeve to take blood pressure. However, much of biomedicine is now based on highly sophisticated technology to study the basic biological processes, to identify disease agents, to develop and test treatments, to diagnose, and to treat diseases and injuries. Electron microscopes, genetic engineering, CAT scans, pacemakers, arthroscopes, and technologically produced drugs are all now routine elements of biomedicine. The reliance on technology is perhaps the one aspect of biomedicine that draws the greatest criticism from advocates of alternative approaches. The technology is seen as dehumanizing and ignoring the emotional, cultural, and spiritual factors that influence health.

SPECIALIZATION

Specialization is reflected in the number of different occupations within medicine, in the major medical specialties, and in specialized treatment facilities. Medicine has evolved from the days when medical healers were either physicians, dentists, or nurses to encompass a very broad range of medical personnel. These include:

Attendant
Audiologist
Dental Hygienist
Dentist
Dietitian
Emergency Medical Technician
Health Aide
Laboratory Technician
Midwife
Nurse
Nurse's Aide
Occupational Therapist
Optician
Optometrist
Orderly
Pharmacist
Physical Therapist
Physician
Physician Assistant
Podiatrist
Psychologist
Radiology Technician
Recreational Therapist
Respiratory Therapist
Social Worker
Speech Therapist

In addition to these people who provide medical care, modern health facilities include other support specialists including medical administrators, accountants, counselors, insurance liaisons, and medical records personnel.

In modern medicine, the general practitioner is largely an occupation of the past. Most physicians are now specialists who treat only certain parts of the body, certain diseases, or perform only certain types of procedures. In American medicine, twenty-four such specialties are recognized with over fifty additional subspecialties subsumed under these general ones:

Allergy and Immunology
Anesthesiology
Colon and Rectal Surgery
Dermatology
Emergency Medicine
Family Practice
Internal Medicine
Medical Genetics
Neurological Surgery
Nuclear Medicine
Obstetrics and Gynecology
Ophthalmology
Orthopedic Surgery
Otolaryngology
Pathology
Pediatrics
Physical Medicine and Rehabilitation
Plastic Surgery
Preventative Medicine
Psychiatry and Neurology
Radiology
Surgery
Thoracic Surgery
Urology

Some subspecialties that are widely known include Sports Medicine, Cardiovascular Disease, Geriatric Medicine, Hematology, Pain Management, and Infectious Disease. Physicians who specialize in any of the specialties or subspecialties receive advanced training in the field and are often certified by the professional organization that oversees the field. In addition to physicians, there are now specialists in other healing professions, including dentists and nurses. Dental specialties include Family Dentistry, Oral Surgery, Periodontics, Endodontics, and Orthodontics. Nursing specialties include first the distinction between Registered Nurse and Licensed Practical Nurse and then specialties such as Pediatric Nursing, Psychiatric Nursing, Nurse-Anesthetist, Nurse-Practitioner, Nurse-Midwife, and Nurse-Educator.

Another form of occupational specialization in biomedicine is that between practitioners, who treat patients, and researchers, who conduct basic research or study diseases and treatments. Some researchers are also practitioners who treat patients, while some researchers are not physicians. These include public health specialists, epidemiologists, neurobiologists, physiologists, anatomists, and kinesiologists.

In addition to occupational and task specialization, biomedicine is characterized by place of treatment specialization. Medical care is offered at physicians' offices, health maintenance organizations (HMOs), hospital outpatient departments, emergency treatment centers, health care centers, hospitals, nursing homes, hospices, mental health facilities, and rehabilitation centers. People may also be treated at home, usually by nurses.

All of these specializations concern the treatment of disease, although in the last few decades the field of preventative medicine or wellness has expanded rapidly. Like treatment, the approaches advocated in wellness programs are based on scientific research. Attention is focused on issues such as diet and nutrition, exercise, weight, self-care, and the environment.

BIOMEDICINE AND CULTURE

While biomedical healers use scientific medicine, cultural factors influence how medicine is actually practiced. One important cultural difference is between medical care in urban centers and medical care in rural areas. In the former, technology plays a greater role, recent innovations are more likely to be available, and a greater range of specialists can be consulted. Similarly, there are variations in biomedical practice across cultures. For example, there are significant differences between how biomedicine is practiced in the United States and in European nations such as Germany, France, and Great Britain. U.S. medicine is considered to be especially aggressive and stresses treatment by exclusion, that is, by taking something out or leaving something out. American physicians use more diagnostic tests, prefer surgery over drugs, use more aggressive forms of surgery, and use vaccinations to wipe out a disease rather than to protect those individuals who may be at risk. Similarly, American dentists clean their patients' teeth more often than European ones. The French, on the other hand, rely more on natural healing and make extensive use of radiation treatment. In general, American medicine is not as good at treating chronic diseases that do not respond quickly to aggressive interventions.

See also ALTERNATIVE AND COMPLEMENTARY MEDICINE.

Larson, David E., ed. (1996) *Mayo Clinic Family Health Book.*

Payer, Lynn. (1988) *Medicine and Culture.*

University of California at Berkeley. (1991) *The Wellness Encyclopedia.*

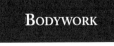 **BODYWORK** Bodywork, or manipulation of the body for healing, is a mode of holistic, complementary medicine that has become increasingly varied and popular in recent years. With a history that goes back to ancient Greece

and China, the combination of specific techniques of massaging muscles, stimulating pressure points, and manipulating tissue is a powerful adjunct to conventional medicine. There are also nonmanual forms of bodywork, which include the martial arts, movement therapies, structural reintegration of the body, and the combined use of physical and psychological methods to heal.

Beneficial effects of bodywork include improved circulation of blood and lymphatic fluid, release of body impurities called toxins, improved muscular and joint mobility, increased strength, relaxation, psychological healing, and enhanced mind/body integration. In the more traditional forms of bodywork that continue to be used indigenously, claims are made for healing everything from birth defects to minor health problems to digestive and pulmonary complications.

MASSAGE

There are three possible origins of the word massage, the most commonly known form of bodywork. The first, from the French "maser" means to shampoo. The second, from the Greek "massein" means to knead. And the last, the Arabic "mas'h" means to press softly. During massage, the somatic (body) tissue is kneaded and pressed to stimulate and revitalize the entire system.

Massage in ancient Greece was promoted by the physician Galen as a treatment for injuries and as preparation for gladiator competition—perhaps the first indication of sports medicine or massage. In ancient China, India, and Thailand, therapeutic massage was done to rejuvenate the body and spirit, as well as to promote healing, using a specific set of points on the body. Chinese acupressure massage, Ayurvedic marma therapy massage, and Thai Nuad-bo Rarn work through these pressure points, which are believed to stimulate energy pathways that circulate the life force through the body.

Massage was done in the time of Julius Caesar for headaches, neuralgia, and paralysis. Roman women and slaves massaged the bodies of returning warriors. Massage was also done in conjunction with bathing to stimulate and refresh.

Lomilomi massage in ancient Hawaii was performed by medical priests called kahunas and was used in childbirth, in preparation for bloodletting, and for rheumatism, asthma, and bronchitis. Babies were massaged to promote health as well as to cure birth defects.

Aromatic and other types of oils have been associated with massage throughout history to smooth the sensation of rubbing the skin and to promote healing. The essential oils of various herbs and flowers have soothing or stimulating effects and, when combined with massage, are used to cure illness, promote relaxation, or enhance feelings of well-being. Marma therapy from Ayurveda uses sesame oil and was done for years as a daily ritual for many Indians. It is still practiced today and is believed to contribute to healing. Egyptian women were massaged with oils by their servants as a beauty ritual. Both the Old and New Testaments of the Bible record the anointing of feet with oils as a gesture of respect and devotion.

Massage and bodywork continue to be an important part of the healing process in most Eastern countries. Acupuncture and acupressure massage never went out of popularity in China, for example, nor did marma therapy in India. Lomilomi is still practiced in Hawaii. But little is heard of bodywork or massage in the West between the time of the ancient Romans and the nineteenth century, perhaps as a result of the rise of Christianity and the association of the body with sin in Christian philosophy.

It reappears in the early nineteenth century, when massage is seen in France and later in Sweden. Peter Henry Ling, a Swedish professor, started a school for teaching massage for healing

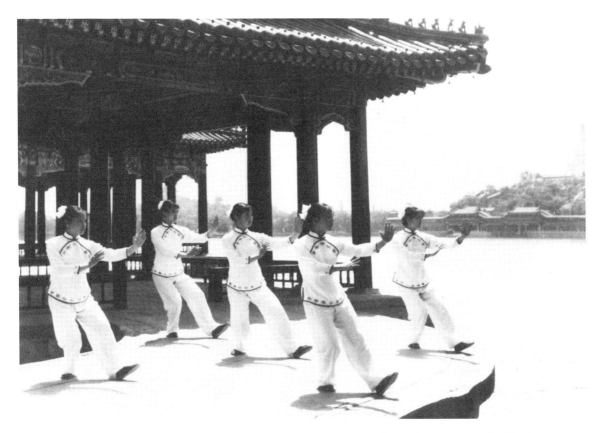

Manipulating the body through movement, massage, or other stimulation to promote healing is called bodywork. Chinese women demonstrate ta'i chi ch'uan, an ancient martial art form, the practice of which is a kind of meditation that promotes healing and grace.

stiff muscles and joints. His technique, known as "Swedish massage," is still used today and consists of a series of repetitive stroking and kneading of the muscles and tissues of nearly every area of the body to loosen the joints and relax the muscles, resulting in an invigorating effect. Swedish massage was introduced in the United States and Britain in the late nineteenth century. In 1894, some American masseuses banded together to form the Society of Trained Masseuses.

Most people enjoy the feeling of massage and of being touched, but bodywork has not been an integral part of the healing systems in the West since the early 1900s, when allopathic medicine took hold. The miraculous ability of powerful drugs to cure specific problems seemed to overshadow the need for attention to the body as a whole. The techniques of physical therapy, which was designed to promote healing through exercises and stimulation of injured body parts, became the "place," medically speaking, where bodywork was done.

Massage was and is now more integrated into the health care systems of Russia, Germany, and Sweden than those of the United States. Massage and bodywork in the United States came to be seen as a luxury for the rich—part of a beauty ritual or an after-sport relaxation. Bodywork as a therapeutic regimen to complement and promote healing of illness became nearly nonexistent for years.

OTHER FORMS OF BODYWORK

With the resurgence of interest in holistic conceptions of health and wellness in the 1960s, bodywork reemerged as a technique for healing the whole body. In the 1990s many Americans use bodywork for relaxation and stress reduction. The number and kinds of bodywork available in the West has mushroomed, and just about every technique performed in the world can be sampled here. There are over eighty different forms.

Some types of bodywork aim to restructure the body, balance the energy, or create smoother pathways for the nervous system. Movement techniques like t'ai chi ch'uan, yoga, dance, and martial arts forms stretch and work the body and contribute to focused concentration and alignment of the body that promote healing.

Some people believe that central to the effect of therapeutic manual bodywork is the mysterious connection of one person to another in the act of touching. Mirka Knaster writes that "we know the world first through our bodies—through our senses, especially touch." (1996: 124) The importance of touch to human growth and development has been explored in many ways, especially in theories of learning. Where infants are concerned, observation and research have shown that premature infants in neonatal intensive care who are touched are more likely to thrive than those who are not, prompting a regular schedule of "handling" by nurses. Babies appear to need to be cuddled and cooed to be motivated to survive, even those in the protective cocoons of incubators. A classic study in 1939 by H. M. Skeels and H. B. Dye investigated the effects of stimulation on the development of infants and young children and found a correlation between lack of stimulation and mental retardation.

Some non-Western cultures regularly massage infants as part of a bath ritual to enhance growth and vigor, correct birth defects, etc. Infant massage is today recommended for infants with developmental difficulties, as well as for healthy infants. To facilitate the emotional bonding of breast-feeding infants to their fathers, massage may also be helpful.

Mental health professionals recommend "a hug a day" to maintain good mental health. Touch can soothe and relax, in and of itself, but another therapeutic effect of bodywork is the awakening of emotionally charged memories. The stimulation of the soma tissues, where the body has stored repressed emotional memories, can bring them suddenly to consciousness. By following an axiom for the healing of psychological disturbances—that the release of repressed emotional trauma heals it—bodywork practitioners may work together with therapists in healing the bodies and minds of clients.

> Somatic [body] tissue functions as a secondary storage facility for the brain. An automobile accident shows us how this takes place. The sound of screeching tires, the sight of an upcoming tree, the touch of an out of control steering wheel are the sensory cues which cause us to hold our bodies tight and to experience fear in the few moments before impact. After impact, the continuing spasms and lingering fear are, in effect, stored images of these original cues. Here muscle spasm is a form of somatic memory arising from three different sources—seeing, hearing and touching.

Bodywork practitioners have observed that when the area of the body that is "holding" the memory is stimulated by massage, the memory may be released to consciousness. Once the emotional memory is released, there is the possibility of healing the incident that caused the trauma. In a sort of circular logic, there appears to be a connection between the release of these emotions and the physical healing of the part of the body storing the memory. Practitioners also speak of energy cysts or stored emotional energies that collect in the body, which dissipate when stimulated and released. These might represent repressed emotional as well as physical trauma.

Different bodywork techniques and practitioners work in various ways with this release of emotional memory. Some practitioners work with clients who want to verbalize and release the pent-up bodily energy that is "behind" the emotions. Specific techniques work with this directly. The ethical question of whether the practitioner is qualified to help patients deal with these notwithstanding, the recommendation is that it is entirely up to the client to express or re-repress these memories. Painful memories are stored because some part of the person cannot deal with them, and professional help is often needed to deal with them when physical stimulation of the body brings them unexpectedly to the surface.

The combination of the relaxing effects of touch and the invigorating effects of the manipulation of body tissue and/or energy centers is an antidote to the lethargy of the sedentary lifestyle of many Westerners. There are many styles of massage for all types of conditions and desired results. More traditional Western techniques include Swedish massage, sports massage, infant massage, geriatric massage, and Russian massage. Structural approaches include Rolfing, Hellerwork, and myofascial release. Functional approaches to bodywork like the Alexander Technique involve relearning how to move and stand comfortably. Eastern approaches include Ayurveda from India, acupuncture and acupressure from China, shiatsu from Japan, and taha from Thailand. Other energetic systems include polarity energy balancing, therapeutic touch, and Reiki.

Bodywork can include movement systems to promote healing and grace, such as t'ai chi ch'uan, aikido, yoga, and martial arts. Combinations of systems include Phoenix Rising Yoga Therapy, Jin Shin Do, and somatosynthesis.

Most bodywork sessions last between sixty and ninety minutes. Some last only fifteen minutes, such as mini-sessions done in chairs, which are becoming more popular in offices. Some forms of Thai massage last three hours.

The following is a partial list of the types of bodywork currently practiced in the United States and elsewhere:

1. **Acupuncture/Acupressure.** Works through the stimulation of 365 points that are believed to exist on twelve invisible energy meridians going the length of the body. Blocked chi, or life force, is dispersed or built up to regulate this flow of energy. Acupuncture uses needles, while acupressure uses the hands and other types of

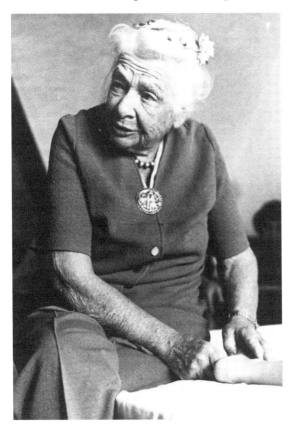

Ida P. Rolf demonstrates structural bodywork that relies on what she called structural integration and is known by its popular name, Rolfing.

massage techniques like squeezing, kneading, walking on the back, and manipulating joints.

2. **Aikido.** Twentieth century martial art form from Japan. *Ai* means harmony in Japanese, while *ki* means life force. Aikido is a nonviolent form of physical discipline that seeks, through focused attention to the form, to eliminate barriers to harmonious, natural movement and self-defense.

3. **Alexander Technique.** By observing poor postural habits and identifying areas of tension, this technique helps people gain an awareness of their bodies and helps them learn easy, natural, and tension-free movement and posture.

4. **Authentic Movement.** A form of spontaneous, self-directed movement exercise, usually done with another person who observes and gives feedback to the mover. The idea is to surrender to inner impulses and explore the images and emotions that drive the movement and that are expressed by it as a way of getting in touch with one's inner thoughts and feelings.

5. **Ayurveda.** The name of the ancient Indian health care system that works on the principle of balancing the doshas, or metabolic energies of a person. Massage with sesame oil is a part of a daily ritual for many Indians.

6. **Lauren Berry Method.** A method of soft-tissue manipulation and deep massage intended to restore the body's inherent balance and alignment.

7. **Bindegewebsmassage.** Works with connective tissue called fascia, which binds bones to muscles and muscles to muscles. Like muscular tissue, fascia constricts with tension. The tissue is worked with crooked fingers in a pulling and pushing motion.

8. **Breema Bodywork.** From the mountains of the Middle East, this Kurdish massage tradition was a part of everyday life for centuries. Movement of the limbs, stretching, bending, and brushes with the hands make it similar to Thai massage, without the use of pressure points.

9. **Chi Kung.** A Chinese technique using breath, meditation, slow movement, and visualization that seeks to increase the life force, or chi. When mastered after many years of study, practitioners can literally throw this energy to repel attackers, without needing physical strength. Chinese doctors use external chi kung to assess the deficient or excess chi in a patient and send in life force. It has been used to treat a number of diseases from gastrointestinal problems to cancer. It is done as a regular meditation-in-motion practice by many Chinese seeking to maintain good health.

10. **Contact Improvisation.** A form of movement, developing out of modern dance, in which a group of dancers works spontaneously to form shapes and patterns in space through points of contact between each other. Trust is a central element, as dancers shift their weight on and off each other at the points of contact.

11. **Continuum.** Seeks to develop awareness of the body as a part of a continuous stream of movement, rather than a set of interconnected parts. Exercises to encourage spontaneous movement and infantile and childhood memories of more fluid movement styles are done to develop relaxing, fluid movement.

12. **Cranio-Sacral Therapy.** Seeks to balance the cranio-sacral system of bones, fluid, and tissues in the skull, spine, and sacrum. The cranial fluid flows through membranes that connect the bones and tissues and has a particular rhythm, which is regulated by this form of manual manipulation.

13. **Dance Therapy.** A form of art therapy that uses movement to assess a psychological problem, work through it, and effect change. Done most often in inpatient hospital settings, it works on the premise that the way we move our bodies reveals how we feel.

14. **Feldenkrais Method.** The self-description of the Feldenkrais method is "functional integration and awareness through movement." The work seeks to rework inefficient patterns of movement through learning. In functional integration, a practitioner helps the client focus on new ways to move limbs and body parts through manual manipulation. In awareness through movement, group lessons are given in highly structured movement sequences to achieve effortless movement.

15. **Hellerwork.** A combination of connective tissue work, movement education, and guided emotional memory of the client's development process. Consists of eleven sessions, which seek to work out difficulties or blocks from infancy to adulthood.

16. **Jin Shin Do.** "The way of the compassionate spirit" is a combination of energetic work, Taoist philosophy, and Reichian theories of how repressed emotion results in inflexible body armor. The technique helps the body relax, aids mind/body integration, and invigorates, while also seeking to teach the release of emotions in an appropriate manner.

17. **Jin Shin Jyutsu.** A system from Japan called "the art of benevolence." Uses twenty-six "safety energy locks" as pressure points to unblock life energy that has become congested through negative thinking and the difficulties of life. Pressure is applied in particular combinations in a system similar to acupressure. The effect is revitalizing and recharges the sys-

tem, but it does not claim to cure illness per se.

18. **Karate.** A form of martial art, once used in combat, but also used as a meditative technique that seeks to help people develop a harmonious relationship with life. The forms of blocking and punching movements combine with sparring and self-defense moves in a particular rhythm and sequence that helps builds physical mastery. The power that results is a result of both physical strength and mastery of balance, timing, and speed. Breaking the form, or going beyond it, is the goal after many years of mastery.

19. **Lomilomi.** A form of traditional Hawaiian massage, once performed by ritual priests called kahunas, that uses rhythmic movements that are both physical and stimulating to the energetic system. Lomilomi means "to break up into small pieces with the fingers." It includes stroking and kneading, walking on the back, gentle pressure with an open hand, and brief pressure on specific points to stimulate the mana, or life energy. Self-massage can be done with a curved stick. It is considered spiritual work and recognizes the power of a divine source working through touch.

20. **Ortho-Bionomy.** Combines elements of the martial arts and osteopathy in working to promote self-regulation and balance. Works at restructuring the posture and body-holding habits.

21. **Phoenix Rising Yoga Therapy.** Using the postures, or asanas, of yoga, a practitioner assists the client in holding the pose past his or her physical limit in an attempt to encourage emotional issues to surface. Verbal dialog then ensues, with the hope of gently integrating the deeply held emotion. The hope is for the practitioner to

assist in the client's mind/body integration and help the client get in touch with feelings, as well as for the practitioner to sense where the client is "holding" emotions, which will be focused on in future work with the client.

22. **Polarity Therapy.** Developed by a Western doctor who studied Eastern energetic approaches like Chinese medicine, polarity is based on the idea of the existence of an energetic system within and surrounding the body and is designed to balance and unblock energy and promote healing. After locating sources of blockage in the body, manual manipulation of the body is done, using anywhere from a light to a heavy touch to restore balance. Occasionally the body is not touched at all, but the energy flowing around the body is moved. A cleansing diet and exercises using polarity yoga are often recommended, as is working with blocked emotional and mental patterns.

23. **Reflexology.** A system generally used in foot massage that incorporates the Chinese idea of energy lines running the length of the body, culminating in the feet and hands. Stimulation of the points in the feet or hands that "reflex" to particular organs or body systems promotes healing by increasing the flow of life force or energy to the area. The bottom of the foot itself becomes a "map" of the whole body, with the center line of the foot representing the waist, etc. Clients report a feeling of relaxation, invigoration, and overall well-being after having received a foot massage. Used as a form of complementary medicine to promote healing.

24. **Rolfing.** Also know as structural integration, this rigorous and sometimes painful method consists of moving the "segments" of the body into alignment. It consists of manipulating the myofascial tissue to lengthen and move freely while massaging muscles and applying pressure to various areas of the body. The goal is to re-align the body on the "Rolf line." It is believed that when the body is properly aligned on this imaginary vertical line going through the body it is working with gravity rather than against it, thus creating ease of movement. Release of chronic tension and emotion is commonly experienced. A series of at least ten sessions is required, and sometimes a few more.

25. **Russian Massage.** This form of massage, well integrated into mainstream Russian medicine, combines elements of Swedish massage and Bindegewebsmassage with a clinical precision. It is used in structural or muscular problems, for recovery from surgery, and with cardiovascular, neurological, and gynecological disorders.

26. **Shiatsu.** An East/West hybrid developed in Japan that combines abdominal massage, acupressure point massage, breathing exercises, and Buddhist philosophy. There are a variety of styles, including some that consist of more Western (Swedish) massage and others that focus on the points along the energy lines or meridians. The most recognized form of shiatsu is the Namikoshi neuromuscular style, which relies on Western analyses of anatomy combined with working the points. Shiatsu became popular in the work world, where short shiatsu massages were given to Japanese workers at their desks. It gained acceptance as a form of medical treatment in Japan, where lifestyle recommendations including dietary changes and corrective exercises are also given. The hand techniques come from an earlier form of Japanese massage called anma.

27. **Somatosynthesis.** Practitioners guide clients on emotional explorations by using the body for emotional clues. Movement and even gentle touch can evoke mental imagery that is used in this process, with the hope of freeing the client from emotional, psychological, and physical problems.

28. **Sports Massage.** Any massage technique that helps athletes to remain free of pain and relaxed and to maintain optimum ease of movement and balance to prevent injuries. Sports massage, which started with nursing the bodies of Greek and Roman athletes, was popularized in the United States following its use by Olympic athletes from Europe and the Soviet Union.

29. **Swedish Massage.** One of the first popular Western forms of medical massage, done using rhythmic manual manipulation of the somatic tissue in stretching, kneading, pounding, and stroking movements. It yields excellent results in promoting relaxation, providing pain relief, and speeding the healing of injuries.

30. **T'ai Chi Ch'uan.** A series of connected movement meditations that sprung from the martial arts tradition in China. Practiced daily by many Chinese as a form of strength-building and balance, both mentally and physically, t'ai chi ch'uan offers a focus to develop and balance the chi, or life force, in one's life. May be done by elders as well as the young.

31. **Therapeutic Touch.** Based on age-old traditions of hands-on healing and developed by a nursing teacher, this technique seeks to complement conventional medicine through interaction with the subtle energy bodies that are believed to exist above the surface of the body. Now accepted as an optional part of a nurse's education, it has elements of Reiki, energetic healing,

and faith healing. Centering, the process of focusing one's energy to become a vessel for the flow of life energy, is done, as well as passing the hands over the energy field looking for areas of imbalance to treat.

32. **Traditional Thai Massage.** A rigorous series of stretches, bends, leans, and joint manipulation that can last three hours. The body is stretched in every imaginable way to stimulate the movement of life energy through pathways called "sen." Rocking movements are used to open the joints and stimulate the body.

33. **Trager Psychophysical Integration.** A system of movement reintegration using a series of rocking, jiggling, stroking, and other motions to relax and soothe the body and reawaken memories of a tension-free body.

34. **Trigger Point Therapy.** A neuromuscular form of therapy that seeks to release the built-up knots of tense muscle and fascia that collect in our bodies after injury and trauma. The sensitive trigger points are released through manual manipulation, and the body is stretched and relaxed to prevent their return.

35. **Yoga.** The physical branch of yoga is done as a series of integrated postures called asanas. These postures are learned and practiced to improve strength, circulation, and coordination, as well as to achieve the union of body and mind that is at the heart of the Hindu philosophy from which it arose. Used by many Westerners as a form of relaxation, the mastering of these postures results in feelings of peacefulness and serenity.

The certification and training for the various types of bodywork vary from state to state. Professional organizations exist for some forms, while others are relatively unorganized. For this reason, word-of-mouth is the most common way to find a bodywork practitioner. Sometimes a massage therapist can be found working in a chiropractor's office, though usually not anywhere near a conventional allopathic physician. Massage therapists are on staff at health spas and hotels, on cruise ships, and in gyms.

Clothes are off for some techniques (Swedish) and on for others (Reiki, Polarity), although the comfort level of a client can sometimes affect this. Trust is an essential element in the practitioner-client relationship, so it is essential that a person seeking bodywork have a good referral and feel comfortable with the practitioner. Competence, confidentiality, and ethics are areas of concern when seeking bodywork. Fees range from barter to $150 per visit, with most falling in the $40 to $75 range. There is usually a course of treatment that lasts beyond one visit.

A bodywork practitioner will usually do a health history and assessment, not as a diagnostic tool but for background. Contra-indications may exist for certain kinds of bodywork, and it should never be used solely as a substitute for conventional medicine.

See also ACUPUNCTURE; AYURVEDIC MEDICINE; REFLEXOLOGY; REIKI; YOGA.

Knaster, Mirka. (1996) *Discovering the Body's Wisdom.*

Chopra, Deepak. (1991) *Perfect Health: The Complete Mind/Body Guide.*

Collinge, William. (1996) *The American Holistic Health Association's Complete Guide to Alternative Medicine.*

Hill, Ann, ed. (1979) *A Visual Encyclopedia of Unconventional Medicine: A Health Manual for the Whole Person.*

Prevention Magazine Health Books. (1989) *Hands-On Healing: Massage Remedies for Hundreds of Health Problems.*

Stillerman, Elaine. (1996) *The Encyclopedia of Bodywork.*

Tappan, Frances M. (1980) *Healing Massage Technique: A Study of Eastern and Western Methods.*

Yamamoto, Shizuko, and Patrick McCarthy. (1993) *Whole Health Shiatsu.*

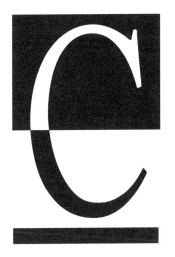

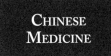

CHINESE MEDICINE Traditional Chinese medicine and modern scientific medicine coexist in the People's Republic of China (mainland China), the Republic of China (Taiwan), and in overseas Chinese communities around the world. Western-trained or allopathic doctors and rural health workers administer medicines and vaccines. Surgery is performed. But the Chinese continue to use techniques of traditional medicine as well.

In the People's Republic of China traditional medicine was at first rejected following the Communist takeover in 1949. During the Cultural Revolution of the 1960s, however, borrowing from the West in both science and culture was rejected and the traditional arts of acupuncture and healing with herbs were reintroduced. In addition to these methods, Chinese believe in "sacred medicine," in which a ritual curer, known as a tang-ki, intercedes with the gods to determine the cause and cure of illness. Divining, exercise, and massage are auxiliary methods to maintain health.

The three major approaches coexist in a sometimes easy, sometimes uneasy way. As we will see, there are religious underpinnings to Chinese medicine that have not been adopted by Communist China. Acupuncture and healing with herbs and foods is secularized in mainland China, while in Taiwan ritual practices associated with traditional medicine are more obvious. And some aspects of Chinese traditional medicine are now recognized for their value in Western nations.

Chinese medicine rests on some basic religious and philosophical beliefs. At the core is the ancient religion/philosophy of Taoism, whose central belief is the underlying unity of all life, with a force of universal energy called chi coursing through it.

Health is believed to consist of the proper amount of chi flowing into and between various organs and body parts. An imbalance of chi anywhere in the body throws off the entire system. As in Indian Ayurvedic medicine, balance is believed to be the key to health. The body is seen as a microcosm of the universe—and the goal is to resonate in balance with it. Diagnosis consists of identifying and rectifying the imbalance, which will have the effect of "curing" the illness. Treatment consists of diverting more energy to those organs with deficient chi, and less to those with too much. Massage, herbs, diet, and acupuncture are techniques that can be used to rebalance chi.

This simple formula gains in complexity as we note the next important concept of Taoism—the balance of opposites called yin and yang that are believed to constitute chi. Yang is thought to be masculine, active, hot, large, and the quality of daytime. Yin is feminine, passive, cold, small, and the quality of night. The union of yin and yang brought the universe into being, according to Taoism, and everything, including people, has a mixture of both. Food, herbs, and organs of the body are all identified as being one or the other and, simplistically, treatment consists of the matching of opposites to achieve the proper flow of the chi. In addition, yang is thought to represent the world of waking consciousness, and yin the parallel world of gods and ghosts. We discuss below how healing in one of these worlds is believed to affect the other.

The next layer in this overall scheme of the natural world is made up of the five elements: wood, fire, earth, metal, and water. Again, all substances are said to consist of some of these, alone or in combination. Yin is metal and water. Yang is fire and wood. Earth is the balance of yin and yang. In the realm of the body, the yang organs are the heart, liver, kidney, spleen, and lungs, while the yin organs are the small intestine, gall bladder, urinary bladder, stomach, and large intestine. Each also has an identification with one of the five elements: spleen and stomach are said to be earth, for example, while the lung and large intestine are metal. The five elements are not believed to be stable. They are constantly changing, with one combining with another to give rise to a third in a fixed cycle. For example, "the liver (wood) controls the spleen (earth) and is controlled by the lung (metal); it also generates the activity of the heart (fire), and its own activity is generated by the kidney (water). These relationships indicate the direction of the flow of chi energy from one organ to another." (Weil 1983: 145)

Diagnosis consists of questioning and observing the patient and of taking his or her pulse. The Chinese physician works many years to master this technique, which involves distinguishing twelve separate pulses from both wrists. He or she places the first three fingers of the hand on both wrists and uses light and firm pressure to gather the separate pulses. The rate of the pulse and its rhythm are important, but there are other subtle qualities that add to a correct diagnosis. Each of the pulses corresponds to one of the twelve "spheres of influence" (loosely cor-

responding to the organ systems). Thus doctors can determine where the excesses or deficiencies in energy exist and which of the five elements are involved, without any invasive techniques.

The fact that the Chinese have developed an "energetic system," or one based on function rather than form, is not surprising when we consider that the Chinese venerate their ancestors and that autopsies were traditionally prohibited, so doctors did not have detailed knowledge of internal human anatomy. What they did discover is the quality and direction of energy or vitality flowing between the twelve spheres of influence. They are believed to exist in a parallel way on the surface of the skin, allowing them to be "read" through the pulse.

HEALING WITH HERBS

Shen Nung, China's legendary god of farming, is believed to have lived about 5,000 years ago. A 52-volume encyclopedia called *Pen Ts'ao Kang-mu*, compiled in the sixteenth century, lists the natural plants and substances that he is believed to have used in traditional healing. The list is not confined to herbs, although these are very important, but also includes animal parts. For example, sliced deer antler is combined with dried seahorses and herbs to make a general tonic believed to be especially good for women after childbirth. Snakeskin and cattle skin are used to treat skin disorders, and the insides of a frog to cure chest congestion. Bones might be ground into a powder and mixed with other ingredients. Tiger testicles were made into a potion to promote virility. One headache remedy contains eight different substances, including herbs, roots, berries, and spices. As in Ayurvedic medicine, different remedies might be given to two patients with the same problem. Age, gender, and the season of the year are taken into consideration.

Some of the ingredients used are being tested by Western scientists to "prove" their value. Ginseng root, for example, has been popular for thousands of years in China. The philosopher Confucius spoke of the plant 500 years before the birth of Christ. The author of *Pen Ts'ao Kang-mu*, Li Shih-chen said, "It would allay fear, expel the evil effluvia, brighten the eye, open up the heart, benefit the understanding and . . . invigorate the body and prolong life." (Ackman 1977: 68) The root was popular in the early colonies of the United States, and it was grown and exported. Chemical analysis has shown that it contains minerals and vitamins and other active medicinal substances. There is evidence that drugs made from ginseng can strengthen the body's immune system and generally tone and increase physical and mental energy. In experimental studies in the former Soviet Union, it has had a positive effect on diabetes, neurosis, and radiation sickness.

In the late 1970s there were 6,000 pharmacies selling herbs in Taiwan and 3,000 traditional doctors. In mainland China, local health care workers called "barefoot doctors" use traditional herbs grown in the area for their treatments in addition to some basic allopathic practices. According to one expert, traditional Chinese medicine consists of 85 percent natural products and 15 percent acupuncture. Herbs are also used as part of acupuncture treatment.

DIET

Dietary changes may be prescribed to balance the yin and yang. Some of the specific qualities of yin and yang in food are as follows: yang is considered to be "hot" and present in the more nutritious foods, such as meats. The qualities of yang are oily, sticky, and of an animal nature. Yin foods are "cold": soups, vegetables, and watery foods like herbal teas. Hot, or yang, foods are used to build the body's resources, whereas yin, or cold, foods are considered to be cleansing and to remove toxins.

ACUPUNCTURE

Acupuncture is the other major method of treatment in China. It is more invasive, involving the insertion of needles into the body at specific points that are believed to control or regulate the flow of chi. The points are configured along invisible lines in the body called meridians. Each organ is connected to a meridian and along each lies a series of points that produce different effects when stimulated. Acupuncture is covered in its own entry in this volume.

ROLE OF RELIGION

The religious roots of traditional Chinese medicine are undeniable. Once all illness was believed to be a result of human misdeeds or of an angry spirit. The remedies were often mixed by priests or temple physicians with incantations and prayer.

Some of this practice continues today, especially in Taiwan, where consulting a tang-ki (curer) about the cause and cure of an illness is as common as going into a pharmacy to fill a prescription. Often a visit to a curer is the last resort—after one consults an allopathic doctor or herbalist with no positive result. Studies have reported a strong need by the Chinese to know the cause of their illnesses, even if there is not an effective cure. It is believed that the sick will gather as much information from doctors as they can to take with them in the event that they have to go to the tang-ki.

One of the many cults in the sacred medical system is called Ong-ia-kong. Ong-ia-kong is the name of the plague god. He communicates his diagnosis and cure through the tang-ki. The tang-ki is selected for certain qualities by older tang-ki; it may not be a choice on the part of the person selected. It is always a man, someone illiterate and willing to go into a trance whenever he is called. He often has a literate assistant who does paperwork for him.

Tang-ki worship involves bowing and offering incense, candles, food, and firecrackers to the statue of the god. The assistant writes information on the back of pieces of blank "spirit" money. Other ritual objects, like red envelopes and a special seal for the god, are arranged. The assistant begins by burning the spirit money and beginning a chant. The tang-ki stands, praying. He then sits and his eyes close. He begins to tremble and his hands beat on his knees. He then begins to jump, still hitting his hands on his knees, and continues for about a minute. Eventually he comes down with his head on the table, his hands clasped above his head. At this point the assistant stops chanting and reads off the cases. The tang-ki speaks in a high, strange voice. When it is time to advise the patient, his voice normalizes, but he goes back and forth into the higher, falsetto voice. He often expresses annoyance at repetitive questions.

People may come in to worship, and stay to chat, offering their own advice. The session may go on for four hours, with the tang-ki in the same position, bent over the table. He may prescribe lifestyle changes and/or herbs. He may refer a patient to another medical system, although he may actually prohibit Western medicine if he feels it will overwhelm the power of the herbs. He also may intuit that there are supernatural forces at work, which may require a particular ritual or exorcism. Any combination of the above may be prescribed.

The most common type of illness is *chhiong-hoan*, which involves having crossed one of the thirteen major deities. One can inadvertently offend the gods, simply, for example, by being born at the wrong time or building something in the wrong place. A sacrifice is usually offered. The second type of illness comes from fear, which results in loss of parts of the soul, which must be reunited to cure the patient. In the third type of illness a fetus god or spirit enters the child in utero. Ong-ia-kong can handle the pains in the pregnant woman's abdomen that may be a consequence of this. Fate is the fourth type, and may be discovered by taking the time of birth to a fortune-teller. The fortune-teller will look for the possible pitfalls in the child's life and set up rituals to prevent them from happening.

DIVINATION

There is a special book that has recorded the various possible situations that a person could be in depending on the position of the elements relative to their life. The book is called the *I-Ching*, or *Oracle of Change*. It is based on the same theory of opposites—yin and yang—as herbal medicine and acupuncture. The oracle tries to calculate the interplay of the possible energies between the yin and yang that brings all things into creation.

The client throws out sticks or coins six times, and each reading indicates an unbroken or broken line. The hexagram that is formed from the lines is broken into trigrams, each of which represents a particular element or energy (e.g., wind, water, the mountain). The resulting hexagram is one trigram over another (e.g., wind over the mountain, or fire on the water), and an interpretation of life is made from this configuration. The fortune-teller is usually a man of middle or old age.

Physiognomy, or "the examining of features," is also used. Interpretations of a patient's personality, behaviors, and past and present lives are "read" from his physical features. Advice is given on how to deal with his problems.

MEDITATION IN MOTION

The Chinese doctor may also encourage a patient to take a form of exercise called t'ai chi ch'uan. Based on a martial arts form, this repetitive, methodical series of forms has a meditative and relaxing effect on practitioners. The goal, once again, is balance, as the chi is raised through movement.

MASSAGE

There is also a form of massage called acupressure that is based on applying pressure to the acupuncture points, which raises and balances the chi. It is based on the same principles as acupuncture but is less invasive.

MENTAL HEALTH

In the realm of mental health, the Chinese do not share the Western notion of personal responsibility for one's problems. Excessive worry or unfulfilled desires are often blamed on forces beyond the person's control, and rest, nourishment, and recuperation are often prescribed.

CHINESE MEDICINE IN THE WEST

Some allopathic doctors have been open to the complementary use of Chinese medicine when treating their patients. The goal of Chinese medicine is for each person to learn how to keep their own balance and good health. According to author and doctor Andrew Weil, the realm of preventative medicine is a natural place for Chinese medicine to fit into the Western medical model. "Because it is chiefly concerned with the energy economy of the body, it is better equipped to deal with illness in its earliest stages. . . . They say that all visible illness is preceded by invisible illness. The idea is that imbalances of energy in the body, if allowed to persist, will eventually cause changes in the material structure of the body. By correcting excesses and deficiencies of energy in vital spheres of function, the acupuncturist prevents invisible illness from becoming visible; that is his primary responsibility." (Weil 1983: 152)

See also ACUPUNCTURE; ALTERNATIVE AND COMPLEMENTARY MEDICINE; HERBAL MEDICINE.

Ackman, Lonnelle. (1977) *Nature's Healing Arts: From Folk Medicine to Modern Drugs*.

Hill, Ann, ed. (1979) *A Visual Encyclopedia of Unconventional Medicine: A Health Manual for the Whole Person*.

Hsu, Francis. (1943) *Magic and Science in Western Yunan: The Problem of Introducing Scientific Medicine in a Rustic Community*.

Kleinman, Arthur. (1978) *Culture and Healing in Asian Societies*.

Kleinman, Arthur, et al., eds. (1975) *Medicine in Chinese Cultures: Comparative Studies of Health Care in Chinese and Other Societies*.

Risse, Gunther, ed. (1973) *Modern China and Traditional Chinese Medicine*.

Tan, Leong T., Margaret Y. C. Tan, and Veith Ilza. (1973) *Acupuncture Therapy: Current Chinese Practice*.

Weil, Andrew. (1983) *Health and Healing: Understanding Conventional and Alternative Medicine*.

CHIROPRACTIC MEDICINE

Chiropractic medicine is a method of drug-free healing that uses manipulation of the joints, muscles, and vertebrae of the spine in combination with nutritional counseling and lifestyle change to cure many painful conditions. In particular, chiropractic manipulation of the spine is recognized as an effective modern treatment for low back pain in some people. Millions of Americans and Europeans see chiropractors every year. In Great Britain, chiropractors are called osteopaths.

The word *chiropractic* comes from the Greek words for hand and practice, and the roots of chiropractic date back to Hippocrates. Damage to the spine caused by poor postural habits, injury, and muscle tension due to stress are corrected primarily through manual adjustments.

The overall aim of this healing technique is to maintain a properly functioning spine, which is the pathway of the nervous system.

ORIGINS

Chiropractic is a natural holistic approach because its aim is to promote proper functioning of the nervous system as part of a preventative health care approach. Its aim in correcting damage to parts of the spine, muscles, and joints is to allow the body to stimulate its own natural healing ability.

The idea that the condition of the spine is an indicator of health goes back to Hippocrates. The spine contains the spinal chord—the neurological pathway through the body. In ancient Greece what we now know to be the nerve impulses were called "vital forces," and the proper flow of the "vital forces" was believed to be the key to health.

Daniel David Palmer developed modern chiropractic in the late 1890s by postulating that "misaligned spinal segments interfere, by way of impingement on nerves coming from the spine, with the passage of . . . nerve impulses." (Hill 1979: 73) Since the central nervous system coordinates all biochemical functions—including our organs, breathing, heartbeat, digestion, sight, movement, etc.—it stands to reason that damage to the nerves would affect those functions. Surrounding muscles and ligaments are affected by improper alignment as well.

According to the American Chiropractic Association, modern chiropractic is based on four theories or principles:

> (1) Disturbances of the nervous system *may* cause disease. Although a number of factors impair health, disturbances of the nervous system—which coordinates cellular activity for adaptation to external or internal environmental change—are among the most important. Disease originates when environmental agents and conditions which unduly irritate the nervous system, and to which the body cannot successfully adapt, produce fluctuations in the pattern of nerve impulses deviating from the norm;
>
> (2) Disturbances of the nervous system may be caused by derangements of the musculoskeletal structure. . . .;
>
> (3) Disturbances of the nervous system may cause or aggravate disease in various parts or functions of the body;
>
> (4) A disorder in a specific organ or tissue will have an effect on the other functions organs and tissues. . . . (Langone 1982: 21)

Here is an example of how this might work: If a person injures his back while picking up a large package, the pressure on the spinal chord may cause a pinched nerve. The injured nerve may or may not be felt, as only some nerves in the spinal column can transmit feeling. Regardless of whether the injury results in pain or loss of feeling, the function of the nerve itself is affected.

That nerve might be part of the pathway of the autonomic nervous system, which controls involuntary actions like digestion and breathing. A pinched nerve that is part of this system can trigger production of stomach acid or spasm in the colon, with ulcer or colitis as the result. A muscle in the bronchial passage may constrict, causing asthma. Any blockage of the nerve impulses has some impact on the automatic functions of the body and may result in disease. Unanswered at this time is the question of how much or how little effect the nerve damage can have on this regulatory system.

The story of the origin of this healing system is that Palmer, a Canadian grocer and dabbler in spiritual matters, happened upon this technique when he persuaded an office janitor to let him manually adjust his spine. The janitor had become deaf after a back and neck injury. After the adjustment, there was a "click" and the man's hearing returned. Palmer continued to experiment and gained many supporters, which resulted in the opening of a school to teach adjustments. Palmer was subsequently jailed for practicing medicine without a license, but his son went on to fame and fortune. His son's frankly commercial interest in building the chiropractic empire and his shoddy educational requirements appalled many.

For many years chiropractic struggled as an untested and condemned form of medicine in the United States. It was and remains more generally accepted in Europe. In the United States it has waxed and waned in popularity. After many years of trying to keep chiropractors from being recognized as healers, the American Medical Association lost its battle against chiropractic in a 1987 court challenge, and chiropractors were allowed to practice in American hospitals.

In December 1994, the U.S. Agency for Health Care Policy and Research recommended spinal manipulation as a primary form of treatment for many acute low back problems. The *British Medical Journal* reported a 70 percent improvement in those given chiropractic treatment over those given normal outpatient care. Now that chiropractic is becoming more mainstream, and its effectiveness in treating some back problems proven, research is going forward to test its effectiveness in treating organic problems and diseases.

PRACTICE

A first visit to the chiropractor will be lengthy and include a detailed medical history and questions about diet and lifestyle. A person's occupation may affect his or her condition, especially if there is manual labor, office work that demands repetitive motion of the hands and arms, or any environment that could lend itself to stress and strain on the muscles or joints. The Doctor of Chiropractic (D.C.) will note standing and seated posture and observe the walk of a patient. A patient's bed may be a consideration.

After the history, a patient will be examined physically. Various tests are performed, including raising the legs, testing reflexes, and moving the body. The chiropractor assesses the range of movement of the affected areas by observation and measurement. He will then palpate or "feel for" the individual positions of a joint, in the next most frequently used diagnostic method. Palpation can take many years to master and includes checks for stiffness, pain, muscle spasm, and restricted range of motion.

Other, more traditional methods are used to identify problems. Subluxation—the name for the lesion of the vertebra that results in loss of alignment and movement—can be identified in several ways. X rays provide a clear picture of abnormalities in spinal position and movement and can reveal subluxation. Magnetic resonance imaging (MRI) can show images of discs, nerves, and other soft tissue. They may also detect disease. Neurological, blood, and urine tests may also be included to round out the diagnosis.

When diagnostic tests are returned, the patient returns for treatment. The most common treatment used by chiropractors is manual manipulation, also referred to as adjustment. The patient may be asked to stand, sit, or lie down, depending on the location of the joint where the abnormality has occurred. The chiropractor then determines the precise amount of force, direction, and pressure needed to mobilize and manipulate the joint.

In mobilization, the joint is moved in such a way as to create traction on the joint, often moving it as far as it will go. Following mobilization, a rapid thrust, using strategically placed hands, causes the release of an immobile joint. This thrust, properly performed, will restore the joint to its proper position and movement. This thrusting action is called manipulation. The sensation to the patient, said to be painless, is described as similar to the feeling of cracking one's knuckles. It is the precise pressure on specific points that causes the release.

Contrary to what one might think, it does not take much force to move a bone. Chiropractors do not have to be unusually strong or large to do adjustments. The following is a description of an adjustment by a chiropractor:

> The position of the doctor is extremely important. If he doesn't get himself balanced and in a proper position he won't be able to make a sharp, quick thrust and a proper adjustment. You have to get your body over the patient to get the greatest amount of leverage, and that means the less force you have to use. Manipulation is an art, truly. There's a science to it, too, of course, because you're talking about anatomy and the structure of the joints. But so much of it is feel. When you put your hands on a patient you'll feel the muscular tone, the amount of resistance. (Langone 1982: 81)

In addition to the spine, adjustments may be done on soft tissue and other joints. The sudden stretching relaxes muscle spasms, improves function, and relieves pain and inflammation. It is believed to be painless because it happens so quickly. Adjustment is taken to the point of pain, but no further. There are a number of different techniques used, including the Palmer Specific and the Gonstead.

Some patients report feeling better immediately, though some are stiff and achy. Occasionally there are headaches, upset stomach, diarrhea, constipation, excessive urination, and a slight rise in temperature. These "recovery symptoms" are similar to the responses to homeopathic remedies—they represent the body's self-correction mechanism. This realignment of the spine can cause temporary discomfort, which usually dissipates shortly.

Each chiropractic session can last from 45 minutes to one hour. A series of treatments may be required to heal the condition. How often and for how long a patient must return depends on the patient's age, the nature of the condition, and the condition of the body's natural healing ability.

In addition to adjustments, adjunct therapies are used. In electrical muscle stimulation, or galvanotherapy, specialized electrical current is introduced by wire through a pad attached with suction cups to the body. A machine generates the current, which is sent to the injured area. The result is the reduction of muscle spasms. Massage, heat, and ice are other treatment options used. Special exercises, nutritional counseling, and lifestyle changes may be recommended to sustain the benefits of the treatment and avoid recurrence.

Conditions most successfully treated by chiropractic medicine include poor posture, which can cause poor digestion and elimination, headaches, disc problems, whiplash, joint pain, scoliosis (abnormal curvature of the spine), and arthritis.

Postural problems may call for a treatment called skeletal balancing. This involves the correction of abnormalities in the skeleton, particularly the pelvis and spine, that can cause many conditions. One condition that causes one leg to be shorter than another is called "short leg" and may eventually lead to back pain.

The treatment for short leg begins with a reflex analysis technique called "challenging." After determining the difference between the two legs by observing the heels of the patient, muscles in the knee area are stimulated by stroking with the hand or by poking with a rubber tipped device called an activator. The leg's reflex is then checked. If there is no response, the pelvis may be a likely next choice. The chiropractor strokes and prods various parts of the skeletal system until he discovers the area of imbalance that is causing the shortening. When the activator strikes at the right place (for example, soft tissue near the bone), the leg releases to its full length.

Treatment of headaches has also been successful. Headaches can be caused by stimulation or prolonged pressure on any of the nerves, arteries, or blood vessels in the skull. Chiropractors believe that most headaches are caused by misaligned vertebrae impinging on nerves or blood vessels. To treat a headache, a patient lies face-down on the table. The chiropractor locates the abnormality in the bone or muscle by turning the head and observing its range of motion while palpating the area. A correctly placed cervical thrust releases misaligned vertebrae, releasing the nerves to their proper position and functioning.

Patients often come for help with disc problems. Discs are the cushions that separate the bones in the spine. The bones, called vertebrae, rock back and forth on the discs. Repeated friction by injury or jarring movement may damage discs. Discs can bulge or rupture and press on nearby nerves, causing pain or nerve damage. Pain may then go beyond the back into the arms, legs, and neck. Painful coughing or sneezing may indicate a disc problem. Manipulation can be done for many disc problems, taking the pressure off the disc and restoring the flow of nutrients to it. Others may require surgery.

Whiplash is caused by sudden jolts to the neck, and is most often associated with rear-end car accidents. Ligaments and muscles are subjected to thousands of pounds of force, causing rupture and compression of discs. Though the most common treatment for whiplash is to wear a protective collar and give it time to heal, disc degeneration and bone spurs may occur years later.

A chiropractor will order X rays to determine if any lasting damage will be done to a whiplash victim. The chiropractor then works with the soft tissue, and when that is healed, manipulation may be done to correct the condition.

Tennis elbow or bursitis is a common condition that is treated well by chiropractic. The bursa is a soft tissue sac that serves to cushion a joint. Its inflammation is called bursitis. If untreated, calcium deposits form and permanently change the functioning of the joint. Gentle mobilization techniques are used to loosen up the muscles in the area first, and then adjustments are made to areas of the spine that may be causing the problem.

Scoliosis can occur in anyone, but it is most common in girls. It is thought to be caused by a muscle spasm that pulls the spine out of shape. An improperly curved spine may crowd the internal organs and hinder circulation. Standard treatment for scoliosis is long-term and tedious: it can involve braces, casts, exercises, and surgery. Early screening may identify scoliosis, increasing the possibility of easy correction. Chiropractors recommend that children be seen by a chiropractor twice a year.

There has been a high level of patient satisfaction reported by patients of chiropractic care. Chiropractic is safe. American Chiropractic Association statistics show that risks to patients are lower than in conventional allopathic medicine. Reported cases of injuries in a twenty-year period just prior to 1980 were fewer than 100, and malpractice insurance for chiropractors is less than that for allopathic doctors.

Doctors of chiropractic must complete about six years of education to earn their degree. This includes two years of college science as a prerequisite to enter a chiropractic college. Most colleges exist independently, but they are now coming under the umbrella of some medical schools. In a three-and-one-half-year program, basic adjustments are taught, including muscle work, trigger points, muscle knots, and proper holding. An internship must be done. Licensing is required in all states, and there is a three-part national board certification. There is some reciprocity between states in licensing. There are professional organizations for chiropractors in most states.

Some health maintenance organizations cover chiropractic, and other health insurance companies may cover it, but it is by no means a standard benefit of health insurance. If its effectiveness can be demonstrated scientifically, it is likely that it will become more available. At this point referrals are usually made for muscle, joint, and back problems rather than for organic disorders.

See also ALTERNATIVE AND COMPLEMENTARY MEDICINE; BODYWORK.

Hill, Ann, ed. (1979) *A Visual Encyclopedia of Unconventional Medicine: A Health Manual for the Whole Person.*

Langone, John. (1982) *Chiropractors: A Consumers Guide.*

Schlagen, Kurt H., D.C. Personal communication.

Weil, Andrew. (1983) *Health and Healing: Understanding Conventional and Alternative Medicine.*

Woodham, Anne. (1994) *HEA Guide to Complementary Medicine and Therapies.*

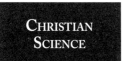 **CHRISTIAN SCIENCE** Christian Science healing is a method of healing through prayer that is practiced by members of the Church of Christ, Scientist. This religion is based on the Christian Bible and seeks to restore the spiritual healing that Jesus Christ is believed to have done during his time on earth approximately 2,000 years ago.

Christian Science's core belief is that faith in the goodness of a loving and all-powerful God, with a focus on the belief that all people are made in God's image, will restore a person to health. Prayer is the method used in healing and may be administered by oneself or a Christian Science practitioner.

The church's founder, Mary Baker Eddy, experienced a healing after being infirm for many years and near death as the result of an injury in 1866. A student of religion and spirituality for many years, she turned to the Bible for solace. She was inspired by the miraculous healings she read about in the Old and New Testaments. She became convinced that, through faith in the healing power of God, she would be healed. She recovered and lived until age ninety. As Eddy began to teach her discovery to others, she continued to study the Bible intently. Her goal became the reinstatement of Christianity with its spiritual element of healing. She wrote continually, but she wanted to "test" her theories on others before she published her ideas. In 1867, with one student, she began a school of Christian Science Mind-Healing in Lynn, Massachusetts. Interest grew so large that she subsequently opened the Massachusetts Metaphysical College in 1881 in Boston. Four thousand students passed through the Metaphysical College in the first seven years of operation. The first edition of her most famous work, *Science and Health with Key to the Scriptures*, was published in 1875.

It was not originally Baker's idea to create a new religion, but most other Christian sects did not appreciate her teaching. In 1879, a group of about thirty people met in Boston to create the First Church of Christ, Scientist. Known as the Mother Church, it is the religion's headquarters and is still located in Boston. Christian Science now has more than 3,000 churches in more than fifty countries. Numerous publications, including the weekly *Sentinel*, which includes articles about Christian Science as well as testimony of those healed through Christian Science, the daily *Christian Science Monitor*, a well-respected international newspaper, and the *Quarterly Bible Lesson*, which includes the weekly selections from the Bible and *Science and Health* to be used in Sunday services, are produced in Boston. Monitor Radio, also based in Boston, covers national and international affairs. For many years the church owned a television station, but, beset by financial difficulties, it closed in June 1992.

Eddy closed the Metaphysical College in 1889 to devote more time to study and writing. She revised *Science and Health*, finishing its current version in 1891. It contains the basic tenets of Christian Science:

1. As adherents of Truth, we take the inspired Word of the Bible as our sufficient guide to eternal Life.
2. We acknowledge and adore one supreme and infinite God. We acknowledge His Son, one Christ; the Holy Ghost or divine Comforter; and man in God's image and likeness.
3. We acknowledge God's forgiveness of sin in the destruction of sin and the spiritual understanding that casts out evil as unreal. But the belief in sin is punished so long as the belief lasts.
4. We acknowledge Jesus' atonement as the evidence of divine, efficacious Love, unfolding man's unity with God through Jesus Christ the Way-shower; and we acknowledge that man is saved through Christ, through Truth, Life and Love as demonstrated by the Galilean Prophet in healing the sick and overcoming sin and death.
5. We acknowledge the crucifixion of Jesus and his resurrection served to uplift faith and to understand eternal Life, even the allnesss of Soul, Spirit and the nothingness of matter.
6. And we solemnly promise to watch, and pray for that Mind to be in us which was also in Jesus Christ; to do unto others as we would have them do unto us; and to be merciful, just and pure.

Mind—with a capital M—refers to divine Mind, as opposed to the lower-case mortal mind. Mind is described as the divine principle, life, truth, and love. Mortal mind is described as "nothing claiming to be something . . . mythology; error creating other errors; . . . a belief that life, substance, and intelligence are in and of

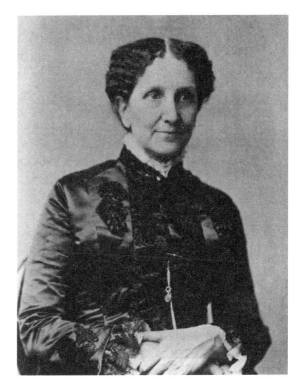

Mary Baker Eddy (1821–1910) was the founder of the Church of Christ, Scientist, and author of Science and Health with Key to the Scriptures (1875).

matter; the opposite of Spirit, and therefore the opposite of God, or good." (Eddy 1875: 592).

Aside from these beliefs, there is little doctrine (belief in the virgin birth and the Resurrection of Jesus are examples), and no ministry. Most issues are left to the conscience of the believer. Lessons drawn from the King James version of the Bible, along with *Science and Health,* constitute the weekly service. Readers are picked from the congregation for three-year terms, and the lessons are determined by the Mother Church in Boston, which produces the *Quarterly Bible Lesson.* On any given Sunday, all branches or congregations, worldwide, will be meditating on the same lesson.

The readings are followed by testimony of those who have experienced healing using

Christian Science principles. A collection of testimonies may be found in the "Fruitage" section of *Science and Health*, in the back pages of the *Sentinel*, and in a collection called *A Century of Christian Science Healing*. Sacraments are not practiced as ritual, but are studied as a Sunday lesson twice a year for their spiritual meaning. Christian Scientists are not baptized with water: baptism and communion are understood as part of the spiritual experience of purifying and sharing daily thoughts and actions. Marriage is recognized if performed by an ordained minister or priest in any other Christian denomination.

Eddy called her religion Christian Science because she believed that the healing occurred through timeless spiritual laws, unchanging truth, and invariable love rather than special miraculous acts. To participate is to believe in the spiritual potential of the present.

Jesus Christ's life "exemplifies the possibility of action outside of and contrary to the limits of a finite material sense of existence. . . . In biblical terms this meant the breaking through of the kingdom of heaven—of the divine order of things—into ordinary sense-bound experience." (Eliade 1990: 7)

Eddy has included a definition of God in *Science and Health:*

> The Great I am; the all-knowing, all-seeing, all-acting, all-wise, all-loving, and eternal; Principle; Mind; Soul; Spirit; Life; Truth; Love; all substance; intelligence. (1875: 587)

And of error:

> Error is a supposition that pleasure and pain, that intelligence, substance, life are existent in matter. Error is neither Mind, nor one of Mind's faculties. Error is the Contradiction of Truth. Error is belief without understanding. Error is unreal because untrue. It is that which seemeth to be and is not. (1875: 472)

And she says of sin:

> All reality is in God and His creation, harmonious and eternal. That which He creates is good, and He makes all that is made. Therefore the only reality of sin, sickness or death is the awful fact that unrealities seem real to human, erring belief, until God strips off their disguise. They are not true, because they are not of God. We learn in Christian Science that all in harmony of mortal mind or body is illusion, possessing neither reality nor identity though seeming to be real and identical. . . . The Science of Mind disposes of all evil. Truth, God, is not the father of error. Sin, sickness and death are to be classified as effects of error. Christ came to destroy the belief of sin. (1875: 472)

CHRISTIAN SCIENCE HEALING

The basis of the religion lies with healing. From the Manual of the Mother Church comes the statement that the Christian Science was founded "to organize a church designed to commemorate the word and works of our Master, which should reinstate primitive Christianity and its lost element of healing." But there are other differences between Christian Science and other Christian faiths. One is that most believe that God created man, that man (Adam) fell, and was redeemed by Christ. They believe that Jesus is God. Christian Science believes that humans—just as Jesus was—are created by God, not as body and soul, but as eternal spirit. Humans are the reflection of God and can heal as Jesus did.

Much of the work in the healing involves restructuring the sick person's inner beliefs that do not correspond with this divine image. According to practitioners, healing occurs when a person, alone or assisted, is able to hold to an entirely spiritual view. The belief is that humans are an entirely spiritual creation, and therefore inherently good. There is no power in the material universe that can affect health if this belief is held, according to believers. Negative "concepts" about the body's ill health that are held in our minds are altered and brought into line with spiritual law as healing occurs.

It is not simply the healing of physical conditions that is asked for. Emotional, financial, and spiritual dilemmas are prayed for as well. Practitioners are paid for their time. Full-time practitioners who publish their names in the monthly *Christian Science Journal* agree to have no other form of income. A two-week course of study with an authorized Christian Science teacher is required, along with a yearly follow-up course.

Healings are called "treatments" and must be requested. A practitioner would consider it unethical to enter into prayer for a particular person without their permission. But one need not be a believer or a member of a branch of the church to obtain a treatment.

The practitioner combines years of personal study and intuition to select prayers that seem to apply to the sick person's situation, and then repeats them. This may be done at the person's side or, most often, without coming into contact with the person, which is called absent healing. When a person asks for a healing, it is hoped that his or her mind and heart are open and receptive to the prayers of the healer. Usually a practitioner is called after a person has tried to heal him- or herself unsuccessfully or, in the case of non–Christian Scientists, after orthodox medicine has failed to heal a condition. The practitioner's role is to help the person hold to their belief in God's power and goodness and to turn thought away from the material sense of the problem.

There is no catalog of prayers for particular physical or emotional problems. The misconstrued belief or misdeed underlying the problem may be different in every person, though the illness itself may be the same. The prayers address the spiritual level. The material world of the body and its illness is seen as an illusion—a kind of nightmare—and it is believed that through leading a spiritual life, one can achieve dominion over it. According to Eddy, "The procuring cause and foundation of all sickness is fear, ignorance or sin. Disease is always induced by a false sense mentally entertained, not destroyed. Disease is an image of thought externalized." (1875: 411)

Sin and its punishment are believed to be the same thing. There is no real pleasure in sin, for the joy of living the spiritual life transcends any earthly pleasures. If a person is knowingly or unknowingly unkind or unloving, the practitioner might try to discover and work with the resolution of the sin.

To counteract the presence of fear, the practitioner tries to replace it with confidence in divine love. Fear is a result of a lack of trust in the divine —often healings involve repetitions of a person's acceptance by God and the protection of God's love. Ignorance may be demonstrated by accepting negative beliefs, even unconsciously. If the mental state of the patient is believing in the presence of the illness, the practitioner will remind him or her of their kinship with God. Reminders of beauty and order and truth are given.

Christian Science believers defy what most of the rest of the world accepts: the laws of material science. The material world is believed to be constantly changing, while God represents a changeless principle. In the chapter "Recapitulation" in *Science and Health,* Eddy says, "There is no life, truth, intelligence, nor substance in matter. All is infinite Mind and its infinite manifestation, for God is All-in-all. Spirit is immortal Truth; matter is mortal error." (1875: 468)

They explain this difference by saying that negativity and illness are the lie behind the truth of God's Kingdom. It is described as an illusion, a screen that we must strip away to find the reality of God's perfect universe at work. "Christ Jesus was a healer. His was not an abstract theology or philosophy. He preached that the Kingdom of God is at hand; he quickened people's moral sense and linked these spiritual truths to safety and health. He healed without drugs or the medicine of his time. He said, 'He that believeth in me, the works I do, shall he do also . . .' Christian Science strives to strengthen the Christian's understanding that Christ Jesus' healings are based on spiritual law. It reveals that this law is just as potent and practical now as it was in Biblical times." (Christian Science Board of Directors 1991: 3–4).

Christian Science is different from positive thinking, or holistic techniques that seek to spiritualize matter by releasing spiritual energy within the body or by bringing the body into harmony. The power in healing is believed to be of God, not in nature or matter, and people partake of it as a part of God's creation. But it is similar to holistic approaches in that it treats the whole person. "Christian Science considers man as a 'whole' and does not neglect healing of apparently unrelated mental, social, financial and moral problems while treating a person with physical difficulty." (Kanami 1991: 48)

CONTROVERSIES OVER CHRISTIAN SCIENCE

Christian Science has raised considerable controversy when healing has not succeeded in a physical cure and deaths have occurred without consulting the orthodox medical profession. There has been legal action as a result of withholding orthodox medical treatment from children, in particular. In cases where orthodox medicine supplies a ready cure, some feel it is wrong to not avail oneself of that treatment or to deny it to dependents. Some adults who were raised with Christian Science have childhood memories of anger and pain at not being treated through orthodox medicine for such conditions.

Although many Christian Scientists say they do not judge those who choose to see a doctor for various ailments, and profess respect and love for the caring of medical professionals, they also believe that belief is at the heart of the treatment. They believe that it is therefore most effective when relied on exclusively. Some point to the fact that many children are lost to failed medical treatment every year, and most of the time no one's right to practice is threatened as a result. They believe that theirs is a system, logical and orderly, and that it should stand on its own merits, specifically the numerous testimonies to healing.

To belong to Christian Science is to have a forever changed view of reality. If one does decide to use orthodox medicine to treat a condition, there is no church action of condemnation. But there may be disappointment and an inner sense of personal spiritual failure. Practitioners do not work side by side with medical professionals because their concepts of healing are so radically different.

See also FAITH HEALING.

A Century of Christian Science Healing. (1966).

Christian Science: A Sourcebook of Contemporary Materials. (1990).

Christian Science Board of Directors. (1991) *Humanity's Quest for Health. Christian Science Sentinel* (Special Issue).

The Christian Science Publishing Society. *The Christian Science Sentinel* (weekly).

Eddy, Mary Baker. (1875) *Science and Health with Key to the Scriptures*.

Eliade, Mircea, ed. (1990) *The Encyclopedia of Religion*.

Gottschalk, Stephen. (1990) "Christian Science." In *Christian Science: A Sourcebook of Contemporary Materials*.

Kanami, Beena. (1991) "Taking Care of Mankind's Needs." *Humanity's Quest for Health. Christian Science Sentinel* (special issue).

Peel, Robert. (1971) *The Biography of Mary Baker Eddy, Vol. II, The Years of Trial*.

Questions and Answers on Christian Science. (1974).

CULTURE-BOUND SYNDROMES

Culture-bound syndromes are disorders of emotional, cognitive, or behavioral functioning (or any combination of the three) that are either caused or shaped by cultural factors. At one time it was believed that these syndromes were confined to traditional non-Western cultures, with each syndrome found only in a single culture or group of nearby cultures and caused by a mix of psychological and cultural factors. For this reason, culture-bound syndromes are sometimes called psychogenic neuroses, ethnic psychoses, exotic psychoses, and culture-bound psychiatric syndromes. Experts now believe that culture-bound syndromes may be found in any society and that there is considerable similarity in certain types of syndromes across cultures. Thus, it is more likely that some syndromes have underlying neurophysiological causes, with the observable symptoms shaped by cultural factors.

Nearly 200 culture-bound syndromes have been described and they can be classified into the following seven categories (Simons and Hughes 1985):

1. Startle Matching
2. Sleep Paralysis
3. Genital Retraction
4. Sudden Mass Assault
5. Running
6. Fright Illness
7. Cannibal Compulsion

STARTLE MATCHING

The startle matching syndrome is found in a number of forms around the world, but it is most often associated with cultures located in Malaysia and Indonesia. Individuals susceptible to startle matching react to a startling event with sudden body movements, blurting out curse words and sometimes matching the movements or words of the person who startled him or her or those of other nearby persons. In some cultures, people are identified as especially susceptible to a startle and they may be purposefully startled for the amusement of others. Key features are shown in this description of latah (as startle matching is commonly known in Southeast Asia) among the Javanese of Indonesia:

> About a month later, Mbok Ti held a small feast in honor of her son's circumcision, and I attended it. All of the neighbors were there, politely drinking tea and conversing with proper subdued tones. A woman came in and Mbok Ti came up to me and said, "Here is a real latah, just watch. . . . With that she exclaimed in a loud voice to the new woman, "*Dag!*" the Dutch greeting, "Good-day." The second latah, Mbok Min, immediately responded, "Dag!" several times, raising her hand automatically each time. When she paused, the first latah, Mbok Ti, started her up again. Then, tiring of the game, Mbok Ti cried out, "*Merdeka!*" the Indonesian slogan, "Freedom!" and Mbok Min imitated her, and again repeated it over and over. . . . It is the custom in Java at one of these feasts, for all of the guests to urge each other politely to eat, saying over and over, "*Mangga!*" "Please eat!" Mbok Min had been sitting at the side for some time without speaking, when suddenly she burst out—this time without being teased—with "Mangga, mangga, mangga!" compulsively repeating the polite word and its accompanying gesture, over and over. People then began to tease her and she grew more and more rattled, and in this upset condition began mixing obscene words in her speech. At one point she offered a cup of tea to someone with the words "Please have some vagina." The word for tea has something of the same sound as the word for vagina. (Geertz 1968: 97)

SLEEP PARALYSIS SYNDROME

The sleep paralysis syndrome, although classified as a culture-bound disorder, actually conforms

75

quite closely to disorders known to Western medicine. The syndrome affects people when they are near sleep and is characterized by an inability to move or speak, although the individual is conscious and can remember events going on about him. Individuals who experience sleep paralysis also report a feeling of disassociation from their body, a heaviness on their chest, anxiety, and exhaustion upon emerging from the state. The following description of the "Old Hag" in a fishing village in Newfoundland indicates some of the key elements:

> It's stagnation of the blood. You think you're bawlin' out but more often you're not. You can see what's goin' on around ya, ya know. Nancy [ethnographer's wife] can 'ag rog ya and my wife too, she's 'ag rogged me plenty o' times. You'll see she comin' in the room and come right down on top of ya and she'll 'ag rog ya. To prevent it put a Bible under your head; I never been 'ag rogged so long as I does that. It's like a stroke I suppose, but the doc can't do nuthin' for it. (Ness 1985: 126)

This account contains one local explanation for Old Hag—someone else causes it to bring the victim harm. Other explanations cite exhaustion and sleeping on one's back that causes blood circulation to slow.

GENITAL RETRACTION SYNDROME

The genital retraction syndrome is best known in Asia, where a number of related conditions are often lumped under the label koro, which means "to shrink" in the Macassaran language of Indonesia. The syndrome is believed to affect men mainly, and its most dramatic symptom is the penis either shrinking in size or retracting into the body. In women, symptoms include a flattening of the breasts and retraction of the external genitalia. Usually preceding and then continuing with the retraction are an overwhelm-

ing sense of fear, panic, and often behavior such as overeating, grabbing one's penis, or seeking medical assistance to end the attack. The following is an example of attacks suffered by a young man in a city in central China:

> The patient, in a state of panic, wandered from one herb doctor to another having vitamin injections. He was told by one doctor that he was suffering from *shenn-kuei* or *yin-kuei*, a sexual defect, and he would eventually die if he continued going to prostitutes. He thought that his symptoms were caused by *yin-kuei*, a disease supposed to be due to poisons secreted in the uterus which penetrate the penis. At this point he quit his job to save his strength; in August 1957 he was referred to the psychiatric clinic by a medical doctor.
>   Almost irresistible sexual desire seized him whenever he felt slightly better; yet he experienced strange "empty" feelings in his abdomen when he had sexual intercourse. He reported that he often found his penis shrinking into his abdomen, at which time he would become very anxious and hold on to his penis in terror. Holding his penis, he would faint, with severe vertigo and pounding of his heart. (Kiev 1972: 67)

As with Old Hag, genital retraction disorders have been viewed by experts as largely caused by psychodynamic factors and shaped by cultural factors. There is, as yet, no clear physical cause.

SUDDEN MASS ASSAULT

Sudden mass assault is a syndrome characterized by an individual who previously seemed to be relatively normal suddenly becoming violent and killing or attempting to kill other people randomly. Often, but not always, the individual then commits suicide. Sudden mass assault is a worldwide phenomenon, although considerable attention has been given to the form found throughout Southeast Asia called *amok*. Experts do not agree on whether mass assault by a person already

 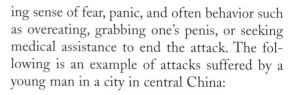

known to suffer from an emotional disorder or already thought to behave abnormally should be included in this category. The attack is usually preceded by an event or series of events that disrupts the individual's life and leads to a severe loss of self-esteem, followed by a short period of unhappiness and feelings of hopelessness. The assault is seen by experts as the behavioral manifestation of those feelings, as indicated in the following example from Papua New Guinea:

> The patient was a healthy young adult male, who originally came from the hinterlands of Abau, Central District. At the time of the act he was working with a building gang on Ferguson Island. He was a foreigner to his workmates, one of whom called him an "Abau bush pig"—a grave insult. One night at about 6:30, the others were in their dormitory reading or lying down, when the patient came in with a 12 in. bush knife and suddenly attacked them, going from bed to bed hacking at them with the knife, mostly in the vicinity of the head and neck. Six died then or later, some with terrible wounds, their heads being almost chopped off. Finally, another man in the vicinity heard the noise and came in with a rifle and one cartridge. The amok attempted to attack him, was fired at, and still did not cease attacking. He was then put out of action by the butt of the rifle and died. (Burton-Bradley 1985: 241)

Running

The fifth category of culture-bound syndromes is called running and covers a number of related disorders characterized by behaviors such as tearing off one's clothing, speaking in tongues, running away, rolling around on the ground, and throwing objects. The attacks, which take the form of a short-lived seizure, rarely cause physical injury to the individual or other persons, although they are often threatening and potentially dangerous. However, since great strength is often exerted, it is usually difficult to restrain the

person. Running syndromes are found primarily in the Arctic regions of Siberia and North America and are commonly called Arctic Hysterias, with *pibloktoq* being the indigenous name. These patterns of behavior were noted by early European explorers of the Arctic and have been studied intensively in recent years. As the following accounts indicate, the particular symptoms often vary from person to person:

> Kalagik is a nine-year-old boy who has been having fits periodically for several years. At times he appears dazed and weak and will gently fall to the ground. He often does this while playing outside with other children. Other times he will fly into a fury, trying to attack one of the other children. One time, he went after a younger brother with a knife, but was restrained by his parents. These attacks are short-lived, lasting only five to ten minutes. Kalagik has no memory for what happens during the attack, but remembers his head "feeling funny" before he blacks out. He also notices that before these attacks his fingers and hands contract, so that he cannot open his hand without prying it open.
>
> Nirik is a young Eskimo woman who for the past six years has had episodic fits of unmanageable fury. These fits last about thirty minutes, during which time she breaks furniture and windows, assaults members of her family, shouts obscenities, and has on occasion tried to rip off her clothes.
>
> Kajat is a man who at the age of fifty-two had his first and only attack of Arctic Hysteria–like behavior. Several months prior to the attack he was noted to be somewhat irritable by the Public Health nurse and by the school teacher. One morning in October he was found by his sons shouting in an irrational way about "a devil" in his house, and had to be restrained from going out of the house with his gun "to shoot caribou" (he said). He broke free and began running around outside the house, grimacing and shouting that he was seeing devils. The people of the village became alarmed that he might harm himself or others. He then went to sleep for twenty-four hours. When

he woke up he sang hymns loudly and kept stating, "I want my wife." Within forty-eight hours his mentation had apparently returned to normal. (Foulkes 1972)

The cause or causes of these behaviors are not known, although it is likely that stress, and especially stress associated with living in the harsh Arctic region, precipitates many of these episodes.

Fright Illness and Cannibal Compulsion

The final two categories of culture-bound syndromes—fright illness and cannibal compulsion—are controversial in that experts do not agree on their classification as culture-bound, and in the case of the latter, the syndrome is no longer believed to exist. The best known of the fright illnesses is susto, which is found throughout Latin America, in the Philippines, and in Latino communities in the United States, with similar disorders reported elsewhere in the world. Although there is variation across groups and individuals, there is also much similarity in the various manifestations of susto. The basic commonality is the belief that susto is caused by the loss of one's soul, which is taken by a supernatural spirit. This condition is manifested in a number of clear symptoms:

> The basic syndrome appears as follows: (1) during sleep the patient evidences restlessness; (2) during waking hours patients are characterized by listlessness, loss of appetite, disinterest in dress and personal hygiene, loss of strength, depression, and introversion. (Rubel 1964: 270)

The cure for susto requires the services of a healer who can contact the spirit that has taken the soul and then convince it to return it to the patient. That susto is so widely distributed throughout Latin America and resembles soul loss in other cultures suggests that it is not a culture-bound disorder.

Cannibal compulsion refers to the windigo syndrome associated throughout the twentieth century with the Algonkian peoples of southern Canada. Windigo is defined as follows:

> The outstanding symptom of the aberration known as windigo psychoses is the intense compulsive desire to eat human flesh. In many instances this desire is satisfied through actual cannibal acts. . . . One who develops this craving for human flesh or is considered to be in the process of doing so is called a Windigo. (Teicher 1960)

Despite this clear definition and numerous reports of the behavior, it now seems clear that the cannibalistic desires and behaviors associated with the syndrome never actually occurred among the Algonkians, although individuals in the community were certainly accused of such desires and behaviors. Thus, windigo is not a culture-bound disorder, but rather is similar to witchcraft accusation in other cultures, in which undesirable individuals are labeled as witches in order to remove them from the community.

Culture-Bound Syndromes in Western Societies

Although culture-bound syndromes have traditionally been viewed as disorders found in non-Western cultures, experts have noted that some disorders fitting the definition of culture-bound syndromes occur in Western contexts but are absent in non-Western cultures. Candidates for the label of Western culture-bound syndromes include eating disorders such as bulimia nervosa and anorexia nervosa; chronic fatigue syndrome; the so-called Type A personality linked to heart disease; obesity; and petism, a disorder found among some elderly people who keep large numbers of cats and dogs in unsanitary conditions, often to the detriment of their own health. From this list, the most likely candidates for a culture-bound classification are the eating disorders, petism, and chronic fatigue syndrome. Both obesity and Type A personality fail to qualify, as these are more patterns of behavior than identifiable psychiatric disorders.

Eating disorders are relatively new and are found mainly in Western societies such as the United States, Great Britain, Canada, and Germany, as well as in Japan. There is also some indication that the disorders are appearing in non-Western cultures, especially among young women exposed to Western culture. It is believed that between 90 and 95 percent of persons with eating disorders are women, and most are adolescents and young women in their twenties. The two primary forms of eating disorder are anorexia nervosa and bulimia nervosa. The former is characterized by an unrealistic desire to be thin and the severe restriction of food intake in order to attain that goal. For those with anorexia, thin is usually defined unrealistically and they have a distorted body image in which extremely thin continues to seem overweight to them. Anorexia is associated with numerous health problems including loss of the menstrual cycle, loss of bone, and heart disease. Unlike anorexia, bulimia does not necessarily involve an obsession to be thin, but rather an obsession with one's body weight and image and compulsive eating behavior that involves overeating and then purging to control one's weight. As with anorexia, it may lead to serious health problems and about 10 percent of people with these disorders die from complications related to them. A third eating disorder is binge eating, which involves overeating that causes physical discomfort at least several times a week for several months.

Behind both bulimia and anorexia is a distorted body image that is the product of a complex mix of individual psychological and cultural factors. The most important psychological component is the distorted body image, which in many women with these disorders involves deep feelings of anger, guilt, and sexual confusion resulting from childhood sexual or physical abuse. It is believed that at least one-half of women with these disorders were abused as children. The cultural factors of importance are the value placed on being thin in Western societies, the unrealistic images of ideal weight portrayed in the media and in advertising, and confusion about the role of women in society.

Chronic fatigue syndrome (called ME in Europe) may or may not be a culture-bound syndrome, as relatively little is known about it other than that it is characterized by a set of symptoms without clear physical causes and that it appeared in the United States, Great Britain, and other Western cultures only in the last few decades. The key feature of the syndrome is long-lasting, extreme physical and mental fatigue that prevents the individual from engaging in normal activities. For some individuals the fatigue may be so severe that he or she cannot get out of bed; for others it may be less severe and may require only that they curtail some activities and take regular naps. From a medical standpoint, chronic fatigue syndrome is diagnosed only when it lasts for more

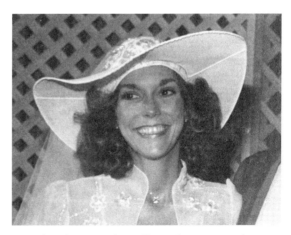

American pop singer Karen Carpenter on her wedding day in 1980. She died three years later of anorexia nervosa, an example of a culture-bound syndrome found in Western societies.

than three months and only when other possible causes of the fatigue such as infection or heart disease have been ruled out. Although there is much variation among individuals, the symptoms most often associated with the syndrome include feeling weak, becoming exhausted following physical activity, a mild fever, muscle aches, anxiety, and unhappiness. The presence of muscle aches, fever, and swollen lymph nodes in some individuals indicates the possibility of a virus, and some people view it as a viral disease, although no virus has yet been identified as the causal agent. In some individuals, the syndrome follows severe emotional stress, although in other individuals there is no such association. This association with emotional stress has led some people to view it as a psychological syndrome resulting from the competitiveness, isolation, and loneliness of Western urban life, and it has been labeled the "yuppie disease." At this point in time, it is not clear whether it has multiple causes or a single cause, whether it is caused by psychological or physical factors or both, or how to cure it, although many symptoms can be controlled with drugs, diet, and rest.

Burton-Bradley, B. G. (1985) "The Amok Syndrome in Papua and New Guinea." In *The Culture-Bound Syndromes: Folk Illnesses of Psychiatric and Anthropological Interest,* edited by Ronald C. Simons and Charles C. Hughes, 237–249.

Foulkes, Edward F. (1972) *The Arctic Hysterias.*

Geertz, Hildred. (1968) "Latah in Java: A Theoretical Paradox." *Indonesia* 5: 93–104.

Johnson, Thomas M., and Carolyn F. Sargent, eds. (1990) *Medical Anthropology: A Handbook of Theory and Method.*

Kiev, Ari (1972) *Transcultural Psychiatry.*

Maine, Margo. (1991) *Father Hunger: Fathers, Daughters, and Food.*

Marano, Lou. (1985) "Windigo Psychosis: The Anatomy of an Emic-Etic Confusion." In *The Culture-Bound Syndromes: Folk Illnesses of Psychiatric and Anthropological Interest,* edited by Ronald C. Simons and Charles C. Hughes, 411–448.

Ness, Robert C. (1985) "The Old Hag Phenomenon as Sleep Paralysis: A Biocultural Interpretation." In *The Culture-Bound Syndromes: Folk Illnesses of Psychiatric and Anthropological Interest,* edited by Ronald C. Simons and Charles C. Hughes, 123–146.

Rubel, Arthur J. (1964) "The Epidemiology of a Folk Illness: Susto in Hispanic America." *Ethnology* 3: 268–283.

Simons, Ronald C., and Charles C. Hughes, eds. (1985) *The Culture-Bound Syndromes: Folk Illnesses of Psychiatric and Anthropological Interest.*

Stoff, Jesse A., and Charles R. Pellegrino. (1988) *Chronic Fatigue Syndrome: The Hidden Epidemic.*

Teicher, Morton. (1960) *Windigo Psychosis.*

Winzeler, Robert L. (1991) "Latah in Sarawak, with Special Reference to the Iban." In *Female and Male in Borneo: Contributions and Challenges to Gender Studies,* edited by Vinson H. Sutlive, Jr., 317–333.

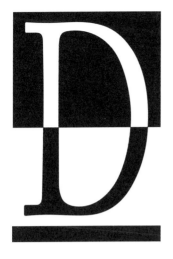

Much about death is universal. All people in all cultures die a biological death. In all cultures people who have died, and those they leave behind, also experience a social death as the dying person leaves the world of the living and his or her future role in the lives of the living is redefined. In all cultures people try to prevent death by treating illness, avoiding dangerous situations, and preventing accidents. In all cultures people believe that humans have a soul and in nearly all cultures people believe that the soul lives on after the body dies. In all cultures death may be viewed somewhat differently depending on the status of the person who has died. Most common in this regard is the death of infants. In many cultures infants who have not yet been defined as members of the group through a naming or other ritual are buried quickly as they are not thought to have been fully alive. Similarly, the deaths of people with certain diseases that are feared, such as AIDS, and the deaths of people by violent means are considered to be different than other deaths. Finally, in all cultures the death of an individual is attended to with various ritualized behaviors that mark the death and the new social status of the deceased.

Despite these important commonalities, there are also some significant variations in beliefs about death across cultures. The major variation is in definitions of death and "being dead." In Western societies there is usually a clear distinction being the states of being alive and being dead. The key markers of death are the end of the physical markers of life, such as heartbeat, respiration, or brain wave activity. In some cultures the distinction is as much, if not more, based on the degree of social rather than physical functioning of the person. At one extreme are some cultures where a person, who is perfectly healthy physically, is defined socially as being dead and is treated as such. For example, some Orthodox Jews consider a person who has married a non-Jew to be "dead" and relatives engage in ritualized mourning behavior and avoid contact with that person in the future. Similarly, some Gypsy groups exile persons who seriously disrupt group activities and define that person as a non-Gypsy and thereby socially dead.

In some cultures a distinction is made between types of death, most often between violent or nonviolent death. The Ifugao of the Philippines, for example, distinguish between ordinary and extraordinary deaths. Classified as extraordinary are those caused by being speared by an enemy, a sudden death by accident, a mother's death during childbirth, and death from a disease called *napu'tut*. The Tiv of Nigeria, for another example, distinguish between violent death and "death on a bed." For the Tiv and many other peoples, violent death is considered troubling because the death is believed to be caused by forces (supernatural or human) beyond human control. Thus, the Tiv seek to dispose of the bodies of those who died by violence quickly, away from the village, and with rites that protect the living. The Tiv also believe that people have some control over their own death and can "decide to die." This applies especially to old people who, regardless of their physical health, may decide that their social role has been fulfilled, make arrangements for the transfer of property, status, and power to their kin, and then die peacefully.

In cultures where people often place themselves at physical risk, the possibility of sudden death is always present. In these cultures, such as the sea-faring Truk of Micronesia, the common view of death is a fatalistic one—"What of it? If I die, it can't be helped." (Gladwin and Sarason 1953: 156). This does not mean, however, that the Truk accept the death of a close one calmly and simply go on with their affairs. Quite the contrary, death is responded to with considerable emotion and ritual on the part of the survivors.

The Santal of northern India take quite a different view and see death as interrupting life. For the Santal, unlike the Truk, death is often unexpected, feared, and always attributed to the actions of supernatural beings, who can easily return and cause two more deaths. As continual efforts to find the causes of deaths are to no avail, the Santal concern about death is reflected in numerous sayings such as "In this life there is eating and drinking and the wearing of clothes. In the next life, who knows what there is?" (Culshaw 1949: 158)

For the Taiwanese, death is not believed to be a surprise, but rather is thought to be predetermined:

> Death, therefore, is met with acceptance and resignation, particularly if the dying person is of advanced age. The onset of illness or sudden debilitation in an elderly person is often taken as a sign of approaching death, so that the family will begin funeral preparations well before death occurs. (Diamond 1969: 45)

The Ifugao of the Philippines are also fatalistic about death and believe it to be predeter-mined, but they are more specific about what forces control death. They believe that death is controlled by the spirits of their ancestors, who want the souls of the living. This does not mean that the spirits can take the souls at will, and they can call upon Imbagaiyan, the Conductor of Souls, to acquire the soul through negotiation:

> Let us go—thy ancestor calls thee.
> I will not, says the soul. It is necessary to prepare for my child's prestige feast.
> Imbagaiyan goes, fetches sugar cane, pounds out the juice in the kopal press, adds it to the rice wine.
> There—the wine is ready. Let us go.
> I will not, says the soul. My fields need weeding.
> Imbagaiyan assembles a large number of women and has them weed the fields.
> There—thy fields are weeded. Let us go—thy ancestor is waiting.
> Kao! says the soul. I will not—there are debts that I haven't collected.
> Imbagaiyan goes and collects the debts. Come, come—thy ancestor awaits thee. (Barton 1946: 170)

The Aymara of Peru differ from these other groups by being resigned to death and seeing it as a natural occurrence that can often end the pain and suffering of someone afflicted with a serious disease. Their care for the terminally ill follows this belief:

> The end of life is taken with resignation and they show great philosophy in those circumstances; they try to impart peace to the dying person and that his departure is in harmony with all, that he does not depart with resentment, and in the final moments, rather than taking care of his illness, they endeavor to ease his mind. (Bouroncle-Carreon 1964: 59)

For traditional Serbs in Europe, death is known to occur because of a change in the physical functioning of the body and the associated departure of the soul from the body. Thus, muscles that continue to move after death are still alive, as is a body still filled with blood, although the soul has departed and the individual is now spiritually dead.

In some cultures, while physical death is recognized, the more powerful belief is that life continues in another world after death. This belief, central to the Hopi religion, is reflected in their origin myths:

> Nearly all the origin myths agree that the first death on earth occurred in the family of the chief who led the Emergence. When the murderer, a witch who is related to the chief, is threatened with punishment, he protests that the victim is unharmed and has merely returned to the Underworld from which mankind had just come forth. When the people look down they see that the dead person appears to be normal and happy, whereupon the witch says, "That is the way it will be. If anyone dies, he will go down there...." At first, according to a First Mesa tale, it was even understood that the dead would have the privilege of returning to earth, but Coyote changed things by throwing a large, flat stone over the *sipapu*. All the people were angry at Coyote for this and drove him away, because only for his action people who died would have been able to revive and walk around on this world four days after death. (Titiev 1971: 107)

As this myth suggests, the Hopi believe that life in the underworld is like life on earth, except that those in the underworld eat on the "odor or soul of the food." The dead are personified on earth by the kachina figures that play a central role in Hopi ceremonies.

Across cultures there are a number of culturally defined behavior patterns associated with particular categories of death or persons who have died. The most significant are death-hastening behavior, gerontocide, infanticide, and rituals associated with death.

DEATH-HASTENING BEHAVIOR

Death-hastening behavior is action or inaction by members of a society that directly leads to the death of another member of the society. Death-hastening behavior can take any one of three forms: (1) failing to support the material needs of an individual; (2) abandoning an individual; or (3) killing an individual. Death-hastening behavior differs from homicide in that death-hastening is socially acceptable, and it differs from capital punishment or death through blood revenge in that the person killed or allowed to die is not accused of or being punished for committing a crime.

Death-hastening actions are taken primarily against individuals who have become a burden to the group and threaten its survival. These are usually the elderly, although death-hastening may also be used with infants (infanticide) and with the disabled. As regards the elderly, death-hastening behavior occurs in about 40 percent of the world's non-Western societies. Death-hastening behavior is one of three ways people treat the aged in cultures around the world. The first way is to support them by supplying them with food and shelter, helping to transport them, affording them respect, and involving them in community activities. The second way is to not support them by forcing them to live alone, insulting them, taking property from them, and treating them as witches. These nonsupportive activities, while lowering the quality of a person's life, do not necessarily lead to death. The third way is to hasten their death. In most societies, elderly people are treated in all three ways, with different aged people treated differently.

The major determinant of whether or not an aged person is the object of death-hastening behavior is whether or not that person is considered by others to be intact or decrepit. In nearly all cultures, a person is considered intact when he or she is productive. A person is considered decrepit when he or she is a social or economic liability, that is, when the individual requires the support of others to survive, support that would otherwise go to others who are productive or that might put the person providing it at risk. Of course, societies vary widely in how they define productivity and liability. In most societies, an aged person is considered productive until a change in his or her health or a change in the society's circumstances causes others to redefine the person as decrepit. Once an individual is classified as decrepit, they are far more likely to be the object of death-hastening behavior. When an individual is considered productive, he or she is more likely to be supported or the object of nonsupportive treatment, but not subject to death-hastening.

Thus, the image of old people floating off into the sea on an ice flow is an oversimplification. While in about 36 percent of non-Western societies some aged are left to die, it is usually only those who are considered decrepit and, therefore, socially acceptable objects of death-hastening behaviors. For example, among the Yanomamö of northwestern Brazil, only the aged who are unable to participate in migrations and the seriously ill who cannot be cured are killed, either by beating with a stick or abandonment in a cave. The Saami (Lapps) of northern Europe in the past killed only the decrepit aged who, like the Yanomamö decrepit aged, could not migrate, in this case in pursuit of reindeer herds. These people were either drowned through a hole in the ice or pushed off a cliff. The latter custom was called *saalekeskoute*, meaning "blessed journey." It is usually family members who kill or abandon their decrepit relatives. While such actions bring personal grief to the participants, they also realize that using extraordinary efforts to keep the person alive will likely drain resources such as food, shelter, energy, and time from others and may put the survival of the entire group at risk.

GERONTOCIDE

Gerontocide is the socially acceptable disposal of the aged through killing or abandonment. Surveys suggest that gerontocide occurs in about 20 to 25 percent of societies. This is a lower percentage than the 36 percent of societies with death-hastening behavior, as death-hastening behavior is a broader concept that includes not only killing and abandoning, but also forsaking and other behaviors, such as suicide by the aged. Gerontocide is found in societies in all regions of the world, except for southern Europe, although it occurred there in the past. It was customary in a greater percentage of societies in North and South America prior to their Europeanization and in Africa than elsewhere in the world. This distribution pattern seems to reflect the more-frequent presence of gerontocide in the semi-nomadic hunting, fishing, and herding cultures that were most common in these parts of the world. Today, gerontocide is no longer customary in most of these societies, as they are now sedentary and integrated, in some cases only marginally, into industrialized economic systems of the nations where they live. For example, the Saami (Lapps) no longer practice gerontocide.

Traditional explanations for gerontocide emphasized the severe climate, nomadic lifestyle, irregular food supply, and weak kinship ties that presumably were characteristic of societies with gerontocide. The Eskimo and Inuit peoples were often cited as a classic example of a gerontocide society and the image of the aged Eskimo willingly drifting off on an ice flow became a popular myth. Recent research suggests that these factors do not cause gerontocide. Rather, societies with gerontocide seem to be ones that are semi-nomadic (seasonal movements following food sources) with a "loose" community structure that does not allow for the sharing of resources to support the aged. In societies with a "tight" structure based on close ties and reciprocal obligations between kin, support for the aged is easier. Additionally, gerontocide is customary only when the aged are defined as decrepit, which may result from a deterioration in their health or a change in community circumstances that prevents them from being socially productive members of the community. For example, the Copper Inuit of Alaska routinely provided the aged with food and clothing and transported those who could not do so themselves from camp to camp on sleds. However, in times of starvation, the aged would be abandoned.

INFANTICIDE

Infanticide is the purposeful termination of an infant's life. In accord with Judeo-Christian beliefs, infanticide has been treated as a particularly abhorrent crime by Western culture for nearly 2,000 years. However, at various times in Western history the penalties imposed have been less severe than those for other types of homicide, and the laws banning infanticide have sometimes been enforced inconsistently. In the non-Western world prior to the imposition of Christianity and Western legal systems, the majority of non-Western societies allowed infanticide for various reasons. In many of these societies, infanticide clearly served as a from of birth control in the absence of other methods that could be used to prevent conception or terminate a pregnancy before birth without harm to the mother. The underlying purpose was to space births so that often scarce resources, including the mother's time and energy, could be given to existing children. A half-dozen cross-cultural surveys place the percentage of such societies at from 53 percent to 78 percent, depending on how precisely infanticide is defined and how the cases are counted. At the same time, of course, there were numerous societies that forbade infanticide. For example, infanticide by

the Ona of the Tierra del Fuego at the southern tip of South America was described by ethnographer Martin Gusinde as "out of the question and inconceivable, so to speak." He then recounts the story of a mother who drowned her daughter and then hid from the group to conceal her crime. When her crime was eventually discovered she was ostracized and then allowed to rejoin the group, although she was now seen as being mentally ill—the only possible explanation for her action. Mental illness is also a common explanation for infanticide in the Western world today, although often without validity and often at the cost of masking the real reasons leading a parent to kill his or her child.

Little is known about who killed the infant, largely because ethnographers wrote little about it, perhaps for fear of getting native people in trouble with colonial officials who considered infanticide a crime. What is known is that in the majority of societies the killing was done by the mother, usually through nonviolent means such as abandonment, smothering, poisoning, or burial. Midwives often did the killing in some societies, while fathers and other relatives did so in a small minority of cultures. In general, however, parents usually killed the infant, a major difference between infanticide by humans as compared to that by nonhuman primates, where the killing is more often done by a male unrelated to the infant.

The reasons commonly given for infanticide in a sample of fifty-seven societies are shown in the chart on the next page.

Infanticide has been explained as a form of after-the-fact birth control, used in a variety of situations as listed above, virtually all of which are circumstances that interfere in some way with a parent's willingness or ability to devote sufficient resources to raising the child. This birth control explanation is supported by the timing of the actual act of killing the infant. In 90 percent of the societies that permitted infanti-

Reason for Infanticide	Distribution
Illegitimate conception (adultery, unwed mother, rape, father from other society or kinship group)	53%
A twin or triplet	40%
Infant unfit (ill, weak, handicapped)	53%
Abnormal birth (breech, premature)	20%
Birth control (too many children, too close birth spacing, poverty)	23%
Infant unwanted (family problems, mother too old)	27%
Infant a girl	17%
Infant a boy	7%
Other	3%

cide, the killing took place before the performance of a birth ceremony. Since a birth ceremony publicly defines the infant as a social being and as fully "human," killing before the ceremony means that the act is not a crime—the infant is not human—and perhaps also makes it somewhat easier emotionally for a mother to kill or lose her child. Other possible explanations, which draw heavily on observations of nonhuman primates such as gorillas, emphasize the use of the infant's body for food (very rare in humans), the role of nonbiological parents (stepparents) who have less biological investment in the infant or child, competition between men that results in their killing one another's offspring, and mental illness on the part of the perpetrator.

Twin infanticide and female infanticide are special forms of infanticide. Twin or triplet infanticide, where only one infant is allowed to survive, occurs in anywhere from 25 to 40 percent of the societies where infanticide occurs. However, the rule is often not rigidly enforced, as among the Guarani of Brazil, where in some communities one of the twins is killed but in other communities both twins are allowed to live.

Whether or not a twin is killed depends mostly on the resources available to the mother to rear two children of the same age. Only when she has much other work to perform and cannot count on child care help from relatives is it likely that a twin will be sacrificed.

Female infanticide, while the subject of much discussion, is not as widespread as many believe, reported in only about 17 percent of societies. Why some societies choose to dispose of female infants more readily than male infants is unclear, although the practice is clearly motivated be a perceived need on the part of the parents to produce sons or at least more sons than daughters. A variety of situations can give rise to this preference for sons. One is the need to produce a steady stream of warriors to battle other communities or societies. Another is a need to produce male heirs when there is much wealth in the family and inheritance is through the male line. Also, in many societies in traditional times, it was easier to replace women by taking women or girls as war captives and then integrating them into the society through marriage than it was to replace men with war captives. Perhaps this is one reason why societies that raided or traded for slaves took far more female slaves than male slaves. And in some cultures, such as China, boys are preferred regardless of any societal needs and are valued more highly than girls.

DEATH RITES

Death rites involve transitions in status for both the individual who has died and members of his or her family and community. For the individual who has died, the rite in nearly all cultures involves movement from the world of the living to the world of the dead. Toward this end rituals are followed carefully to insure that the deceased reaches and enjoys a happy existence in the world of the dead. The motivation for insuring the well-being of the deceased is two-fold. First, it reflects real concern for the soul of the deceased. Second, it reflects in many societies a belief that spirits of the dead can influence the living and that if the spirits fail to reach the afterworld or are unhappy there, they will make life unpleasant for their descendants on earth. For some of the survivors, the rite often involves a transition in their social roles and statuses in the family and the community: a son may now become head of the family, a daughter the head of the household, a wife a widow who must remarry her deceased husband's brother, a member of the village council may now become the community leader, the heads of the village kin groups may now compete for village leadership, and the kin group may

have to decide on the disposition of the property of the deceased. In some cultures, however, the line between the world of the living and dead is blurred and, after death, the deceased is defined as an ancestor, who continues to influence the lives of his living descendants. In these cultures, such as China and Korea where ancestor worship is an important aspect of traditional religion, funeral rites include additional rituals designed to make the deceased an ancestor. These rites are often spread over one or more years, and the position of the grave and the body in it are important considerations. All of this ritual activity is meant to smooth subsequent relations between the deceased ancestor and his living

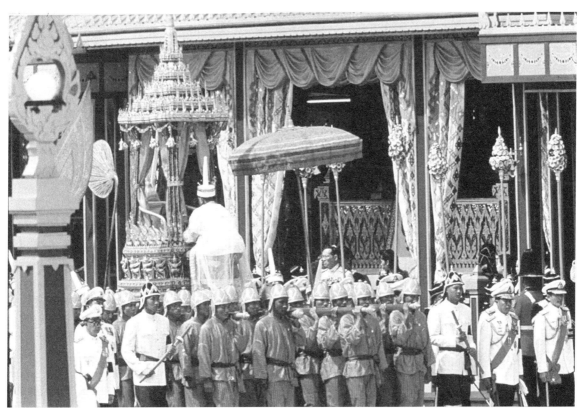

King Bhumibol Adulyadej of Thailand attends to the ashes of his mother contained in an urn during Buddhist funeral rites in Bangkok in 1996. Such rites following death mark the transition for an individual and for the family and community from life to death.

descendants. And, of course, ritual worship of ancestors continues in the home and community as a regular activity.

Across cultures, death rites serve a number of functions:

1. Disposal of the body and other physical objects associated with the deceased
2. Provision of material and emotional support to the survivors
3. Public announcement of the death
4. Public recognition of the new status of some of the survivors
5. Rule setting for the appropriate mourning behavior and period of mourning
6. Renewal of ties among family and community members
7. Affirmation that the family and community will survive despite the death of one of its members

Perhaps the two most striking features of death rites across cultures are that (1) in nearly all cultures substantial numbers of people attend the rites and (2) in 75 percent of cultures it is customary to have a final funeral rite that occurs at some time after the first rite. In some cultures the final rite takes place later in the year as part of a community rite for all who have died in the previous year; in other cultures there is a series of rites culminating in a final rite; and in others there are two rites, with the second ending the formal mourning period.

While there is much variation across cultures in the details of death rites, there is also some commonality, as the body is always disposed of in some way, the immediate family is always involved in the rite, the supernatural is invoked, there is community involvement, a religious specialist conducts the rites, rituals are followed carefully, there is a defined mourning period, and there is considerable individual variation permitted in mourning behavior. Death rites among the

Chippewa of the Great Lakes region display many of the general features of death rites across cultures, as described below.

Immediately after death the body was washed, dressed in fine clothing, and adorned with beads and the hair was braided. His face, moccasins, and blanket were painted in brown and red designs to assist them in joining the "dance of the ghosts where the northern lights are shining." The body was laid out and buried with a few objects of personal value and other objects that would be needed on the four-day journey of the soul to the hereafter:

> My father was buried with his jackknife and pipe, the Grand Medicine Man who buried him requesting this and saying that his soul might crave those articles and not leave at once for the Hereafter. (Densmore 1929)

The death rites were conducted by members of the deceased's Medicine Society, who comforted the family and spoke to the spirit of the deceased, advising it on how to have a safe trip to the hereafter. Communication with the spirit often began with a statement such as "Your feet are now on the road of souls." The body was then wrapped in birch bark or placed in a wood coffin and set in a shallow grave. Relatives danced around the grave and it was then filled, food was placed on it, and a fire was kept burning for four nights. The fire was to assist the spirit in keeping warm, and food placed on the grave was allowed to be taken by the poor, relatives, and friends for their own consumption. The body was generally placed with the feet to the west, the direction of the soul's journey. The grave was then covered with bark, cloth, or a small shelter, and food was placed there periodically, including the first harvests of maple sap and berries. A clan totem was placed on the grave upside down as a marker of both death and the deceased's clan identity.

While certain ritual behavior was required of all mourners, there was much freedom for individuals to express their personal grief and some cut themselves, others wailed loudly, and others wailed not at all. Widows and others who chose to do so publicly displayed their status as mourners for one year by wearing old clothing, cutting their hair short or wearing it unbraided, and painting their face black. Once a year a ceremony of "restoring the mourners" was held and those in mourning were comforted and given gifts and brightly colored objects that terminated the mourning period. Close relatives might also elect to keep a "spirit bundle" of the deceased, which at its center contained a lock of hair cut from the deceased wrapped in birch bark to which other objects such as blankets, moccasins, and beads might be added over the course of the year. Such bundles were more often kept by women for a deceased child or husband and were unwrapped one year after the death at a feast and the core of hair and birch bark wrapping were buried next to the grave of the deceased.

See also SUICIDE.

Barton, Roy F. (1946) *The Religion of the Ifugao.*

Bohannan, Paul, and Laura Bohannan. (1958) *Three Source Notebooks on Tiv Ethnography.*

Bouroncle-Carreon, Alfonso. (1964) "Contribucion al Estudio de los Aymaras." *America Indigenista* 24: 129–169, 233–269.

Child, Alice B., and Irvin L. Child. (1993) *Religion and Magic in the Life of Traditional Peoples.*

Counts, Dorothy, and David Counts. (1985) *Aging and Its Transformations: Moving toward Death in the Pacific.*

Culshaw, W. J. (1949) *Tribal Heritage: A Study of the Santals.*

Daly, Martin, and Margo Wilson. (1988) *Homicide.*

Densmore, Frances. (1929) *Chippewa Customs.*

Diamond, Norma. (1969) *K'un Shen: A Taiwan Village.*

East, Ruppert, ed. (1939) *Akiga's Story: The Tiv Tribe as Seen by One of Its Members.*

Gennep, Arnold Van. (1960) *The Rites of Passage.* Originally published in 1909.

Gladwin, Thomas, and Seymour B. Sarason. (1953) *Truk: Man in Paradise.*

Glascock, Anthony P. (1984) "Decrepitude and Death-Hastening: The Nature of Old Age in Third World Societies." *Studies in Third World Societies* 22: 43–67.

Glascock, Anthony P., and Richard A. Wagner. (1986) *HRAF Research Series in Quantitative Cross-Cultural Data. Vol. II: Life Cycle Data.*

Granzberg, Gary. (1973) "Twin Infanticide—A Cross-Cultural Test of a Materialistic Explanation." *Ethos* 4: 405–412.

Gusinde, Martin. (1931) *The Fireland Indians. Vol. 1. The Selk'nam, On the Life and Thought of a Hunting People of the Great Island of Tierra del Fuego.* Translated from the German by Frieda Schutze.

Hausfater, G., and S. Blaffer Hardy, eds. (1984) *Infanticide: Comparative and Evolutionary Perspectives.*

Jenness, Diamond. (1922) *Report of the Canadian Arctic Expedition, 1913–1918, Vol. XII, Part A.*

Kemp, Phyllis. (1935) *Healing Ritual: Studies in the Technique and Tradition of the Southern Slavs.*

Langer, William L. (1974) "Infanticide: A Historical Survey." *History of Childhood Quarterly: The Journal of Psychohistory* 1: 353–365.

Levinson, David. (1989) *Family Violence in Cross-Cultural Perspective.*

Maxwell, Robert J., and Philip Silverman. (1989) "Gerontocide." In *The Contents of Culture: Constants and Variants; Studies in Honor of*

John M. Roberts, edited by Ralph Bolton, 511–523.

Minturn, Leigh, and Jerry Stashak. (1982) "Infanticide as a Terminal Abortion Procedure." *Behavior Science Research* 17: 70–90.

Rivers, William H. R., ed. (1926) *Psychology and Ethnology*.

Rosenblatt, Paul C., R. Patricia Walsh, and Douglas A. Jackson. (1976) *Grief and Mourning in Cross-Cultural Perspective*.

Schaden, Egon. (1962) *Fundamental Aspects of Guarani Culture.* Translated from the Portuguese by Lars-Peter Lewinsohn.

Sokolovsky, Jay, ed. (1990) *Culture, Aging, and Society*.

Titiev, Mischa. (1971) *Old Oraibi: A Study of the Hopi Indians of Third Mesa*.

DIET AND NUTRITION

Since everyone must eat to live, food is one of the earliest forms of medicine. Herbal remedies and natural food remedies handed down over the generations were used universally before the advent of modern medicine. The ancient Greeks, Romans, Chinese, Indians, and Middle Easterners all used food to heal the body, as did virtually all traditional cultures. When modern science was able to isolate the active ingredients of such remedies, and they became the standard treatments, the use of food in healing became a source of ridicule and was considered an "old wives' tale" in Western culture. While doctors have always known the importance of giving the body its proper nutrients to maintain health, actual healing using food went out of favor in the West with the advent of allopathic medicine.

In other cultures the use of herbal remedies and systems of healing that incorporate food—such as Ayurveda in India, Chinese medicine, and humoral medicine in South and Latin America and Africa—continue to thrive. In Western societies since industrialization, there has been a trend toward foods that are heavily refined for reasons of taste, ease of preparation, and preservability (which meant profitability for the producers of food). This does not mean, of course, that only Westerners produce and eat refined food. So, too, do other peoples. For example, bitter manioc, a staple food in South America and parts of Africa, must be processed to remove a bitter poison before it can be eaten. Similarly, Indians of the western United States had to leach poisonous chemicals from acorn flour before making it into cakes. However, the process of refining food in the West is more often for appearance and taste and can decrease the nutritional and energetic integrity of the food. The food becomes separated from its natural context, and the parts that are removed are often the most nutritious.

Food is equated to "fuel" in American culture, and for many people the difference between "regular" and "super high octane" has to do with taste rather than nutritional content. The introduction of chemicals to crop fertilizers and food preservatives has added to what many feel is a downward spiral in the quality of American nutrition. Instead of promoting health, some feel that modern nutrition, with its high fat and high sodium content and toxic additives, actually contributes to chronic disease.

Since the 1960s there has been a movement in the West to return to healing with food. The natural foods diet, the use of specific diets in healing illnesses such as cancer and heart disease, and energetic, holistic models like macrobiotics seek to restore food as an important component in maintaining health and well-being and even curing disease.

The hunter-gatherer ancestors of modern humans ate more fiber, carbohydrates, calcium, and vitamins than we do, less fat and sodium, and virtually no dairy products. While the biological makeup of humans has remained roughly the same, the variety of nutrients available in foods obtained from hunting and gathering in the wild is nowhere near the same. The advent of agriculture and the development of technology for the acquisition, preparation, preservation, and storage of food have made the kinds of food we eat radically different from those of our ancestors.

Our narrow food base, largely coming from wheat, rice, potatoes, and corn (eaten more often than the next twenty-six most-often-eaten foods combined), and our reliance on meat and dairy foods lead to deficiencies in essential nutrients, to an oversupply of energy, and to obesity and other diseases of the affluent world.

When people started working in factories rather than on farms, they acquired their food from greater distances, resulting in loss of quality, variety, and freshness during transportation. Refining and preserving foods to prolong their shelf-life also resulted in a loss of nutrition, while industrialization caused pollution to the natural environment in the form of coal dust and lead as well as in newly created toxic chemicals like polychlorinated biphenyls and dioxin. Toxic chemicals enter the water supply through the air (acid rain) and by direct dumping, and they are passed on to animals and humans through the foods that are grown nearby. Though there is much research to be done in this area, many governments have outlawed some pesticides. There is concern among proponents of natural foods that even if some of these chemicals do not directly cause illness, they may be stored in the cells of our bodies, build up over time, and contribute to disease.

Poor nutrition reduces the effectiveness of the body to ward off disease. When disease does occur, the result may be the interruption of the digestive process, either by poor absorption or by reduced appetite. Modern proponents of healing through diet feel that despite our apparent longevity compared with earlier times, our lives are not qualitatively better and that the loss of the integrity of whole food is a strong contributing factor. Nutritionist Annemarie Colbin believes that learning difficulties and behavior problems of children may be rooted in degenerating nutrition:

> Childhood problems that were rare a generation ago are now so prevalent that they are called "the new morbidity": learning difficulties, behavioral disturbances, speech and hearing difficulties, faulty vision, serious dental misalignment. . . . It is my profound conviction that a great many of our more serious health problems today stem not only from bad food or pollution, but also from the chemical treatment of minor physiological adjustments. (Colbin 1986: 15)

FOOD ACROSS CULTURES

The human need to obtain food to eat is a fairly obvious cultural universal and cultures vary widely in the methods they use to obtain the foods that are regularly eaten. People may obtain food by either gathering it directly from nature or by altering nature so as to produce food. Although rare today, for nearly all of human existence (over 2 million years) humans and their ancestors have subsisted by gathering—hunting for animals; collecting plants, insects, and shellfish; and fishing. About 8,000 years ago agriculture and the herding of domesticated animals appeared in the Middle East and eventually spread to all regions of the world. Today, nearly all people in the world live on food that they produce themselves through horticulture, agriculture, aquaculture, herding, or ranching or that others produce and they purchase.

Across cultures there are a number of commonalities in eating behavior and nutrition:

1. The consumption of a large number of essential nutrients
2. The development of an individual cultural cuisine consisting of staple, secondary, and

complementary foods and customary behavior for the preparation and consumption of food

3. The consumption of a mix of both vegetables and meats
4. The movement of food from the place
where it is obtained to where it is stored
5. The storage of food
6. The use of technology to acquire and prepare food
7. The sharing of food
8. The division of labor between men and
women in the acquisition, storage, and
preparation of food
9. The existence of food taboos that apply
to specific foods at all times or only at certain times and that apply to all people or
only to certain categories of people
10. The use of food for nonnutritional purposes such as sacrifice or offerings

Across cultures there is considerable variation in what people eat and what they prefer to
eat. However, within this considerable variation
there is much regional patterning of consumption, as throughout human history the natural
environment has been the major determinant of
what foods grow in a particular environment and
therefore what people have available to eat. However, environment is not the only determining
factor and people often avoid certain foods for
social and religious reasons, even when the food
is readily available. The foods people eat can be
divided into three groups—staples, secondary
foods, and complementary foods. The ten most
frequently consumed foods in these three categories in a sample of 383 non-Western cultures
are shown in the accompanying chart.

The information in these lists, of course,
masks the considerable variation in food consumption among cultures and even within regions. However, the lists do point out that
humans by-and-large eat more vegetables than

Staple Foods	Cultures
Maize (corn)	171
Rice	161
Manioc (cassava)	106
Fish	105
Millet	94
Bananas/Plantains	84
Sorghum	68
Taro	52
Sweet Potato	51
Wheat	46

Secondary Foods	Cultures
Chicken	363
Squash	222
Beef	196
Maize	187
Pig	180
Goat	166
Sweet Potato	163
Banana	160
Fish	139
Beans	137

Complementary Foods	Cultures
Chili Pepper	171
Salt	151
Sugar	62
Fish	57
Ginger	54
Coconut	41
Garlic	40
Sesame	38
Bees and Honey	36
Palm Oil	35

meat and mainly eat foods that they produce
rather than those that they gather.

Another salient issue in diet and nutrition is
what people prefer to eat in contrast to what they
actually eat. Not all staples and secondary foods
are necessarily the preferred foods in cultures
where they are regularly consumed. For example,
maize is the staple in 171 cultures, yet its overall
preference rating is low and it is considered only
acceptable. On the other hand, rice, which is the
staple in 161 cultures, is rated highly and is generally preferred or highly preferred.

DIET AND HEALTH: ALTERNATIVE AND COMPLEMENTARY APPROACHES

There are roughly three categories for the current, and seemingly endless, varieties of healing diets: those based on a mechanical model, those based on a holistic model, and those based on a metabolic model. Some approaches seek to modify a condition of imbalance in nutrients (e.g., diabetes—mechanistic), others seek to restore the body's balance and innate ability to heal (raw foods diet—holistic), and still others seek to make digestion more harmonious by working more closely with the body's metabolic processes (humoral—metabolic). Some are a combination of two or even three of these general approaches.

In the last forty years, mainstream medicine has prescribed diets for various conditions—low fat and cholesterol diets for heart disease, weight-loss diets, diets for hypoglycemia and diabetes. These also represent a "mechanistic" approach to using food for healing, in that the substances added or taken away just seek to replace a nutritional "part" that is missing—or make the "machine" work more smoothly.

The return to natural foods healing, on the other hand, is holistic. The whole is greater than the sum of its parts. It incorporates the idea that disease reflects more than the illness of just one part of the body, but instead is a reflection of a total condition of the organism. It sees health as a return to a stabilization or equilibrium for the entire organism—and the use of whole, natural medicines to stimulate it. Colbin explains holism in terms of "living systems theory": "Living systems are unstable—constantly exchanging energy and matter with the environment. There is a strong tendency to homeostasis or restoring balance." A living system is "an aggregate of physical elements and parts, plus an organizing energy field that makes the separate parts cohere and establishes them as a system." The holistic model looks at homeostasis and the health and well-being of that "organizing energy field," which is affected by internal and external stimuli, to the key for health.

Colbin and other proponents of natural foods believe that foods, being live material, have a "life force" that is negatively affected by the addition of chemicals, refinement, and even cooking and freezing. And, at the very least, they say, the nutritional content of foods is negatively affected by these same forces. A holistic model of healing with natural foods is one that draws on available information about the inherent properties of a natural food to address deficiencies in the body, but with the understanding that it is the unadulterated state of the food, with its nutrients and life force intact, that will stimulate the body's inherent ability to heal itself.

The metabolic model views certain foods as interacting with the process of ingesting, digesting, and eliminating foods in particular ways. Viewing digestion as basically a building up and breaking down process that engages the body's metabolism has attracted a number of approaches. In humoral and macrobiotic approaches, a healing with opposites, yin and yang, hot-cold dynamic is believed to exist. Some foods create "heat," others "cold" in terms of the body's utilization of them. Foods that are "hot" help the body to build itself up while "cold" foods tend to aid the elimination of toxic materials. They are thus administered accordingly.

The following is an overview of the basic categories, with examples of each.

Mechanistic Approach

In this view, adopted concurrently with the Industrial and Scientific Revolutions, the body is viewed as a series of interlocking parts, much like a machine. In the most basic mechanistic approach to maintaining health with food, the building blocks of food—proteins, fats, carbohydrates, water, vitamins, and minerals—comprise, in their proper proportions, the fuel that keeps the machine running.

The basis of this approach is that you eat all the building blocks and you get good nutrition. It does not matter if your source is whole or processed food. Replace what is lost, repair what is "broken."

Proteins build and repair the organs of the body and are indispensable for growth and development. They are found in eggs, milk, fish, meat, and beans. Combining plant foods, such as rice with beans, or cheese with whole grain breads can also create a complete protein. Fats carry vitamins and provide the body with quick energy. Sources of fat include meat, butter, cheese, cream, eggs, margarine, nut butters, and oils. Carbohydrates are found in bread, pasta, potatoes, beans, fruit, and starchy vegetables. Water helps to move nutrients to the areas of the body that will utilize them.

Vitamins are essential for many metabolic functions: they are necessary to build and protect the body, assist in healing, and prevent disease. The following vitamins and minerals are considered essential for good health:

Vitamins

- Vitamin A—Promotes good eyesight and helps keep the mucous membrane resistant to infection. Best sources: liver, sweet potatoes, carrots, kale, cantaloupe.
- Vitamin B1 (thiamin)—Prevents beri-beri. Essential to carbohydrate metabolism and health of nervous system. Best sources: pork, enriched cereals, grains, soybeans, nuts.
- Vitamin B2 (riboflavin)—Protects skin, mouth, eyes, eyelids, and mucous membranes. Essential to protein and energy metabolism. Best sources: milk, meat, poultry, cheese, broccoli, spinach.
- Vitamin B6 (pyridoxine)—Important in the regulation of the central nervous system and in protein metabolism. Best sources: whole grains, meats, fish, poultry, nuts, brewer's yeast.

- Vitamin B12 (cobalamin)—Needed to form red blood cells. Best sources: meat, fish, poultry, eggs, dairy products.
- Niacin—Maintains the health of skin, tongue, and digestive system. Best sources: poultry, peanuts, fish, enriched flour and bread.
- Folic acid (folicin)—Required for normal blood cell formation, growth, and reproduction and for important chemical reactions in body cells. Best sources: yeast, orange juice, green leafy vegetables, wheat germ, asparagus, broccoli, nuts.
- Other B vitamins—biotin, pantothenic acid.
- Vitamin C (ascorbic acid)—Maintains collagen, a protein necessary for the formation of skin, ligaments, and bones. It helps heal wounds and mend fractures and aids in resisting some types of viral and bacterial infections. Best sources: citrus fruits and juices, cantaloupe, broccoli, brussels sprouts, potatoes and sweet potatoes, tomatoes, cabbage.
- Vitamin D—Important for bone development. Best sources: vegetable oils, wheat germ, whole grains, eggs, peanuts, margarine, green leafy vegetables.
- Vitamin K—Necessary for formation of prothrombin, which helps blood to clot. Also made by intestinal bacteria. Best sources: green leafy vegetables, tomatoes.

Minerals

- Calcium—The most abundant mineral in the body, works with phosphorus in building and maintaining bones and teeth. Best sources: milk and milk products, cheese, blackstrap molasses, tofu.
- Phosphorus—The second most abundant mineral, performs more functions than any other mineral and plays a part

in nearly every chemical reaction in the body. Best sources: cheese, milk, meats, poultry, fish, tofu.

- Iron—Necessary for the formation of myoglobin, which is a reservoir of oxygen for muscle tissue, and hemoglobin, which transports oxygen in the blood. Best sources: lean meats, beans, green leafy vegetables, shellfish, enriched breads and cereals, whole grains.
- Other minerals include chromium, cobalt, copper, fluorine, iodine, magnesium, manganese, molybdenum and potassium, riboflavin, thiamine, and zinc.

Viewing nutrition in this way, as the fuel for the machine, is the most common use of nutrition in allopathic approaches. The proper amount and kind of nutrients combine to provide the correct fuel for the machine, thus assuring optimal performance. In the United States, the U.S. Department of Health and Human Services and the Department of Agriculture issue dietary guidelines for a recommended diet for the American public. In 1990, these were their recommendations: (1) no more than 30 percent of calories from fat, or about sixty-seven grams of fat in a 2,000-calorie diet; and no more than 10 percent of calories, or twenty-two grams of fat, from saturated fats; (2) maximum alcohol consumption of about one drink a day for women, two for men; (3) daily consumption of three to five servings of vegetables; two to four servings of fruits; six to eleven servings of pastas, cereals, or breads; two to three servings of milk; and two to three servings of meat, poultry, fish, and eggs. (Serving sizes: vegetables, one cup of raw leafy greens or one-half cup other kinds; fruit, one medium apple, banana, or orange; grains, one slice of bread, one cup of pasta or one ounce of cereal; milk, one cup or one and one-half ounces of cheese; meat and poultry, two to three ounces of cooked lean beef or chicken without skin.)

A mechanistic approach to healing with diet can be found in the use of nutritional supple-ments in that what is prescribed is that which is deficient. Many mainstream physicians recommend a daily multiple vitamin with minerals to ensure that all of the building blocks are covered. Since the 1960s, proponents of natural foods have stressed the importance of natural vitamins and mineral supplements. There has also been interest in and some research done in the medicinal properties of megadoses of certain vitamins and minerals.

Orthomolecular medicine is the "preservation of good health and the treatment of disease by varying the concentrations in the human body of substances that are normally present in the body and required for good health." It is sometimes called megavitamin therapy. An example of this is Nobel Prize–winner Linus Pauling's claim that high doses of vitamin C could prevent and cure the common cold. Some research supports this and the use of other vitamins and minerals in curing and preventing both physical and mental illnesses, but other research suggests that this approach has little impact.

There is controversy, even among proponents, about the proper use of vitamin supplements, considering the intricate balance of overall nutrition and the nutrients themselves. "The purist will claim that any deficiency must be made good by careful selection of those foodstuffs rich in the missing vitamin as well as the avoidance of those elements that interfere with its availability to the body. Proponents of supplementation are of the opinion that in some cases barrow-loads of foodstuff may have to be consumed in order to get the quantity of vitamins necessary." (Hill 1979: 147)

Some deficiencies caused by vitamin depletion include: night blindness from lack of vitamin A, skin and hair problems from lack of the B vitamins, poor growth and anemia from lack of folic acid, sore gums and low immunity to infection from lack of vitamin C, and premature aging and sterility in males from lack of vitamin E. Taking large doses of individual vitamins to self-medicate for these conditions is not advised—megadoses of some vitamins, particularly the fat soluble ones, are harmful to the body, while others simply pass through the system.

Mineral supplements include cobalt, copper, iodine, iron, zinc, calcium, chlorine, magnesium, phosphorus, potassium, sodium, and sulfur. Some signs of mineral depletion include anemia, loss of energy, brittle bones, and loss of weight and appetite. Like vitamin supplementation, adding minerals to the diet is delicate: some minerals should be taken with others to be absorbed prop-

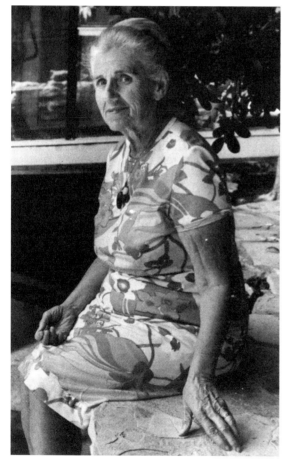

Herbal and natural food remedies have long been associated with health and healing. Adele Davis, author of several popular books on nutrition, emphasized consuming whole, fresh, and natural foods.

erly and megadoses should be avoided unless prescribed. Calcium, for example, needs magnesium and vitamin D to be properly absorbed. Taking iron supplements interferes with the absorption of other minerals, but vitamin C enhances the absorption of iron.

Raw juices are used by some to supplement diet. They are assimilated quickly and are high in all nutrients and roughage. Fruit juices are seen as cleansing the body, and vegetable juices are rebuilders. Freshness is a high priority, and a special machine is needed to create the juices. Juices can be made from a single fruit or vegetable, such as apple or carrot. A sample of a blend of juices is equal quantities of apple, carrot, and beet. Certain fruit and vegetable juices are purported to have medicinal value: cabbage for the digestive system, apple for soothing the nerves.

The Western mechanistic model of healing includes the training of specialists for virtually every organ and system in the body. If a person has a problem with his heart, he goes to a cardiologist. All efforts are made to help the heart function again, mostly through medication or surgery or other techniques that are applied directly to the heart or to the circulatory system, which connects the heart to the rest of the body. Only in the last thirty years has diet become a major part of preventing and recovering from cardiac illness.

The mechanistic theory of nutrition includes specific diets to prevent or control conditions. Factors that increase the risk of heart disease are elevated serum cholesterol, elevated serum triglycerides, obesity, hypertension, poor eating habits, and a sedentary lifestyle. When these conditions are observed in patients today, it is standard procedure to recommend a corrective diet that is low in fat and cholesterol. Diets low in fat and cholesterol reduce the chances of blood becoming blocked in the arteries that move blood away from the heart.

Adele Davis, whose classic, *Let's Eat Right to Keep Fit*, was published in 1954, gained a popular following and became a bridge between the mechanistic model and the holistic model. Her analysis of food deficiencies and nutritional practices in the West were mechanistic in that they sought to recover what was lost nutritionally in processed foods, but in her emphasis on whole, fresh, natural foods she foreshadowed the holistic model.

Taking their cue from Davis and the many other authors in the budding diet and nutrition fields, proponents of whole foods began to publish suggested diets to aid in the healing of illness. Many of these have not been exhaustively researched or proven effective. They are suggestions based on anecdotal and some research evidence. In most cases, they are not considered to be harmful, especially when considered an adjunct to standard medical treatment.

The following recommendations from *Prescription for Natural Healing* are meant to help the body prevent and recover from cancer. They are presented here as an example of the mechanistic approach, but the authors recommend whole, unadulterated food:

> Include some of the following in your cancer prevention or cancer therapy program: black radish, dandelion, echinacea, Jason Winters tea, pau d'arco, red clover, and suma.
>
> Many with external cancers responded well to poultices made from comfrey, pau d'arco, ragwort, and wood sage. . . .
>
> Drink beet juice (from roots and tops), carrot juice (beta-carotene), and asparagus juice often. Grape, black cherry, and all dark-colored juices are good, as are black currants. Also beneficial is apple juice, if it is fresh. Fruit juices are best taken in the morning, and vegetable juices are best taken in the afternoon. . . .
>
> Eat onions and garlic. . . .
>
> Do *not* consume the following: junk foods, processed refined foods, saturated fats, salt, sugar, or white flour. Instead of salt, use a kelp or potassium substitute. A small amount of blackstrap molasses or pure maple syrup acts as a natural sweetener in place of sugar. Use whole wheat or rye instead of white flour. Eliminate alcohol, coffee, and all teas except for herbal teas.
>
> Do not eat any animal protein—*never* eat luncheon meat, hot dogs, or smoked or cured meats. As your condition improves, eat broiled fish three times a week. Restrict consumption of dairy products; a little yogurt, kefir milk, or raw cheese occasionally is enough. Do not eat any peanuts. Limit, but don't eliminate altogether, your intake of soybean products; they contain enzyme inhibitors. (Balch and Balch 1990)

Holistic Approach

A holistic model of healing with natural foods is one that draws on available information about the inherent properties of a natural food to address deficiencies in the body, but with the understanding that it is the unadulterated state of the food, with its nutrients and life force intact, that will stimulate the body's inherent ability to heal itself. The basis of holism is that the whole is greater than the parts. The whole food diet, the raw food diet, and most forms of vegetarianism are examples of holistic approaches to diet. The Hay, Ayurvedic, and macrobiotic diets are partly holistic as well, but will be discussed as metabolic approaches.

The whole food diet includes fruit, vegetables, grain, and edible seeds. They are often consumed raw, or with as little cooking as possible. A whole food diet would eschew sugar, which is refined from its natural state in sugar cane or beet, and use honey or molasses, sweeteners which retain their original forms. Whole food is usually organically grown—without chemical fertilizers, pesticides, or herbicides. There is also a preference for traditional plants rather than those produced through genetic engineering.

Whole foods contain many more nutrients than the refined versions. According to Colbin:

> Fragmentation affects food. When wheat is refined into white flour, for example, not

only does it lose its bran and germ, but some twenty nutrients are lost or greatly reduced. Enriching the flour—which entails returning four of those twenty nutrients—does not solve the problem. Not only are the added nutrients fewer in number than those present in the original whole wheat; they also lack the energy they had when they were simply part of a living, growing plant. (1986: 39)

Raw foods are consumed so that there is no loss of nutrition through preparation, heating, or freezing. The water content of raw foods is of better quality and is higher in fiber.

The raw foods diet includes eating the outer shell or skin of most fruits and vegetables, because the part of the plant closest to the skin contains a higher concentration of vitamins (the introduction of more and more pesticides to fruit and vegetable agriculture has put a damper on this for many health enthusiasts.) Loss of vitamins and minerals from vegetables into cooking water resulted in the popularity of steaming and baking as preferred methods of food preparation. About 80 percent of the raw food diet consists of fruit and vegetables, 10 percent is protein and 8 percent cereal grains. The preponderance of fruits and vegetables creates an alkaline environment in the body to which some attribute better health.

Some believe that a proper whole food diet will correct imbalances in the body, allowing the body to cure itself of certain conditions and illnesses. Naturopathic physicians often prescribe whole food diets and herbal remedies from nature, believing in the inherent ability of the body to heal with corrective help from mother nature. They also screen for food allergies and other obstructions to proper digestion (toxins from pesticides, etc.) because they see proper digestion and elimination as setting the tone for optimal health.

Whole food supplementation may be used with foods high in nutrients. Some of the most commonly used whole foods medicinal remedies

include apple cider vinegar, honey, molasses, wheat germ, brewer's yeast, and ginseng, a general tonic root grown in China, Korea, and Russia.

Although vegetarianism is somewhat new to the West as a philosophy or style of diet (becoming a trend over the last forty years), it has been practiced in many parts of the world for centuries. Spiritual disciplines, including Buddhism, Hinduism, and some forms of Taoism, require a meatless diet. Just as people in the West considered meat a sign of affluence, Asians viewed meat as lowering the spiritual potential of the individual, and the upper classes there were more likely to be vegetarian.

The cruel practices that are used in raising and slaughtering animals for beef and veal, especially, are part of the explanation that Western vegetarians give for their decision. Animals are often raised in restricted surroundings, unable to range. They are fed enormous amounts of grain, and growth hormones may be used. The nutrition content of the amount of grain used to raise animals for food is several times higher than the end result of the meat, leading many to say that meat-eating is ecologically wasteful and expensive. Half the total grain consumption of the world is fed to domestic animals.

Many believe that meat has a stimulating effect on the nervous system, while vegetables have a calming effect. Red meat is virtually eliminated in diets designed to prevent and control heart disease due to its high fat and cholesterol content. Recent research suggests a relationship between red meat consumption and some forms of cancer.

Some vegetarians eat dairy and eggs and are called lacto-ovo vegetarians. Lactarians eat dairy, but no eggs. The raw foods diet and the Natural Hygiene diet are strictly vegetarian, as is the standard vegetarian diet. Adherents to these are also called vegans. Some vegetarians are not strictly whole food eaters—they eat prepared, processed, and refined foods.

Metabolic Approach

The metabolic structure of digestion and elimination corresponds to a building up and breaking down cycle. The body takes in nutrition and converts it into energy that is used to build and strengthen cells for all of the bodily functions. It breaks down what is not usable and eliminates it.

It has been observed by many cultures that certain foods aid in the build-up process and others in the break-down. This observation led to a dynamic approach to using food in healing called humoral medicine.

Humoral medicine is found in Africa, China, Latin and South America, Australia, and elsewhere, particularly among indigenous peoples. Some anthropologists believe it is rooted in the ancient Greek medicines (the origin of the word "humoral" is from the Greek word for the four bodily humors) and others believe that it appeared independently in other cultures. The basis of the healing is using foods to heal illness by assessing whether a "hot," or building-up food, is needed, or rather, a "cold" breaking-down food. Illnesses are classified according to whether they are "hot" or "cold" and the opposite remedy (in most cases) is applied.

This idea of maintaining a dynamic balance of opposites in the body is seen in the modern philosophy of macrobiotics. A Japanese philosopher named George Oshawa developed a belief system based on the study of opposites most common in Asian medicine, yin and yang. These opposing forces, the yang being forceful, outgoing, and "hot," and the yin being receptive, passive, and "cold," are believed to hold the universe together.

In the realm of diet, macrobiotics (meaning large life) seeks to ingest in a balanced way that is consistent with those forces in the natural environment. Foods are classified into yin and yang based on factors including growth and structure. Oshawa reversed some of the properties of yin and yang to align them more closely with Western thinking, according to Colbin, but the interplay of opposites is the critical element that makes the diet work for many people. The following describes the properties of yin and yang in vegetables (Hill 1979: 133):

Yin	Yang
Growing in a hot climate	Growing in a cold climate
Containing more water	More dry
Fruits and leaves	Stems, roots, and seeds
Growing high above the ground	Growing below the ground
Causing an acid reaction in the body	Causing an alkaline reaction

Colbin explains, "What interests us most in Oshawa's macrobiotic philosophy is his classification of foods into relative stages of yin-ness (expansiveness) and yang-ness (contractiveness). Alcohol, sugar and fruits were on the furthest extreme of yin, while meat and salt were on the furthest extreme of yang. Grains, most notably brown rice, were placed in the middle, as the most balanced food. Healthful eating meant always, continuously, striving for a balance between opposites of the yin and the yang, the expansive and contractive." (Colbin 1986)

Grains are the most important element in the macrobiotic regime, making up about 50 percent of total food intake. The grains include brown rice, whole wheat, millet, oats, barley, buckwheat, maize, and rye. Vegetables comprise about 25 percent. Dairy foods are avoided, but soy products and animal products like fish are used occasionally. Sea vegetables like seaweed are high in nutrients and are used as an important supplement to the primarily grain and vegetable diet. Macrobiotics is not a strictly vegetarian diet; it seeks to balance. Fish may be eaten, although poultry is avoided. Refined flour and sugar, and any processed foods, are avoided. Fruits are eaten occasionally as desserts, but are not a primary staple in the diet. Some vegetables are avoided entirely: eggplant, potatoes, tomatoes. Coffee is also avoided.

Macrobiotics was popularized in the West by Michio Kushi, whose Kushi Institute trains cooks and those who want to eat in this way. Anecdotal claims for cures from hemorrhoids to cancer have been made; if true, it is not clear from a scientific standpoint how the diet works. It is an austere diet, which requires an initial investment of much time and energy in preparation and adjustment of the body.

Viewing the acid/alkaline balance of the body is another metabolic approach. William Howard Hay popularized a diet in the 1930s that suggested a ratio of 20 percent acid-forming to 80 percent alkalinizing foods. Dr. Pavlo Airola, another nutritional pioneer and naturopath, subscribed to this theory as well. The idea is that our diets are so full of acid-forming foods that it is disrupting our digestive function. The acid-saturated digestive tract is conducive to constipation, which some feel may contribute to chronic degenerative illness.

Acid-forming foods include alcohol, sugar, honey, fats, oils, white flour, beans, whole grains, cereals, fish, meat, poultry, and eggs. According to Colbin, alkalinizing foods are coffee, fruits, land vegetables, potatoes, sea vegetables, tamari, miso, salt, green beans, and coffee. Buffer foods are ice cream, yogurt, butter, tofu, milk, and cheese.

The combining of foods is an important aspect of the Hay diet. Green vegetables and protein or starch is recommended, but protein and starch (meat and potatoes) is not. Proteins may be eaten with fruit, and starches with fats, but not starches and acid fruits. It is believed that one of the pair of these incompatible foods interferes with the digestion of the other.

Food combining is an essential ingredient of the Natural Hygiene diet, which seeks to prevent disease by lowering toxicity in the system. In addition to food combining, several other recommendations are made regarding the overtaxation of the digestive system. It is recommended that one not eat when tired, and only when hungry, because digestive power is less at these times, and putrefaction of food possible. Fasting is recommended during illness. Natural Hygiene methods were popularized in the *Fit for Life* diet.

Ayurveda is an ancient Indian system of health based on interrelating metabolic principles called doshas. There are three doshas, and everyone is a mixture, but is predominant in one. The Ayurvedic diet is prescribed based on the identification of one's dosha and sub-dosha, and balance achieved by eating the foods that "feed" the deficient dosha.

DIET AND NUTRITION TODAY

The return to healthier eating and natural foods by the affluent West is only one part of the diet and nutrition story. In many less developed nations people struggle with severe poverty and malnutrition. Nutritional deficiencies in some cases can be attributed to poverty alone. In some, soil depletion has been caused by the economic domination of cultures that disrupted the natural food production system by appropriating land for the development of cash crops. Even if these countries are no longer dominated by others, the economy continues to function in a similar way, so that much of the available land is used to produce a limited number of crops. This reduces the variety of foods for the native population and leaves farmers with only small plots to produce a variety of their own products.

Natural and whole foods are still eaten in many parts of the world and healing with herbs and foods continues. But the infatuation with things Western contributes to the problem of malnutrition. For example, African mothers used infant formula in places where the impurity of the water (which was mixed with the formula) caused dehydration and disease in infants who would have been much better off drinking breast milk. An international boycott against the producer of the formula, for their aggressive marketing, finally put an end to the practice. It is ironic that the affluent West is obsessed with loosing weight, when the developing world cannot get enough.

Fasting, the act of denying the body food, is often prescribed in natural food regimes as a way to rest the digestive system while the body's natural healing mechanism does its work in fighting infection or disease. While not recommended without medical supervision, the old adage "starve a fever" is one expression of the commonality of this technique. Some advocate fasting as a spiritual exercise. Often there is a gradual reduction in food, and herbal teas taken, and a gradual introduction of food when the "fast" is over.

The unhealthy side of fasting comes in the form of the food disorder anorexia nervosa, a disease that occurs mostly in teenage girls from comfortable backgrounds in the industrialized world. Anorexics starve themselves. The disorder is treated as a psychological illness and is associated with perfectionism, low self-esteem, and a preoccupation with cultural norms of thinness. Bulimia is another disorder, which involves vomiting food after it is eaten so that there will be no weight gained, often after a "binge," or great intake of food. These disorders are serious—many anorexics eventually starve themselves to death. They often have such a distorted body image that when they see themselves in the mirror, even when they are seriously underweight from not eating, they see a "fat" person.

More Americans than ever were overweight in 1996, despite a weight-loss-obsessed culture, in which dieting is a social norm. Sedentary couch-potato lifestyles add to the problem. There are high-protein diets, high-fiber diets, fruit and vegetable juice diets, restricted diets, the mono diet (only one food is eaten), and the Bircher/Benner diet, among many others. Many psychologists believe that food is used as a substance that gives comfort and energy to those who are lonely, depressed, and anxious. Feminist scholars have examined the role of food for women who are not able to express their selves in the context of traditional relationships. Overeaters Anonymous is a spiritual program based on the model for Alcoholics Anonymous, which helps people examine and correct the reasons for compulsive eating or "food addiction."

See also ALCOHOL AND DRUGS; AYURVEDIC MEDICINE; CHINESE MEDICINE; HERBAL MEDICINE; HOLISTIC HEALTH AND HEALING; HUMORAL MEDICINE.

Balch, James F., and Phyllis A. Balch. (1990) *Prescription for Nutritional Healing.*

Bogin, Barry. (1991) "The Evolution of Human Nutrition." In *The Anthropology of Medicine*, edited by Lola Romanucci-Ross et al., 158–195.

Chernin, Kim. (1985) *The Hungry Self: Women, Eating and Identity.*

Colbin, Annemarie. (1986) *Food and Healing.*

Currier, Richard L. (1966) "The Hot-Cold Syndrome and Symbolic Balance in Mexican and Spanish-American Folk Medicine." *Ethnology* 5: 251–263.

Davis, Adelle. (1954) *Let's Eat Right to Keep Fit.*

Eaton, S. B., and M. Konner. (1985) "Paleolithic Nutrition." *New England Journal of Medicine* 312: 283–189.

Hill, Ann, ed. (1979) *A Visual Encyclopedia of Unconventional Medicine: A Health Manual for the Whole Person.*

Human Relations Area Files. (1964) *Food Habits Survey.*

Lappe, Francis Moore. (1970) *Diet for a Small Planet.*

McElroy, Ann, and Patricia K. Townsend. (1989) *Medical Anthropology in Ecological Perspective.*

Stanfield, Peggy. (1986) *Nutrition and Diet Therapy.*

DISABILITIES When discussed across cultures, it is impossible to define disability and categorize people as disabled because the notion of "being disabled" is a cultural construct. That is, while being sightless or hearing impaired or lacking a limb or movement of some body parts is an observable biological reality in any society, which of these are defined as disabilities and how disabled people are perceived and treated is a cultural construct and therefore varies widely from culture to culture. In the United States, for example, disabled people note that their physical impairment is often less a difficulty for them than the social impairment that results from their being defined as less than human. There has been very little research on disability across cultures and therefore the examples below point to the considerable variation rather than to any known cultural patterns.

Across cultures there is considerable variation in how disabilities and the disabled are perceived. In some cultures, disabilities are classed with illnesses and death and seen as natural, and disabled people are treated accordingly, as in rural Korea:

> Why not laugh at illnesses, death, and deformity, I once heard a Corean argue.
> It does not make people any better if you sympathize with them; on the contrary, by so doing you simply add pain to their pain, and make them feel worse than they really are. Besides, illnesses help to make up our life, and it is our duty to go through them as merrily as through those other things which you call pleasures. We people of Cho-sen do not look upon illnesses, accidents, or death as misfortunes, but as natural things that cannot be helped and must be bravely endured; what better, then, can we do than laugh at them? (Savage-Landor 1895: 95)

In other cultures, disabilities are seen as supernatural punishment, as with this account from rural Taiwan:

The daughter of Landlord Lau had a mentally retarded son. In a seance where a "hell trial" was held, it was determined that the woman in a previous existence had been a fox fairy who was the assistant of a Taoist magician. The magician was kind to the fox, but the two of them had done many evil deeds to other people, and because of this they had been sentenced to be reborn in a later existence as mother and son. mThe magician was made to be born retarded, so that people would be able to trick him and take advantage of him, just as he had done to other people when he was a wily magician. The mother had the duty of caring for the magician in the form of the retarded son, just as the magician had cared for her. (Seaman 1983: 101)

This same belief is found in Central Thailand where Buddhist priests attribute physical disability to bad karma from a previous life. For the Toradja of Indonesia, blindness may be caused as a punishment for theft:

> It is said that there are people who can make someone blind as punishment for theft. For this they go to work in the following way. They place before them a bowl of water and spit into it their saliva, which has been stimulated by chewing pieces of a certain kind of wood. Then they cover the bowl with the piece of *foeja* [beaten tree bark] and place a sirih quid next to it. Now, with a Cordyline leaf, they beckon the soul of the thief to come closer. After having stared into the bowl for some time, they think they see an eye; they stab it with the finger, and then the thief is supposed to become blind. Sometimes the water in the bowl is made to undulate, so that little eyes of foam form on the piece of foeja. These eyes are pierced with a needle. If one of them is pierced, then the thief becomes blind in only one eye. The To Pakambia people are said to have developed this art so far that they can even blind iguanas that steal their eggs and chickens. (Adriani and Kruyt 1951: 292)

In some cultures, disabled people are socially defined as having special powers or abilities and thus occupy unique social roles. In rural Korea, for example, some blind men for over 1,000 years have been *pongsa*, a distinct group of diviners who tell fortunes, select sites for buildings and graves, pray for rain, and place curses. Their special ability is based on the belief "that the blind have another kind of sight, 'eye sight of mind.'" (Knez 1960: 150)

Similarly, the Tiv of Nigeria do not see losing one's sight as an impediment to developing supernatural powers. In fact, the blind are expected to develop this ability and may develop more such power than a man with sight. Enhanced supernatural influence is also attributed to some disabled people by the Amhara of Ethiopia who view religious healers called *debtera* as especially successful because they are often disabled or dwarfs. These healers often live together in church-affiliated communities. Among the Kanuri of Nigeria, the blind are afforded a specific role within the occupational caste structure. Just as some craftsmen such as potters, matmakers and well-diggers live in their own neighborhoods, the blind live in their own neighborhoods where they make rope and are managed by a blind official who reports to the senior blind official in the capital.

The formation of distinct communities by the disabled, while not a widespread phenomenon, does occur in a number of societies in addition to the Kanuri and Amhara mentioned here. In the United States, for example, there is a distinct community of the deaf on Martha's Vineyard in Massachusetts and in Israel the blind form a distinct cultural group who live in some ways outside of Israeli society. In these communities the disabled use their own language and ways of life.

In other cultures, however, having a disability disqualifies one from certain social roles. For example, the Ashanti of West Africa did not permit someone who had lost a finger, toe, or extremity or who was born with an extra toe or finger to become a chief. Similarly, a Wolof chief in Senegal will be removed from his throne if he loses his sight, a fact supporters often attempt to conceal from political rivals: "The blindness of the damel De Thialao being publicly disclosed, brought about his downfall at the age of 30 or 35 at the most, to the great displeasure of all the ayors." (Rousseau 1933: 97) However, while one category of the disabled may be discriminated against, others may be favored with special roles in the same society. For example, while the Ashanti disqualified some disabled from being chiefs, most hunchbacks served as heralds who served the chiefs, although not all heralds were hunchbacks. The herald was a central figure in the Ashanti royal family and wore a cap decorated in red or gold. He served the chief as a representative to other chiefdoms, as a tax collector, sanitation inspector, doorkeeper, and court jester. Thus, the herald was an honored individual in Ashanti society and the divine origin of the herald was noted in drum language (Rattray 1927: 279):

> The creator made something,
> What did he make?
> He made the Herald.
> He made the Drummer
> He made . . . the Chief Executioner.
> Come hither, O Herald, and receive
> Your black monkey-skin cap.

As regards the treatment afforded the disabled, in many cultures it seems that the situation is much the same as that with the elderly. So long as one is able to care for oneself and is not a burden to others, a disabled person, like an elderly one, will be supported. However, if one is perceived as being a burden, they may be abandoned, as indicated by this story regarding the Mbuti of Central Africa:

> There once was a Pygmy named Butuwa. He was in the forest, and was sleeping with his wife, children, and old mother. His

mother had no legs. In the middle of the night Butuwa said to his wife: "Mother is sleeping soundly; get the children together and let's go away." So they quietly picked up their belongings, and, together with their children, they crept away. They walked and walked and walked.

Early in the morning the old woman woke up. She said: "Where is everybody? Oh! They are a bad family, they have gone off and left their legless old mother to die. I will follow them." So saying, she stood on her head and walked and walked and walked until she caught up with them, walking on her head. She was very angry with them for having deserted her, and told them how bad they were to have left her alone in the forest. That night they all went to sleep together.

In the middle of the night the Pygmy said to his wife: "Now mother is really asleep: get the children together and let's go away." So they collected the children, picked up their belongings, and stole away. They walked and walked and walked.

Early in the morning the old woman woke up, and she was very, very angry to find that her family had deserted her again. So she stood on her head and she walked and walked and walked, until she caught up with them, walking on her head. She told her son how mad she was. She was very cross indeed. Her son went off into the forest and gathered some honey, and then he got a very bad worm and put it into the honey. He returned to the camp and said: "Don't be angry with me, mother. Look, I have brought you some fine honey." And the old legless mother ate up the honey, worm and all. And the worm ate up the legless old mother's stomach, and the legless old mother died.

Butuwa left and went to another camp where they had relations. When they got to the camp, their relations asked: "What news; where is your mother?" "Oh! She died," said Butuwa. "That's too bad," said the others. (Turnbull 1965: 265)

Adriani, N., and Albert C. Kruyt. (1951) *The Bare'e-Speaking Toradja of Central Celebes (the East Toradja)*. Translated from the Dutch by Jenni K. Moulton.

Bohannan, Paul, and Laura Bohannan. (1969) *A Source Notebook on Tiv Religion in 5 Volumes.*

Cohen, Ronald. (1966) *The Kanuri of Bornu.*

Deshen, Shlomo. (1992) *Blind People: The Private and Public Life of Sightless Israelis.*

Groce, Nora. (1990) *Everyone Here Spoke Sign Language: Hereditary Deafness on Martha's Vineyard.*

Ingersoll, Jasper C. (1969) *The Priest and the Path: An Analysis of the Priest Role in a Central Thai Village.*

Knez, Eugene I. (1960) *Sam Jong Dong: A South Korean Village.*

Murphy, Robert. (1987) *The Body Silent.*

Rattray, Robert S. (1916) *Ashanti Proverbs.*

———. (1927) *Religion and Art in Ashanti.*

Rousseau, R. (1933) *Senegal in Former Times: Study on Cayor, Notebooks of Yoro Dyao.* Translated from the French by Ariane Brunel.

Savage-Landor, A. Henry. (1895) *Corea or Chosen: The Land of the Morning Calm.*

Seaman, Gary W. (1983) *Temple Organization in a Chinese Village.*

Turnbull, Colin. (1965) *The Mbuti Pygmies: An Ethnographic Survey.*

Young, Allan L. (1971) *Medical Beliefs and Practices of the Begemder Amhara.*

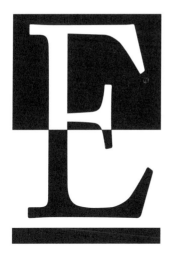

crease, or redirect the flow of chi. The system of acupuncture points, believed to exist on twelve invisible, magnetized lines of energy running the length of the body, is part of the Chinese system. After a pulse diagnosis, and questions regarding the patient's complaint, specific points are chosen into which needles are inserted to regulate the flow of chi. These points "reflex" to the organs and other parts of the body that need attention. Acupuncture has proven effective as an anesthetic and is commonly used in China during surgery. It has been found effective in treating migraine headaches, gynecological problems, and other problems.

This system of activating energy points is the basis of Chinese acupressure massage as well, and it appears in many other cultures. Pressure-point massage in Japan is called Jin Shin and shiatsu, in Hawaii it is incorporated into traditional Lomilomi massage, in Thailand as Nuad-bo Rarn, in the Indian medical tradition of Ayurveda as marma, and in traditional Kurdish massage as sen. In all of these approaches, massage of the points is used to awaken and stimulate an invisible energy pathway that will result in greater health and well-being.

In the West, since the time of the Greeks, a number of scientists have tried to isolate and identify a life force under strict scientific conditions, but they have failed to reach a level of accuracy that was satisfactory to the majority of scientists. Today's proponents of bioenergetic energy fields call it "subtle" energy. Dr. Randolph Stone, an American naturopath, studied ancient healing systems of China and India and believed that the body had negative and positive poles with a magnetic field surrounding them. He developed a form of bodywork called polarity energy balancing to repolarize the body after it is depleted through injury, trauma, and stress. His technique, while not officially sanctioned by the medical community, has been practiced since he published his book *Energy—The Vital Principle in the Healing Art* in 1948. In it, the electromag-

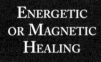

ENERGETIC OR MAGNETIC HEALING

The idea that the human body operates within an electromagnetic field has been suggested for centuries. In ancient Indian and Chinese cultures, prana and chi, respectively, were the names given to the divine energy that supports and holds life. This energy was not simply an abstract idea—it was an observable and manipulable substance that regulated one's health and well-being. In ancient Greece it was called the vital energy, in Europe, among naturopaths especially, it was called the vital force. The American psychologist William Reich called it orgone, and the Russian Victor Inyushin called it bioplasma. However it is referred to and whether it actually exists or not, healers have been manipulating it, with various results, for centuries.

The basis of Chinese medicine is the balancing of the opposing energies of the chi, called yin and yang. It is in the maintenance of this ebb and flow that one maintains good health, according to the Chinese. When out of balance, a number of techniques are used to increase, de-

netic energy of a practitioner is conveyed through the hands to the client to repolarize the body. It also consists of manual stretching of the body, dietary recommendations, and exercise-polarity yoga.

Other techniques that have emerged that manipulate bioenergy are therapeutic touch, a form of laying on of hands and manipulation of the energy field to speed healing. Developed by Dolores Krieger, a nursing professor, this technique is now an accepted part of nursing education in the United States. It does not use the energy point system, but works with energy outside the body, called the aura or human energy field. Practitioners center themselves and ask to become a channel for divine energy. They scan the energy field looking for blocks, disturbances, or heat. They work with the blocked areas, smoothing and balancing the energy field. Though critics attribute its effectiveness in producing more rapid healing and demonstrable physiological changes to the placebo effect, some studies have shown its effectiveness when clients were not aware of what was happening to them. Dr. Robert O. Becker, a pioneer in the study of bioelectricity, explains what process may be at work:

> Since we know that the body uses electrical control systems to regulate many basic functions and that the flow of these electrical currents produces externally measurable magnetic fields, it does not require a great leap of faith to postulate that a healer's gift is an ability to use his or her own electrical control systems to produce external electromagnetic energy fields that interact with those of the patient. The interaction could be one that "restores" balance in the internal forces or that reinforces the electrical systems so that the body returns toward a normal condition. (1990: 108)

Barbara Ann Brennan, a former astrophysicist, developed a system of working with the human energy system. Her publication, *Hands of Light,* describes the relationship of life energies to health, life, and healing. She began a school for healers and describes seven levels of the human energy field that exist in layers starting with the physical body, and the sensations of pleasure and pain that are felt. She also draws on the Indian concept of the seven energy centers in the body, called chakras in Sanskrit. In her system, she combines the spiritual, emotional, and physical arenas. What is understood as a measurable phenomenon—the human energy field to scientists—Brennan describes in much more esoteric detail as the repository of past-life experiences, emotional trauma, and grief, among other things.

Brennan refers to the aura as the broader concept of the human energy field and bases much of her teaching on the clairvoyant higher sense perception of established healers to describe the aura in all of its complexity and interrelationship to the emotional and spiritual realms. Though the human aura has been described by many spiritual adepts and is believed to be the halo that we see around saints in religious art, science stops here. After the layer of the physical body, the second level is associated with the emotional life and the third with the mental or rational side of life. The fourth level contains our human relationships and the fifth divine will. The sixth is the spiritual body and the seventh divine mind. Brennan's school accepts the perceptions and intuition of healers, spiritual leaders, and philosophers and integrates these "knowings" into her work. Her work includes use of channeled information from noncorporeal beings.

The intersection of a measurable energy field with the perceptions of the highly sensitive psychics and healers who have experienced this energetic phenomenon around the body forms the basis of energetic healing. Energetic healing is also being conducted on a telepathic level in Reiki and faith healing with the concept of distant healing. The telepathic communication of healing from one person to another or, as in prayer, that moves from the petitioner to God to the recipient is also being explored. There is some scientific basis to the efficacy of prayer in speedier recoveries from surgery. Dr. Larry Dossey, co-chair of the Panel on Mind/Body Interventions at the Office of Alternative Medicine at the National Institutes of Health, believes that prayer has the power to heal.

The Gentle Winds Spiritual Community in Maine has developed a series of tools, which they say were channeled from some benevolent force in the universe, that will heal the trauma that exists in the energetic bodies of human beings. All that is required is to hold these tools and the system will more naturally draw to it the life experiences it needs to live a more balanced, healthy life. These claims are backed up by anecdotal evidence only, and the community freely admits they do not understand the workings of the tools. Thus, the notion of energy fields within the body, though used across cultures in some healing approaches, remains controversial.

See also MAGNET THERAPY.

Becker, Robert O. (1990) *Cross Currents: The Perils of Electropollution, the Promise of Electromedicine.*

Brennan, Barbara A. (1993) *Light Emerging: The Journey of Personal Healing.*

Brennan, Barbara Ann. (1988) *Hands of Light: A Guide to Healing through the Human Energy Field.*

Carreiro, Mary. (1987) *The Psychology of Spiritual Growth, A Gentle Winds Book.*

Dossey, Larry. (1993) *Healing Words: The Power of Prayer and the Practice of Medicine.*

Krieger, Dolores. (1995) *Therapeutic Touch.*

Siegel, Alan, and Phil Young. n.d. *Polarity Therapy: The Power That Heals.*

ENVIRONMENTAL DISASTERS

Environmental disasters are events that change the environment so seriously that the lives of a large number of people are disrupted. Individual victims of a disaster commonly experience it as an event beyond belief and are left feeling out of control over their own lives. It is the number of people affected and the large amount of damage done that distinguish a disaster from an accident or an emergency.

Environmental disasters can be classified as being caused by either nature or humans and as being either quick onset or chronic. Natural disasters are precipitated by environmental events that are not the result of human actions. However, human acts of omission or commission before, during, or following the environmental events themselves turn the damage caused by these events into disasters and result in large numbers of people suffering serious disruptions to their lives.

Quick onset natural disasters are often referred to as "acts of God," a conceptualization that tends to free human beings from responsibility for the damage the disaster causes. A belief in the supernatural basis of natural disasters is common across cultures. Muslims believe that disasters befall those who act immorally. The Santal of India attempt to end a drought by appealing to the deities and by making offerings to them when the rains come; they respond to epidemics of disease in the same way. The Central Thai, who suffered from cholera, smallpox, and other epidemics until the arrival of Western medical treatment in the twentieth century, blamed these outbreaks on the "Epidemic Ghost," who was believed to come from a different ethnic group such as the Lao. The Ghost is still believed to cause animals such as water buffalo to fall ill, and farmers will seek a cure by sacrificing a chicken to the Ghost. In the Western world, up to the Lisbon Earthquake of 1755, natural disasters were attributed to supernatural causes. Only after 1755 did scientific explanations replace supernatural ones.

The major quick onset natural disasters are earthquakes, tsunamis, volcanoes, floods, hurricanes, fires, insect infestations, and disease epidemics. Less widespread disasters include ice and hail storms, frost, avalanches, and floods caused by the collapse of glacial dams. Not all societies or even all regions within a societal territory are threatened by all natural disasters. For example, the western United States is more prone to damage resulting from earthquakes and fires, the Midwest to floods, and the southeast to hurricanes. However, some societies are subject to the effects of many damage-producing natural events. For example, between 1900 and 1990 the Solomon Islands in the South Pacific experienced sixty-one earthquakes, forty-two volcanic eruptions, thirty-seven hurricanes, seventeen tsunamis, eleven floods, eight storms, three droughts, and three landslides. The hurricanes and droughts caused the most hardship, resulting in 134 and 106 deaths respectively. The other six types of events caused only 20 combined deaths.

As was the case in the Solomon Islands, hurricanes cause the most deaths of all types of natural disasters. They generally strike heavily populated floodplains, where farmers prefer to live because the soil is rich and the land is often free or inexpensive.

The amount of damage caused by earthquakes is influenced by the soil and rock conditions under buildings and the materials used in building construction. In industrialized nations, buildings in earthquake-prone regions are built with foundations, reinforced supports, and flexible structures that can withstand earthquakes. Therefore, earthquakes cause relatively limited damage and result in few deaths in these nations. Elsewhere in the world, however, dwellings are often built of mud and sticks and straw or of stone with no foundations and are, therefore,

quickly destroyed by earthquakes. If the dwellings are in use when the earthquake strikes, such as during the night, loss of life can be extensive.

Tsunamis are giant ocean waves—caused by earthquakes or underwater volcanoes—that cause extensive damage when they hit shore communities. Like hurricanes they can also cause considerable erosion of sand and soil.

Most volcanoes are found in the zone called the "ring of fire," which includes Japan and East Asia, the west coast of North and South America from Alaska to Chile, and islands in the Pacific Ocean. The most damaging volcanoes occur in tropical regions with fertile soil that attracts large populations. The volcanic eruption of Mount Lamington in northern New Guinea in 1951, for example, killed about 4,000 Orokaiva and caused another 5,000 to be evacuated. Volcanoes can also cause avalanches.

Floods are caused by excessive water and are made worse by various human-induced conditions such as deforestation. Floods cause considerable damage, and often many deaths, because many people live in river deltas or along rivers, where rich soil is found for farming. A special kind of flood is the lake rupture (called *jokulhlaup* in Iceland and *tshoserup* in Nepal) caused by a glacial dam giving way and allowing the water behind it to rush through the valley below. Such lake ruptures not only cause extensive damage but may also alter the environment by eroding river banks or even rerouting rivers.

While insect predation and disease are not usually considered natural disasters since they arise in human beings' biological rather than physical environment, they too can cause considerable damage to crops and human life. For example, a mealybug infestation in northern Zambia from 1985 to 1989 caused shortages of cassava, which led to famine and ultimately to a shift to the growing of corn instead.

Human-induced disasters involve human actions (or failures to act) that cause damage to the environment, in turn damaging humans and their communities. Quick onset human-induced disasters include those caused by oil spills such as the *Exxon Valdez* spill off the south coast of Alaska, technological accidents such as the gas leak at the Union Carbide plant in Bhopal, India, or the leak of buried chemical waste at Love Canal in upstate New York, and nuclear accidents like that at Chernobyl in the former Soviet Union.

Chronic human-induced disasters now are the greatest threat to cultures around the world. Rather than just threatening one region, these processes have the potential to effect the entire world. At this point, the effects are not fully known and experts disagree about how damaging they may prove to be. For example, environmentalists claim that global warming will produce food shortages early in the twenty-first century, although many economists say that agriculture can be adjusted and there will be no food shortages. Major, chronic human-induced disasters include greenhouse-induced climate change, ozone depletion, desertification, deforestation, depletion of fisheries, depletion and pollution of fresh water, salinization of irrigated land, and soil erosion.

The greenhouse effect is caused by carbon dioxide pollution, which limits the reflection of solar heat back toward the sun. It might eventually raise the temperature by about two to three degrees Celsius and lead to other unpredictable climate changes that will effect agriculture.

Stratospheric ozone depletion is a thinning of the ozone layer, which helps protect the earth from ultraviolet radiation from the sun. A major health consequence is skin cancer.

Desertification is the transformation of agricultural or grazing land to desert, thus rendering it no longer usable for food collection or production. Desertification occurs most often in arid or semi-arid regions and is caused by the overgrazing of herd animals and by nonsustainable agri-

cultural practices. Among its results are droughts, famine, migration, poverty, and ethnic conflict.

Deforestation is the harvesting of large tracts of trees in such a manner that the soil is left bare. It results from the cutting of wood for lumber, the clearing of forests for other uses such as farming or herding, pollution, mining, fire, and drought. The effect on peoples living in forests being deforested, which is occurring mainly in tropical regions, is disruption of their traditional ways of life, involvement as low-paid laborers in a wage-base economy, migration, illness, and death. The effects on the environment include floods, erosion, and a loss of many species of animals, birds, and other living things in the forest.

Overfishing is the taking of more fish than can be replaced naturally. The depletion of fish resources results from the "tragedy of the commons"—the overuse and misuse of the oceans because they are open for use by all and therefore can be overfished by those who derive limited benefits from maintaining the resource and thus are not inclined to do so. Depletion results mainly from modern, industrialized fishing methods rather than traditional techniques.

The depletion of water resources is due to water pollution by industry that makes fresh water unsafe for human use. Water-based disasters are also caused by the construction of large dams such as the Aswan Dam in Egypt or the Akosombo Dam in Volta, which required the relocation of much of the local population and subsequent changes in their economic, political, and social systems.

Salinization results from irrigation without adequate drainage in which salts drawn up through the wet soil leave deposits on the surface, rendering the land useless for agriculture.

Erosion, which can result from both natural and human-induced disasters, is the wearing away of soil. It can leave the land unsuitable for human exploitation.

HUMAN FACTOR IN DISASTERS

The human role in disasters becomes clear when one considers the effects of disasters in three different societal situations—traditional societies, economically developing nations, and economically developed nations.

The greatest damage caused by disasters in traditional societies is the loss of their food supply. While this loss may be only temporary, in many situations in the past it would take months or even years before the indigenous subsistence system could be rebuilt. Until that time, the people would either have to move elsewhere or suffer from famine. For example, heavy frost periodically destroys the sweet potato crop of the Fringe Enga in New Guinea, who before the availability of government aid would then migrate to lower elevations and live with the Central Enga for up to six years until they could reestablish productive sweet potato gardens. In northern Zambia, when a mealybug infestation from 1985 to 1989 destroyed the cassava crop, the people lived in famine and eventually adjusted by switching to the growing of corn. In the Mortlock Islands in Oceania, the greatest damage caused by hurricanes is the inundation of inland freshwater taro swamps with sea water. The salt in the sea water causes the crops to die, destroys boundaries between plots, and results in the loss of years of work put into creating the rich swampland plots. In good years with plenty of rain, it takes from six to twelve months for the salt water to be replaced by fresh water before reconstruction can begin. In general, before aid from outside sources such as the national government, United Nations, or nonprofit organizations was available, people in traditional cultures dealt with disasters by eating less, diversifying their subsistence practices and diet, sharing, reducing community size, raiding other societies for food or land, moving elsewhere, or living with kin.

In the twentieth century, disaster relief is more and more provided by nonindigenous organizations, and recovery efforts are directed and supported by government agencies. The underlying philosophy of many of these efforts and programs is that the indigenous subsistence economy is not capable of sustaining the society after disasters and that it must be modernized. Thus, natural disasters in traditional societies now speed along the modernization process and leave communities dependent on outside sources of assistance, capital, and political support. Among major changes are the drawing of the culture into a market economy; the replacement of kinship ties with ties based on employer-employee or seller-buyer relations; women leaving the home to work outside the home; men migrating to cities or towns for wage labor; changes in agricultural practices such as multi-cropping, food storage, and the planting of disaster resistant crops; and changes in local leadership in which younger men with experience outside the community replace the traditional elders. Some experts see these changes as damaging to the traditional ways of life of these cultures while others argue that in the modern world system no traditional culture can be self-sufficient.

Disasters such as earthquakes in Peru and Central America, hurricanes in Bangladesh, and drought in the Sahel of Africa often cause large-scale damage in developing (Third World) nations. There is often enormous loss of life beyond what is found in traditional societies (because they have small populations to begin with) and developed nations (because they have effective warning and evacuation systems and safer buildings) and massive destruction of dwellings. These two results of disasters are linked because in many developing nations large populations aggregate in specific locations where land is free or cheap and the soil suitable for farming. Also, in many developing nations dense settlements, called squatter settlements, are built by poor migrants from rural sectors on the outskirts of cities, often on unstable hillsides. Thus, the combination of a large, dense population living in poorly constructed housing in areas prone to natural disaster events such as hurricanes or earthquakes makes wholesale damage inevitable. For example, on 29 April 1991, a hurricane (called a cyclone in South Asia) struck the delta region of southern Bangladesh killing 67,000 people, mostly poor farmers and their children. There are a number of reasons that so many people died, all having to do with human behavior rather than the storm itself. First, 97 percent of the houses built of straw and mud could not withstand the high winds. Second, the high population density of nearly 9,000 persons per square hectare placed many people at risk. Third, the storm shelters provided by the government were too few and inadequate. Fourth, the people did not fully understand the warning signal system. In the system, eight, nine, or ten signals all meant the same thing—great danger. But many people believed that fewer signals meant less danger so that when the first warning was with ten signals and the second with nine, many thought the danger had decreased. Fifth, the people did not take the warnings seriously because of false alarms in the past. Sixth, some people refused to leave their homes because of fear of looting in their absence. Seventh, people did not believe a severe storm would hit in April. And eighth, some groups, such as women and children in their homes, were placed at especially high risk and suffered the greatest loss of life.

Disaster relief efforts in developing nations tend to be highly politicized. Often the government attempts to downplay the extent of the disaster so as to not scare off tourists or investors. Also, governments may not ask for help from international organizations so as to conceal government incompetence or corruption. Post-disaster recovery efforts are also highly politicized, as those in power direct a disproportionate amount of aid to their constituents, developers and investors seek access to lucrative replacement projects, poor farmers are displaced from their land, and out-of-power political parties use the handling or mishandling of the situation by the party in power as an issue to attract the support of voters.

In both traditional and developing nations, disaster relief efforts may make the disaster worse by stressing short-term solutions that create long-term vulnerability to disasters. For example, government intervention and support programs weaken indigenous support programs such as kin ties and trade patterns and also make the local communities dependent on the bureaucratic services provided by the government. As indicated above, the provision of these services is often influenced by political considerations. For example, a hurricane struck the Mortlock Islands in 1976 and caused varying amounts of damage to different communities, ranging from nearly complete destruction to little damage. However, the communities with the least damage got the most relief for two reasons. First, communities with power in the central government were sent more aid. Second, local officials who distributed relief supplies sent more to the districts where they had relatives. Thus, in these societies and nations, the local culture and political process can strongly influence aid efforts.

Developed nations are affected least by natural disasters. Property damage is the major result, with relatively few deaths and no food shortages. Recovery is managed by the government (local, state, and national), private organizations, and insurance companies. The major problem in providing assistance is coordinating the actions of the numerous agencies and companies involved in the effort. Developed nations, unlike traditional cultures and developing nations, experience no long-term societal changes.

See also FAMINE.

Abbink, Jon. (1993) "Famine, Gold and Guns: The Suri of Southwestern Ethiopia, 1985–1991." *Disasters* 17: 218–225.

Aptekar, Lewis. (1994) *Environmental Disasters in Global Perspective.*

Belshaw, Cyril S. (1951) "Social Consequences of the Mount Lamington Eruption." *Oceania* 21: 241–252.

Blong, R. J., and D. A. Radford. (1993) "Deaths in Natural Hazards in the Solomon Islands." *Disasters* 17: 1–11.

Brower, Barbara A. (1987) *Livestock and Landscape: The Sherpa Pastoral System in Sagarmatha (Mt. Everest) National Park, Nepal.*

Button, John. (1988) *A Dictionary of Green Ideas.*

Hansen, Art. (1994) "The Illusion of Local Sustainability and Self-Sufficiency: Famine in a Border Area of Northwestern Zambia." *Human Organization* 53: 11–20.

Homer-Dixon, Thomas F. (1994) "Environmental Scarcities and Violent Conflict: Evidence from Cases." *International Security* 19: 5–40.

Marshall, Mac. (1979) "Natural and Unnatural Disaster in the Mortlock Islands of Micronesia." *Human Organization* 38: 265–272.

Mukherjea, Charulal. (1962) *The Santals.*

Mushtaque, A., et al. (1993) "The Bangladesh Cyclone of 1991: Why So Many People Died." *Disasters* 17: 291–304.

Stern, Gerald M. (1976) *The Buffalo Creek Disaster: The Story of the Survivors' Unprecedented Lawsuit.*

Textor, Robert B. (1973) *Roster of the Gods: An Ethnography of the Supernatural in a Thai Village.*

Torry, William I. (1978) "Bureaucracy, Community, and Natural Disasters." *Human Organization* 37: 302–308.

———. (1978) "Natural Disasters, Social Structure and Change in Traditional Societies." *Journal of Asian and African Studies* 13: 167–183.

———. (1979) "Anthropology and Disaster Research." *Disasters* 3: 43–52.

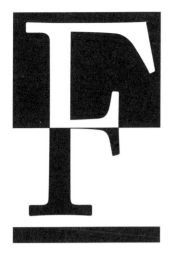

least a two-way street, in that the person requesting the healing must believe in order for the power of the gods to work. Even if the petitioner believes, as most Western people do today, that illness is not caused by God, they must believe that God has the power to heal it.

Faith healing appears early in ancient Greek culture as a cure for any number of illnesses, from barrenness to blindness. Patients were put to sleep through hypnosis or herbal medicine, ministered to by priests in the meantime, and woke up "cured." Whether there was actual surgery done during the ritual while the patient was sleeping is debated, but often the patient spoke of cathartic dreams and visions. The belief is that they were cured through the intercession of the gods, who were believed to have caused the illness in the first place. The power of suggestion is believed by many psychologists to be an important component to faith healing.

The early New Testament of the Christian Bible contains many stories of healings by Jesus Christ and his followers. Faith was an integral part of these healings to the extent that a delay in or the failure of healing was attributed to lack of it:

> The centurion's servant was healed because of the faith of his master; a paralyzed man was healed on account of the faith of his friends; the woman with an issue was made whole by her faith. . . . On the other hand, the lunatic boy's cure was delayed through want of faith. . . . On one occasion Jesus did not and could not put forth His power because of the want of faith of the people. (Hastings 1908–1926: 698)

In Christian healing the devil is often reported to be the agent of illness, and healing is the exorcism of the devil or devils within a person. This is somewhat of a variation on the mischievous gods of the Greeks both creating the illness and offering healing.

Faith healing lost some of its ardor for Christians during the Protestant Reformation,

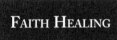

FAITH HEALING The use of the supernatural in healing is a cultural universal. As the use of the supernatural in healing in traditional non-Western cultures is covered in the articles on Healers and Health Care Systems, among others, this entry focuses on supernatural healing—often called faith healing—in a Western context.

In both Eastern and Western religious traditions, there is a belief that illness may result from losing favor with God or the gods. Appeals are made both for assistance in the diagnosis of illness, as to the tang-ki god of Taiwan, where the priest intermediary requests the nature of and medicine for the illness, and for full spiritual and physical healing, as promised by Christian Science. The physical, emotional, mental, and spiritual lives are believed to be connected, and maintaining a good relationship with a higher, more powerful being is considered crucial to one's total well-being.

Faith healing may be described as "the power of the gods joined to the faith of the sufferer." (Hastings 1908–1926: 698) It appears to be at

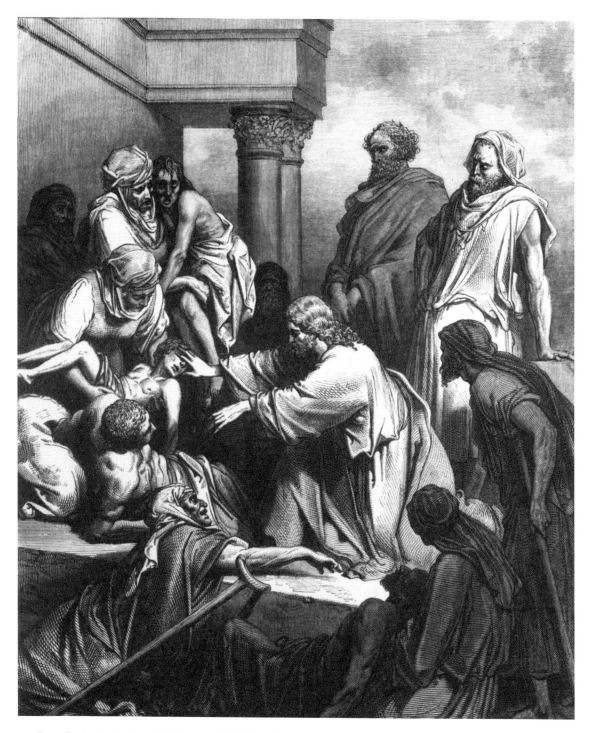

Jesus Christ heals the blind, lame, and sick in a nineteenth-century European engraving by Gustave Doré.
Healing through faith in a god is widely accepted among many cultures and religions.

but resurfaced in the Pentecostal movement of the early twentieth century. Emotionally charged meetings often include "witnessing" the power of God coming through the faithful, speaking in tongues like the early disciples after the death of Jesus Christ, and laying on of hands in prayer to heal as Jesus did. The body of the faithful became the vessel for the words and healing energy of God to pass through. These meetings are not seen in most Protestant churches, but did take hold in many fundamentalist sects. In other, more mainstream denominations, both Protestant and Catholic, people with gifts of healing appear from time to time. Prayer continued unabated, of course, in more conventional services, as a personal conversation with God, with requests for healing included.

In the East, the ancient Chinese concept of health and illness spread to neighboring nations. The basis of it is that the dynamic relationship of opposite forces called yin and yang creates the life force, or chi. The Chinese believe that it is the responsibility of each of us to maintain this balance between opposites to constitute health. Chi is the life force that underlies the universe. Faith healing intersects with this dynamic, balancing approach to healing in that the creative life force energy that the Chinese call chi is what is believed to be "channeled" by faith healers. In fact, an energetic system surrounding the body has been observed and worked with in the act of laying on of hands. In Japan, the technique of Reiki and in the West the technique of therapeutic touch work with this energy. In a process called centering, the healer asks that the body be a channel for divine energy to heal.

The purest form of faith healing in the West is Christian Science. Its founder, Mary Baker Eddy, sought to revive the art of healing as it existed in the time of Jesus. Faith in an all-powerful God capable only of good, with a petitioner's thoughts aligned only to divine purpose, is the prescription for healing. Testimo-nies to Christian Science healings are included in Eddy's book *Science and Health with Key to the Scriptures.* A personal experience of a Christian Scientist follows:

> For several weeks I was bothered by a painful pinched nerve in my shoulder. After inquiring, I was told that massage would soothe it momentarily, that chiropractors wanted X-rays but couldn't assure a cure, and that surgery might help. One evening the pain became so severe that I got out the dictionary and looked up "nerves." The word communication is used. I used a concordance to *Science and Health* and found all the passages that referred to nerves. All the words used communication. Pondering each passage I had the feeling that there was something that I had forgotten, something on the tip of the tongue waiting for recognition. I reached out in thought, waited some moments, and the phrase "The communication is only from God to man" crashed into my mind. I felt like I was meeting a loved child after a long absence. "I knew that," I said out loud. That night the pain ceased and I slept peacefully. The pain has not returned in nine years.

The process of faith healing is mysterious, invisible, and ineffable. But its effects are measurable. Prayer, which has been described as directing the power or energy of God through words and thoughts to the soul of the sufferer, has actually been studied by researchers. Dr. Larry Dossey, co-chair of the Panel on Mind/Body Interventions at the Office of Alternative Medicine at the National Institutes of Health notes:

> Experiments with prayer showed that prayer positively affected high blood pressure, wounds, heart attacks, headaches, and anxiety. . . . Remarkably the effects of prayer did not depend on whether the praying person was in the presence of the organism being prayed for, or whether he or she was far away; healing could take place either on site or at a distance. (1993: 201)

Dossey is thoroughly convinced of the efficacy of faith healing:

> Scientific evidence supporting spiritual healing is considerable. In addition to the 131 controlled experiments on prayer-based, "spiritual" . . . healing reviewed by Benor, which showed statistically significant results, psychologist William G. Braud reviewed 149 experiments . . . [and] found that approximately half of these studies were statistically significant. . . . Why are these findings—almost three hundred studies dating back to the early 1960's—ignored or rejected by most scientists? (202)

Dossey believes that cognitive dissonance—an inability to reconcile these results with their Western materialistic training—combined with the nonscientific nature of religion and mysticism and resistance to change are among the reasons for resistance on the part of doctors to acknowledging the healing power of prayer. Most allopathic doctors acknowledge that there are unexplainable cures for terminal illnesses and categorize them as spontaneous healings. But little has been done to try and understand why these occur.

With the resurgence of interest in Eastern philosophy and beliefs and the embracing of holistic health, spiritual healing is becoming more "mainstream." Among even the more rationally or logically oriented Protestant congregations, healing services are appearing. The following was adopted from the United Methodist Book of Worship and was used in a service at the Congregational Church in Monterey, Massachusetts:

> The root of the word *healing* in New Testament Greek, *sozo*, is the same root as that of the words *salvation* and *wholeness*. . . . We believe the greatest healing of all is the reunion or reconciliation of human beings with God. When this happens, physical healing sometimes happens. Mental and emotional balance is often restored. Spiritual health is enhanced. Relationships can heal. We believe that this reconciliation is available to individuals, families, groups, even nations. We believe that God makes all things new. We believe that healing is not magic, but an expression of the great mystery of God's perfect love. We cooperate in God's healing work through our simple willingness to taste that perfect love. . . .

Faith healings are attributed to items that have been touched by the saints, called relics, to certain sacred places, and to gifted individuals. The most famous healing site in the Western world is Lourdes, France, where the Catholic faithful believe that the mother of Jesus appeared to some peasant children. Thousands of people travel there yearly in search of healing. Some healings have occurred, but many psychologists believe that the healings that occurred there were more a tribute to the tenacity of the sick in getting there than to any divine intervention. Apparently there is a correlation between the length and the hardship of the journey and the efficacy of the cure. Psychological excitation is another factor: "There is probably no stream in Britain which could not boast of as high a proportion of cures as the stream at Lourdes if patients came in the same numbers and in the same psychological state of expectant excitement." (Weil 1983: 172)

Some people believe that healing is latent in every person and that it simply takes the right stimulus to elicit it. This, however, begs the question of how people who did not even know they were being prayed for seemed to benefit from prayer, as in the research mentioned earlier. Whether it is the power of suggestion, the receptivity of a latent healing ability deep in the subconscious, or an actual channel of energy into which a believer can tap, faith healing continues to be turned to as a means of psychological and spiritual, if not always physical, comfort.

According to spiritual teacher and writer Marianne Williamson:

The experience of spirit breaks through illusions of our guilt and separateness. It is radically committed to the natural goodness and inherent one-ness that lie at the center of who we really are. When too far from the blaze (of spirit) we are cold and spiritually lifeless. We are less than human without that heat. Our connection to God is life itself." (1994: 32, 33)

See also CHRISTIAN SCIENCE; HEALERS; THEORIES OF ILLNESS.

Dossey, Larry. (1993) *Healing Words: The Power of Prayer and the Practice of Medicine.*

Eddy, Mary Baker. (1875) *Science and Health with Key to the Scriptures.*

Hastings, James, ed. (1908–1926) *Encyclopedia of Religion and Ethics.*

Montgomery, Ruth. (1973) *Born to Heal.*

United Methodist Book of Worship (1992).

Weil, Andrew. (1983) *Health and Healing: Understanding Conventional and Alternative Medicine.*

Williamson, Marianne. (1994) *Illuminata.*

FAMINE

Famine is "reduction in a normally available food supply such that individuals, families, and eventually whole communities are forced to take up abnormal social and economic activities in order to ensure food." (D'Souza 1988: 7) Famine is the extreme form of starvation. Starvation is the physical condition that results when an individual consumes food that does not provide adequate calories. Endemic starvation is the situation where some members of a community or society suffer undernourishment in times when the food supply is considered to be at normal levels. A survey of food conditions primarily in the nineteenth and early twentieth century in 186 nonindustrialized cultures indicates that in about 13 percent of cultures some people suffered from endemic starvation. Epidemic starvation is episodic and affects a larger percentage of the community population. Short-term starvation epidemics last only a few days to several weeks and were reported as occurring in 7 percent of cultures in the world survey. Seasonal starvation occurs at specific times each year and takes the form of shortages of particular types of food, changes in consumption practices such as eating less or eating foods not otherwise eaten, and worry about not having enough to eat. The survey indicates that seasonal starvation occurred in 34 percent of cultures around the world. Famine is a form of starvation that is indicated by a high death rate and the disruption of customary activities. Famine is reported as having occurred in 68 percent of cultures.

Famine can be described in terms of its severity, persistence, and recurrence. Severity means the extent of disruption to community life. Famine of limited severity takes the form of people having to eat less-preferred foods, preparing foods in different ways such as mixing grain husks with the grain when it is ground, restrictions on sharing food, people moving elsewhere in search of food or aid, and the acceptance of food from relief agencies or other communities. More severe famine takes the form of entire families or even the entire culture moving to a locale with food or employment opportunities, riots, stealing, and epidemics of starvation-related diseases. At least on some occasions famine has been limited or severe in 48 percent of cultures. Persistent famine is famine that occurs more than once in the recent past in a society and occurred in 26 percent of cultures. Finally, famine that recurs more than once in a 100-year period is described as recurrent and occurred in 5 percent of cultures.

Famine is such a disastrous occurrence that it does not disappear readily from the human memory. For example, Bengali men in a 1940 survey classified themselves by whether they were born before or after "72"—the Bengali year 1272 in which terrible famine took place. Similarly, the Hopi keep the unlikely possibility of famine in their minds through stories old people tell of the last major famine, which occurred from 1860 to 1862. Famine is taken so seriously because it not only results in much death, but also disrupts for generations the social core of communities where it occurs. The following description indicates some of the social and economic costs of a potato famine in Highland Scotland in the 1830s and 1840s:

> In the thirties epidemic and famine began to take their toll. Destitution became widespread and there was no system of relief beyond the moral obligation of the proprietors to provide grain. The marriage rate fell. In Kilmuir the average annual number of marriages fell from twenty-one to six. Sub-division [of land] was forbidden, but it was too late. (Ducey 1956: 127–128)

Five years of famine ended the growth of population. The emigration of large numbers and the death of untold members must have seriously disrupted the patterns of interaction within the extended family and the township. Although the proprietors made a final effort to help their tenants, ruining themselves financially, they had forsaken their people. The ministers were no longer able to contribute to group solidarity, because the symbols and values they upheld reflected the attitudes of the landlords and lacked significance for the people.

Similarly, the extinction of the bison and the resulting famine led to massive cultural change for Plains Indian groups such as the Blackfoot in Montana:

> The unsuccessful hunts of 1883 and 1884 marked the end of the subsistence pattern on which the Blackfeet had built their cul-

ture. The Indians scoured the region for food, and moved in around the Agency to ask for help from the Agent. In Blackfeet culture, those who had food shared it during times of want; the Agent supposedly had food and as a leader he was now expected to validate his status by caring for those who had none. The United States government had acknowledged responsibility for the Blackfeet in the 1855 and subsequent treaties, but Agency supplies were inadequate to meet famine conditions. Up to one-fourth of the Piegan perished during the winter 1883 to 1884.

> The Indians had to find a new and meaningful subsistence base, new ways in which to express old values and to maintain their prestige and status. At the same time, the government, upon which they were dependent, pressed them to accept new value and prestige systems. (McFee 1971: 59)

A final and especially dramatic report of the social effects of famine is reported for the Truk of Micronesia in the early twentieth century:

> Although the natives had sufficient food supplies in normal times, or could have, nevertheless times of famine are not unfamiliar to them. Causes of famine might be a typhoon or a long drought. A lack of rain for three or four months can be disastrous for the islands, since, with the thin layer of humus, all the plantings die. In such times of famine many cases of death always occur; the families broke up, because everybody was only concerned with saving his own skin. The people cut down the coconut trees and ate the heart, which resulted in the death of many. There was no longer any order. Looting, theft, and murder were the order of the day. Especially clever ones carried some soil onto very high trees and raised some tobacco there.

> An old saying gives the following advice for famine: "*nugu sebi, nugu neif, nugu lul.*" Protect the bowl, the knife, the coconut cord. That is, one who has a bowl can make himself *mogemog* (arrowroot) when other foodstuffs are exhausted. . . . But anyone who also has the other two things besides the

bowl, he can climb the coconut palms, cut the blossom stalk, fasten a bowl to it, and thus procure for himself the fortifying palm wine. This gives him a chance to struggle through until better times come. (Bollig 1927: 182)

Throughout human history famine has been associated with rural populations like those covered in the survey noted above and with peasants in nation-states. The victims of the largest famines have been peasant farmers such as the 3.25 million who died in India in the famine of 1899 to 1901, the 16 to 30 million who died in the China famine beginning in 1931, the 1.8 million who died in the Bangladesh famine of 1973 to 1975, and the millions who have died in the famine affecting the Sahel region of Africa since the early 1970s. This pattern through human history of people who produce their own food being most impacted by famine suggested to some experts in the past that famine was the result of environmental changes that led to food shortages. However, it is now clear that famines in modern times are rarely caused by changes in environmental conditions or by natural disasters that produce food shortages. Instead, they are caused by economic, political, and social factors that lead to unequal distribution of food, with some groups having less access to food than do other groups. Thus, famine can and does occur in a region or nation where there is adequate food; the problem is that not all people have equal access to the food.

CAUSES OF FAMINE

The interaction of three factors leads to famine: (1) the physical environment, (2) the sociopolitical system, and (3) the economic system. The physical environment provides the context in which famine occurs, with environmental change leading to food shortages one possible factor in causing a famine to occur. Rainfall variability is a major factor, as either too little rainfall, causing drought, or too much rainfall, causing flooding, can lead to a food shortage that may eventually become a famine. Other environmental factors include insect predation, which destroys crops; animal diseases, which kill herd animals; erosion and lowering of soil fertility caused by overcropping and overgrazing; and deforestation caused by logging and conversion of forest into agricultural land.

Given that the environment provides the context for famine and that certain environmental events may set the process in motion, the basic cause of famine is the system of property ownership and exchange in a society, which may under certain conditions prevent the flow of food to certain segments of the society. Thus, famine is not caused by an individual's ability to produce food but rather by restrictions on an individual's ability to acquire food through purchase or trade. Sociopolitical factors that can restrict access to food include ethnic discrimination by the government against certain groups, warfare in which one society destroys or blocks the food supply of another nation, government famine relief policies and practices that fail to get the food to those most in need, and cultural beliefs and practices about sharing. At the economic level, whether famine occurs or not and how severe it becomes are influenced by the food production system, rural non-food production system, urban non-food production system, and the food delivery system. These four economic subsystems interact with one another in the context of the physical environment and under government control (through laws, policies, and taxation) to create an economic system that either functions in a way that prevents famine or allows famine to occur for a segment of the population.

The food production system includes agricultural practices and technology, the size of the crop, the timing of the crop, labor, and land ownership, all of which can impact on the ability of food producers to produce a harvest of the correct size for the market at the right time. The rural non-food production system includes secondary economic activities such as fishing, which are susceptible to environmental uncertainty and therefore may not always be available as secondary sources of income. The rural non-food production system also includes people who live in the rural region such as blacksmiths or shopkeepers who purchase rather than produce their own food. These people may be the victims of famine when their rural customers experience bad years. The urban non-food production system controls the flow of money to the rural sector through food purchases, loans, and land ownership and also provides a haven for those fleeing famine. The food delivery system includes traders who act as middlemen between the rural food producers and merchants, the merchants, and the actual transportation infrastructure—the railways, shipping, and highways themselves.

Across cultures in the modern world, under optimal conditions, food produced in the rural sector flows through the food delivery system to the mainly urban markets, and money flows from the urban markets back to the rural sector, with a balance between supply and demand so that those in the rural sector earn enough to purchase food. However, if environmental variables, such as too much or too little rainfall, warfare, ethnic discrimination, low demand for a food, oversupply that drives down prices, or some other factor, disrupt the adequate flow of food to the urban sector or money to the rural sector, famine may result.

The famine of 1943 in the Bengal region of India near the city of Calcutta is an example of the interplay of the forces that create the conditions for a famine, determine how famine is dealt with, and reveal the consequences of famine across cultures. In 1942 the Japanese controlled most of nearby Burma and the British, who then controlled India, were preoccupied with the threat of Japanese expansion into India. Of the 60 million Bengal residents, 44 million were farmers whose staple food was rice. However, crop yields had been poor since 1934 and only in 1937 were imports of rice not needed to feed the Bengal population. At the same time, the British stored masses of rice for use in the war effort. In 1942 the winter crop was poor in most locales and destroyed in some by a hurricane and floods. As a hedge against anticipated shortages, the farmers kept a third more for themselves and thus sent that same third less off to be sold. Finally, in April 1943 the government pulled some 25,000 boats out of the water in response to the Japanese threat. These actions meant that rice farming in delta areas ceased. All of these events and actions served to drive up the price of rice and by May 1943 it had risen 600 percent in the Bengal market. The farmers began to suffer and sought alternative sources of money and food and tried to lower their demand for food. They sold family and personal ornaments, the doors and iron roofs from their homes. They took to collecting foods such as wild grasses and snails that would not be eaten in better times. Widows were asked to leave the homes of their deceased husband's brothers, families split up, children were abandoned, and some were left at the gate of the homes of the wealthy. The effects of the famine spilled onto the streets of Calcutta as people fled there in search of food, shelter, and employment. They lived on the sidewalks and in rail yards and were given food by private and government relief organizations, but they also acted in ways otherwise unheard of—they ate dogs, foraged in garbage dumps, and sold their children, and Hindus and Muslims exchanged food with one another. By July 1943 at least 100,000 people had moved to Calcutta. Despite reports that hundreds of people were dying in the villages every week, in November and December 1943 and January 1944, the police, following a new law, sent over 43,000 people back to the rural areas. In January nearly 23,000 people died. It was not until October 1943 after months of public denial, that the government admitted that "Bengal is in the grip of an unprecedented famine." Finally, by the end of the year the combination of famine, cold weather, and a shortage of clothes and shelter added malaria and cholera to the disaster. In early 1944 a good crop came in and all returned to pre-famine conditions, with the Governor of Bengal noting that "I am convinced that there is plenty of rice in Bengal for all the people of Bengal. The difficulty is that it is unevenly spread. . . . Our task is to spread the butter evenly on the bread." While the famine may have ended, it was still common twenty-five years later for villagers to find skeletons in their rice fields.

CONTROLLING THE EFFECTS OF FAMINE

In the contemporary world, the short-term effects of famine such as malnourishment and disease are mainly dealt with through the intervention of international organizations who import food and distribute it to those living in famine conditions or through the migration of those suffering from famine to other regions where food is available. However, the success of such efforts is more often determined by local, regional, national, and international politics than by the needs of the famine victims, the availability of food, or the condition of transportation systems. In Ethiopia and Somalia in the 1980s and 1990s the problem in obtaining relief was not a shortage of food but a combination of indifference outside the region and local political conflicts that channeled food to some groups but not others. However, since all cultures and communities are affected by external political, economic, and social factors as well as resource variability, it seems unlikely that most communities in developing nations can be entirely self-sufficient and can survive in times of famine

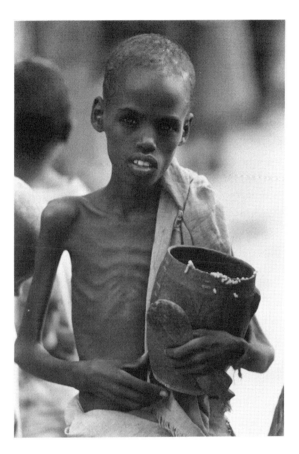

A Somali boy suffering the effects of famine clutches a spoon and bowl containing rice and beans distributed by the Red Cross in 1992.

without outside help. One group that did manage to survive on its own is the Suri of Ethiopia. After several years of difficult circumstances, they suffered a severe drought and famine beginning in late 1984 and lasting into 1991. The drought destroyed their sorghum and corn crops, decimated their cattle herds, and forced many Suri to migrate to Sudan. By late 1991 they had recovered, without any outside aid, and their traditional economy was restored with fields of sorghum and corn, cattle herds back to pre-1985 size, and many people returned from the Sudan. For the Suri, however, the key to their success was the mining of gold in their territory, which could be sold to purchase food, seeds, fertilizer, cattle, and automatic rifles to keep neighboring groups away. Thus, by exploiting a new resource, they restored their traditional economy and built a defense system to protect themselves from human predators. Across cultures, however, few groups have such new resources to exploit to deal with famine.

Many experts believe that a number of basic economic and political changes are needed to prevent famines in areas of the world such as North Africa, where famine is frequent. These measures include increasing food production in those regions, creating markets for the sale of food produced in the regions, building and maintaining roads, creating a demand for food outside the local community, and providing family farmers with adequate amounts of land, water, and technical support.

See also DIET AND NUTRITION; ENVIRONMENTAL DISASTERS.

Abbink, Jon. (1993) "Famine, Gold and Guns: The Suri of Southwestern Ethiopia, 1985–1991." *Disasters* 17: 218–225.

Bollig, Laurentius. (1927) *The Inhabitants of the Truk Islands*. Translated from the German.

Culshaw, W. J. (1949) *Tribal Heritage: A Study of the Santals*.

Desai, Meghnad. (1988) "The Economics of Famine." In *Famine,* edited by G. Ainsworth Harrison, 107–138.

Dirks, Robert. (1993) "Starvation and Famine: Cross-Cultural Codes and Some Hypothesis Tests." *Cross-Cultural Research* 27: 28–69.

D'Souza, Frances. (1988) "Famine: Social Security and an Analysis of Vulnerability." In *Famine,* edited by G. Ainsworth Harrison, 1–56.

Ducey, Paul R. (1956) *Cultural Continuity and Population Change on the Isle of Skye.*

Hansen, Art. (1994) "The Illusion of Local Sustainability and Self-Sufficiency: Famine in a Border Area of Northwestern Zambia." *Human Organization* 53: 11–20.

Harrison, G. Ainsworth, ed. (1988) *Famine.*

Keen, David. (1994) "In Africa, Planned Suffering." *The New York Times* (August 15): A15.

McFee, Malcolm. (1971) *Modern Blackfeet: Contrasting Patterns of Differential Acculturation.*

Morehouse, Geoffrey. (1972) *Calcutta.*

Seavoy, Ronald E. (1986) *Famine in Peasant Societies.*

Segal, Gerald. (1993) *The World Affairs Companion.*

Sen, Amartya. (1981) *Poverty and Famines: An Essay on Entitlement and Deprivation.*

Titiev, Mischa. (1971) *Old Oraibi: A Study of the Hopi Indians of Third Mesa.*

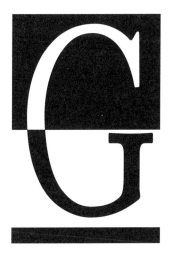

In his world survey of sexual behavior, Edgar Gregerson noted that "Whatever the reason, people in many different societies have felt and still feel that the genitals should be altered in one way or another by cutting, piercing, hacking, or slicing, or by inserting objects." Modification of genitals of one's children, relatives, and neighbors is culturally approved, and in many societies, required behavior around the world. Mutilation of the genitals of war captives, slaves, and other outsiders is also a fairly common aftermath of war and raiding. In Western and Westernized societies, male circumcision is currently the only common genital modification, and it is usually performed in a medical setting when the infant is young. In traditional non-Western societies, genital operations were and are commonly performed in the community and often, for boys, as part of a ceremony marking their entrance into adulthood.

Male genital mutilations come in three major forms:

1. Circumcision is the removal of the foreskin and is the most common genital modification. It is estimated that 50 percent of the men in the world today have been circumcised. It is required of Jews and customary for Muslims, and circumcision of male babies is a routine medical procedure in some Western societies, including the United States. In non-Western societies circumcision usually occurs later in life, commonly at puberty when boys are initiated into adult status. Some social scientists suggest that circumcision is found primarily in societies where boys develop a strong attachment to their mothers and a weak attachment to their fathers. Circumcision plus other stressful and traumatic activities as part of initiation rites presumably allow the boy to break his emotional ties to his mother and assume a male identity.

2. Superincision (supercision) is the slitting of the foreskin lengthwise, without removal. It occurs only in a few Polynesian societies.

3. Subincision is the slitting of the underside of the penis lengthwise to the urethra. It is found almost exclusively among a few aboriginal cultures in Australia. These are all cultures located in territories inhabited by kangaroos, the males of which have two-headed penises. It has been suggested, both by the people themselves and anthropologists, that subincision is an attempt to imitate kangaroos.

Other forms of male genital mutilation are bleeding the penis without permanent modification, removal of one testicle (hemicastration), complete castration, nipple excision, and inserting objects under the foreskin. All of these only occur under special circumstances and usually only for a select group of boys or men.

Unlike male modifications, female mutilations are not regularly incorporated into initiation ceremonies and they are usually performed on girls before they reach marriageable age. Female genital mutilations come in four major forms:

1. Ritualistic circumcision is the nicking of the clitoris and involves no gross mutilation.
2. Circumcision, or Sunna (the Muslim namc), is the removal of the clitoral precipice and less often the removal of the tip of the clitoris also.
3. Excision, or clitoridectomy, is the removal of some or all of the clitoris and sometimes part of the labia minora.
4. Infibulation, or Pharaonic circumcision, is the removal of all of the female genitalia and the sewing shut of the remaining edges of labia majora, leaving only a small opening for the passage of urine and menstrual fluid. At the time of marriage, the opening will be enlarged to allow sexual relations.

Female genital mutilations occur in forty nations and many more cultures within these nations, primarily in Africa and the southern Middle East. Estimates place the number of African women who have experienced genital mutilation at nearly 100 million. Although current interest in these operations is focused on African cultures and nations, such operations have been used elsewhere. For example, from about 1890 to the late 1930s clitoridectomies were surgically performed in the United States as a "cure" for masturbation. Unlike male modifications, female modifications often cause serious health and emotional problems. Girls may die from the operation or from complications such as infection, women experience chronic health problems such as urinary tract infections, painful intercourse and childbirth, inability to experience orgasm, and menstrual pain, and the society often must bear additional health care costs.

The severity of the modifications and the resulting problems for women has led to a loud and ongoing debate about the legitimacy of such operations and efforts to end the practice. On one side of the debate are those who see the mutilations as motivated by sexual inequality and male control of women, a position supported by the use of these operations in cultures where women are considered to be inferior to men and where men control female sexuality. Advocates for the banning of female mutilations also see them as a violation of the human rights of girls and women, and women have been granted political asylum in the United States in order to avoid returning to their homeland, where they will be forced to submit to genital mutilation. The pain, physical risk, and control of female sexuality involved in female genital mutilations is indicated in this description of excision as practiced by the Somali:

> The excision of girls may take place a few days after birth or at about the age of two or three or about the age of seven. It is done by women. One fact is to be noted here, for it is characteristic: excision is followed by what has inaccurately been called "stitching." After the clitoris has been cut off, the two sides of the organ are made raw and joined with actual hooks made of thorns. Only a very small opening is left. Gum is spread upon the wound to facilitate the healing process, and the flesh soon grows together. It is established that the women are not "stitched," but rather "welded." This operation, which is extremely painful, is followed at the time of marriage by a re-opening which is no less painful. Without hesitation, one may regard this quite simply as an attempt to guarantee virginity in the most extreme manner possible and with complete disregard for the consequences of such precautions (fatal accidents, absence of normal muscular reactions at childbirth which forces the midwife to enlarge the opening with a dagger, etc.). (Leroi-Gourhan 1953: 13)

Various efforts by both private and government organizations have sought to end female mutilations in Africa through legislation, public pressure, and education, with mixed results.

On the other side of the debate are those—usually men in the cultures with operations but also some women as well—who argue that the operations are a major symbol of ethnic identity and a matter of ethnic self-determination, and that they are therefore not subject to control by outsiders. The role of such operations in cultural identity is indicated by excision as practiced by the Dogon of West Africa:

> A respected woman operates on all the girls of the class on the same day in the dune, the house reserved for adolescents, which they occupy together, often even before having been excised. The children will remain in the dune during their seclusion for three weeks; they will be very well fed and will rest. Old women take care of the ones newly excised; until cicatrization is complete, the wound is treated by being bathed with warm water. Instruction concerning women more particularly is given during this period.
>
> At the end of the seclusion, the matron who operated on the girls shaves their heads. Bathed and with their bodies coated with sesame oil, the adolescents make their re-entry into social life by promenade in the streets of the village, where they will be welcomed with special songs. (Palau-Marti 1957: 67–68)

The view of the those who seek to end the operations is that change must come from within the cultures and nations themselves, through a combination of public attention, education, legislation, and the support of political leaders.

Doorkendoo, Efua. (1995) *Cutting the Rose: Female Genital Mutilation, the Practise and Its Prevention.*

Frayser, Suzanne. (1985) *Varieties of Sexual Experience.*

Gregerson, Edgar. (1982) *Sexual Practices: The Story of Human Sexuality.*

Hosken, Fran. (1982) *The Hosken Report; Genital and Sexual Mutilation of Females.*

Leroi-Gourhan, Andre. (1953) *French Somaliland.* Translated from the French by Bernard Scholl.

Levinson, David. (1989) *Family Violence in Cross-Cultural Perspective.*

McLean, Scilla, and Stella Efua Graham, eds. (1983) *Female Circumcision, Excision, and Infibulation: The Facts and Proposals for Change.*

Palau-Marti, Monserrat. (1957) *The Dogon.* Translated from the French by Frieda Schutze.

Slack, Alison T. (1988) "Female Circumcision: A Critical Appraisal." *Human Rights Quarterly* 10: 437–486.

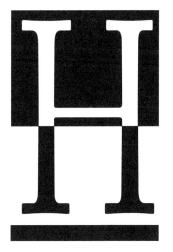

supernatural forces that cause illness. Magico-religious healers differ from professional healers in that they do not have formal training and that they attribute illness to supernatural forces. Like professional healers, however, they are paid for their services and often enjoy considerable prestige in their communities. Third are informal healers, whose status as a healer is based on their status as a caretaker in the family or community.

While it is useful to classify healers into these three categories for discussion purposes, it is also important to note that in actual day-to-day life in most societies, the definitions of who is a healer and what type of healer he or she is may be more complex. A major source of complexity is that in many societies one finds all three types of healers. For example, Saraguro Quichua in Ecuador choose among *curandoros* (ritual healers), herbalists, midwives, pharmacists, nurses, physicians, and female relatives when seeking medical care. And even in a nation such as the United States, where one health care system—scientific medicine—is dominant, dozens of magico-religious and informal treatment options are available and commonly used. For example, a woman may choose among an obstetrician, family practitioner, nurse midwife, lay midwife, or granny midwife when giving birth. Some of the factors that determine which type of healer an individual chooses are discussed in the entry on Health Care Systems.

HEALERS Healers are individuals who are socially defined as able to cure illness, and they are featured in health care systems in all cultures. Allopathic physicians, Ayurvedic physicians, chiropractors, Chinese herbalists, shamans, and the leaders of healing cults are all healers, even though they may believe in different explanations for illness, use different healing methods, and achieve their status as healers in different ways. Across cultures, the broad array of healers can be classified into three general categories. First are healers, often referred to as "professional healers," who engage in healing as a full-time occupation, whose status as a healer is based on knowledge and skill acquired through formal training, and who are paid for their services. Often these healers base their practice on scientific medicine, although in many cultures professional healers such as herbalists base their practice on other theories of illness. Second are magico-religious healers, often referred to as "folk healers," whose status is based on their ability—which may be innate or acquired—to control the

PROFESSIONAL HEALERS

Professional healers are the primary type of healer in societies with large, settled populations, such as most modern nations. However, they are also found in many less complex non-Western cultures where healers such as herbalists, midwives, and bonesetters are consulted because of their knowledge and skill in treating illness. This knowledge and skill is acquired through learning—often by means of an apprenticeship—and through practice. The diffusion of Western medicine in the twentieth century now means

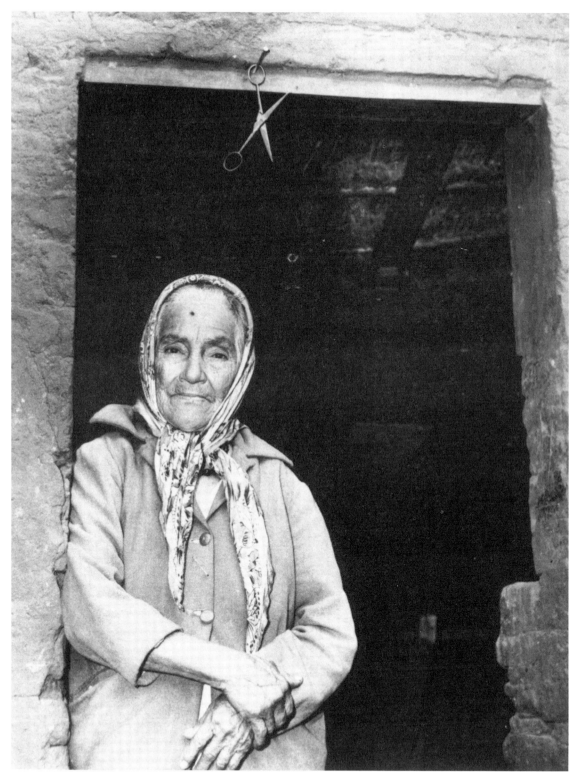

Professional healers, magico–religious or folk healers, and informal healers exist in all societies. Here a Paraguayan midwife stands in a doorway that displays a pair of scissors, a tool and symbol of her profession.

that, in nearly all cultures, scientific medicine as practiced by physicians, nurses, midwives, and other health care personnel is one component of the health care system. The status of these practitioners rests on their possession of knowledge, equipment, and drugs that can be used to successfully treat many illnesses. Across cultures, however, such healers are most often consulted for acute illnesses such as infections, which they are often able to treat quickly and successfully. Chronic illnesses are more often left to traditional specialists such as herbalists, magico-religious healers, and informal healers.

MAGICO-RELIGIOUS HEALERS

Across cultures there are a number of types of magico-religious healers. Some, such as shamans, shaman/healers, and magical healers, devote all or much of their attention to treating illness. Others, such as priests, mediums, and sorcerers, might also treat illness, although much of their activity is concerned with other matters. In many cultures there is more than one type of magico-religious healer, with each specializing in certain types of illness. For example, the Aymara of Peru consult six different types of magico-religious healers, all of whom use magic to cure illness: magician, sorcerer, doctor, diviner, chiropractor, and midwife.

Shamans

Shamanism is a system of religious and medical beliefs and practices that centers on the shaman, a specific type of magico-religious practitioner. Shamanism rests on the belief that many events on earth are caused by supernatural forces and that, therefore, human contact and control of the supernatural is necessary to control life on earth. The shaman is the individual who specializes in contacting and controlling the supernatural. What anthropologists call classic shamanism is customary among the indigenous peoples of Si-beria and Central Asia and is characterized by the shaman being a charismatic male, a master of the supernatural spirits, concerned mainly though not exclusively with curing disease, and serving a client base composed of particular families or communities.

During the nineteenth and twentieth centuries classic shamanism was severely repressed by the Russian, Soviet, and Chinese governments and in some cultures disappeared, in others survived only in limited form, and in others went underground. Since the mid-twentieth century there has been a revival of shamanism and a broadening of the meaning of the concept to include related magico-religious practices elsewhere in the world. In the former Soviet Union, the end of Soviet rule has led to a revival of shamanism in some Siberian cultures as part of a broader pattern of cultural revitalization. In Korea, where shamanism was also repressed, it has been revived as a marker of indigenous Korean culture, although nearly all Korean shamans are now women rather than men.

The conceptualization of shamanism has also been broadened by social scientists and others to include related practices that rely on an altered state of consciousness or possession trance and thus one now speaks of Cuna, Tibetan, Malay, and !Kung shamans in Panama, China, Malaysia, and Botswana. Some experts argue that many of these other religious-healing systems are not shamanism as the key element of shamanistic control of spirits is missing.

In the last several decades, and particularly in the 1990s, elements of shamanism have appeared in the New Age movement, especially such practices as chanting and drumming, which are seen as tools for achieving a deeper state of personal spirituality and for preventing illness by reducing the stresses of daily life. The New Age movement has drawn both from classic shamanism and from similar customs among various Native American cultures in North and South America.

Shamanism as a religious-healing system has a number of key elements: (1) the shaman himself—his characteristics, initiation and training, and life style; (2) the illnesses addressed by the shaman; and (3) the curing seance. The discussion below focuses on these topics, with examples provided from classic Yakut shamanism in Siberia.

The Shaman

Shamans may be male or female, old or young, and benevolent or harmful. The key characteristics are that shamans control supernatural spirits and that they use that power to cure illnesses caused by these spirits as well as to influence or communicate with the spirits about other earthly concerns such as the weather. Shamans also must be brave, smart, creative, and willing to alter their behavior by behaving in ways required of their status.

The Yakut distinguish between male (*oyun*) and female (*udahan*) shamans and white-creative (*Ajy ayuna*) and black-harmful (*Abasy oyuna*) shamans. The white shaman looks like other people and uses no special means to communicate with the creator spirit, who is asked to help in matters such as infertility. He or she is incapable of causing harm and of little use in curing illness caused by evil spirits. The black shaman more closely fits the image of the classic shaman—he intervenes between spirits and humans to cure illness caused by spirits. The power of the individual shamans varies according to the power of the different spirits they control. The black shaman can also compel the spirits to cause others to fall ill. Although he or she may be consulted for other reasons, the Yakut shaman is mainly occupied with curing illness.

Yakut shamans trace their qualifications to the spirits:

His name was An-Argykl-Ojun. He was powerful and performed great miracles. He raised the dead, and gave the blind their eyesight back. This fame eventually also reached Aj-Toen (God, the Lord). He sent a messenger to the shaman to ask in the name of what god he did those miracles and whether he believed in him, Aj-Toen. An-Argykl-Ojun (the important shaman) replied three times he did not believe in God but performed miracles by his own strength and power.

Aj-Toen became angry at that and ordered the shaman to be burned. However, Ojun's body consisted of countless vermin, and one little frog managed to be saved from the flames. The powerful demons who still give shamans to the Yakuts are descendants of this little frog. (Krauss 1888: 171)

For the Yakut shaman-to-be the initiation is a public ritual, directed by an older shaman on a hill. The public nature of the ritual suggests the future role of the Yakut shaman in treating all members of the community. These oaths indicate the type of catastrophes the Yakut feared and the central role Yakut shamans played in curing disease:

I promise to be a protector of the unhappy, a father of the miserable, and a mother of the orphans. I shall honor the demons who live on the tops of the high mountains, and swear that I shall serve them with all my strength. I shall honor, bow to, and serve the highest and most powerful of them, the demon who commands all demons, the master of the three demon sibs who live on the tops of the mountains; him whom the shamans call Sostuganach Ulu-Toen (the frightful, terrible one); his elder son Ujgul-Toen (the insane one), his wife Ujgul-Chotun (the insane woman), his younger son Kjakja-Curan-Toen (the loudly speaking one), his wife Kjakja-Curan-Chotan, and their numerous family and servants, through whom they send the people diseases, accidents, breakings of legs, and the podagra. I vow to save those who have been affected by these diseases, by sacrificing a cream-colored mare.

I shall profess and worship, bow to, and serve Ulu Toen's younger brother, the demon Chara-Surun-Toen (the black raven), his son

Alban-Buran-Toen (the resourceful venturer), his daughter Kys-Salisaj (the virgin who walks), who prompts people to commit manslaughter, suicide, and calumny. I promise to help rid these people of their passions by offering the said demons a black horse.

I shall profess, worship, and bow to the demon Altan-Sobiraj-Toen (the brazen basin), his wife Altan Sobiraj-Chotun (the one with the biggest brazen arrow), their daughters Timir-Kuturuk (iron tail) and Kejulgaı Darchan (the important, great, lopping woman), who send mankind chronical abscesses. I shall help free the sick by sacrificing some (Arago) liquor, and offering the demons a motley searnew, as a gift of honor.

I shall profess and worship, and bow to the ancestor of these demons who is known as Kjun-Zelerjuma-Sakryl-Chotun (the horrible foe of the sun) who has tables full of holes, and 52 servants. She sends people the passion game and drinking, robbery, plundering, abject deeds, and suicide. I shall try to heal those who are obsessed with these vices. I shall kill a red-spotted young mare who is an ambler, and twist heart and liver of the mare round my neck; I shall perform shaman magic to propitiate the goddess.

I shall profess and honor the demon above the demons of the six sibs who live in the place where the sinners' souls are sent to; I will bow to the one who is known among the shamans as Talirdach-Tan-Taraly-Toen (he who drags into ruin), his daughters Sorocho-Chotun (the wind-driven female beauty), and San-Chotun, and his countless servants who send men and cattle epidemic diseases. To propitiate them I shall offer them a sorrel-spotted mare.

I shall profess, honor, and bow to the demon Bor-Malachaj-Toen (deformed earth) and his wife Bor-Malachaj-Chontu who send mankind various diseases and, especially, death. If in a family children should die, I will implore these demons for mercy, and offer them a black cow with a half-white head.

I shall profess, honor, and bow to the demon Archach-Toen (the sick one) and his wife Archach-Chontun, who send mankind consumption. I shall heal the affected by offering a blackish brown cow.

I shall profess and honor the demon Njas-Elju (cart-horse, death) and his wife Yeryk-Chotun (the sick one) who send the people falling sickness and Siberian pestilence. I shall try to heal those who have been affected by these diseases by offering an eel-pout and a trout.

I shall profess, honor, and bow to the demon Kytaj-Baksy-Toen who gives the Yakuts resourceful smiths and powerful shamans. When Kytaj, angry with a smith, sends him a disease, I promise to kill a red cow in his honor, to spread the blood over all the forge tools, and to burn the heart and liver to ashes in the chimney. If I should be affected by this disease, another shaman will sacrifice for me and propitiate the demon.

I shall profess, honor, and bow to the daughter of the demon, Tamyk-Choton (the haughty one). She sends mankind mental diseases of various kinds. Those who have been affected by such disease I shall heal by sacrificing nine ermines, nine snow-weasels, nine fitchews, and nine pigeons; I vow to catch them alive, to adorn them, and to release them entirely.

I shall profess and bow to, I shall honor the shaman woman Tajaktach-Njacaj (the feeble one with the reed), her husband Atyr-Chataj (the eagle) and his countless family and descendants, who send the people oppression of the chest. Those who have been affected by this disease I shall try to save by sacrificing a light-red cow with but one horn.

I shall acknowledge, honor, and bow to the heavenly shaman Kybilyr Ojun (the white swan), his sister Kytalyktyr-Kyrbyky (the swan of the acute wings), and their mother Soruktach-Sodor (the charitable ruler), who send the people deafness and every kind of ear disease. Those who have been affected by it I shall try to save by offering a red cow with but one horn (*agar mostach kugas*). (Krauss 1888: 170)

This oath serves as a "job description" for the shaman as it lists the diseases he is expected to prevent and cure, the spirits involved, and the procedures used to control the spirits.

Once a man or woman becomes a shaman he or she is expected to appear and behave in ways that mark him or her as different than other members of the community, that reinforce his or her powers, and that protect him or her from harm. These include food taboos especially on shellfish during certain months, sexual continence for long periods, and fasting for days before conducting a seance. The shaman's wife and some relative might also be expected to honor these taboos and restrictions. The shaman also has to obtain and protect his or her ritual paraphernalia—most importantly the masks that represent the animals whose souls he or she controls and his or her drums and rattles.

Yakut shamans, along with blacksmiths, are the most respected people in the community. Because villages might be far apart, shamans travel about and are sought after:

> As soon as a shaman arrives somewhere, news of his arrival will be quickly spread over the entire neighborhood. Curious people, and those who hope to be relieved from the ailments, will crowd together at the spot to see the shaman and to inquire of him about the future. (de Laguna 1972: 72)

The shaman is seated in the place of honor, fed well, and might demand from his or her client an offering of meat or sacrifices to the spirits and gifts to himself or herself before conducting the seance.

The Seance

A seance is a ritual in which the shaman is possessed by a spirit or travels to the spirit world and serves as a medium of communication between humans and the spirit world. The shamanic seance is a magical performance in which the shaman uses a combination of power over the spirits, knowledge, physical strength and stamina, performing talents, and an altered state of consciousness to convince the audience of his or her

powers and to achieve the goal of the seance, which is often to cure a sick person. Believers in the power of the shaman attribute any success he or she has to his or her powers. Skeptics, while admitting that the altered state of consciousness takes place, attribute any success to the placebo effect in which patients get better because they are getting attention and expect to be cured and to the healing cult nature of curing seances.

Yakut seances involve soul travel to the supernatural world, communication with evil and benevolent spirits, healing rituals, and animal sacrifice. The shaman, patient, and audience all operate on the belief that healing will result if the spirit responsible for the disease is satisfied with the sacrifice. If the spirit is not propitiated, the shaman can do no more to save the patient. After he or she is fed and honored and his or her help requested, the Yakut shaman begins the work of contacting the spirit world. As with all magical rituals, shamanic seances require that the shaman follow the required procedures exactly.

> He . . . approaches the fireplace at its front side, throws fat into the fire as a sacrifice for the spirits, grasps the fat smoke with open hands and brings them to his mouth to make believe that he is swallowing them and so gets control over the spirit whom he wants to address with his intercession. Then he takes the drum, sits down before the fireplace on a reindeer skin of good quality, and takes a whip which is adorned with fringes of horse hair and motley rags, or with tails of small game, colored with alder bark. The skin is turned toward the fireplace so that the head is next to it. The shaman now beats his drum and tries to divert the spirits' attention towards himself by sounding a long ay, he yawns devilishly opening his mouth, sounds three times the cry of the ember-goose (cek, cek, cek), apes three times the cry of a stork, three times that of a cuckoo, and three times that of a raven.
>
> Then he calls upon the squint-eyed (*inistjaga*), deformed (*keltjagjaj*), lame

(*dogolon*) devil (*jugjug emjagjat*) and curses himself by assuring Satan [the evil spirits] of his devotion, promises to be a faithful servant, and asks him to obsess [possess] him. Now he rises, supposing that he now has communication with the devil, that the latter has obsessed him, and that he himself is now in command of the devil's power and might. He calls upon the white bird (*jurjunas*): May this become my place; may green grass grow on here; I have given myself to your life and blood, of Satan. You root of every evil and mishap (*ytyk eljuterde*), so he continues, you monster of the eight feet, I have joined you, so lend your aid in accomplishing the wishes. I have come from the *sjurdjach-kjaptjach, sjugja-toenton*, the terrible god of the hatchet, and from *kini-sjurgju-jutjanjan-sjurgjuju*, in order to save him by means of the salutary tool. But you, she-shamans of the fiery lashes, who live in the nether world, do not come to the upper world to fight or curse me. I have sat down on the navel of the earth in order to give protection to the sick. I am well aware of my faults, but suppose I were without faults and give way. Your three black shadows, of devil, have come upon me, so I beg you, help me. Look, I am offering you such an animal, so help my misery. (Krauss 1888: 173–174)

Upon returning from the trip to the upper or lower world, the audience questions the shaman about the condition of the patient and the chances of a cure. This report is followed by the healing ritual, which may take a variety of forms depending on the illness, patient, and circumstances. A common element is the offering and picking of an animal that will satisfy the spirit who has entered the patient's body and caused the disease. An acceptable sacrifice will cause the spirit to leave and the patient will be cured. One healing ritual takes the following form:

The shaman approaches the patient's couch and cries three times above the head of the latter: Just tell me what kind of sacrificial animal you want; only leave the patient. The spirit who lives in the sick person replies through the shaman: If you offer me a *sadzaga* (a cow with a white-spotted back) or a *bulur* (a dun horse), I shall quit the patient. The animal is offered. For this purpose, ten very small larches and one birch are needed. One larch and the birch are placed before the tent, one behind the other. Nine notches are made into the first larch. The other nine are placed around the first two in a semi-circle. On the southern side they are twisted with a linen cord, which is hanged with motley rags and horse-hair.

The animal to be offered is bound on the tree which has been notched (*salama*); the shaman, going to heaven, addresses Aj-Toen asking pity from him. He says: As men feel pity towards the patient, and since the old mothers (*chotottur*) have given back his soul to him (*kul*), accept the animal instead of his soul. After he has cried three times and spat at the animal (the patient spits, too), the animal is allowed to run to the flock. Then the shaman continues: Look here it is, accept it, give deliverance. I have accepted it, the devil replies through the shaman, and the patient will recover within seven, eight, nine days.

The shaman sings that the devil is at once precipitating into the nether world (*ojbontimirja*) with the ember-goose; there he delivers the animal offered for slaughter. For concreteness's sake the shaman takes a little board (which may be interpreted as a table), carves a round hole in it, puts a bit of meat on it, and throws everything into the fire. Then he lights the mane of black horse three times, inhales the smoke, and asks somebody of the present to cut the fire below his head, and give him a drink of water and sour milk (*umdan*), of the water of this world. Now he takes three twigs, beats the drum with them, and exercises the last survivals of the devil: Those of you who have fallen from above, go up; those of you who have come from below, go down, you devils! Exhausted by the movements on all sides, and giddy, he sits down, wet with sweat. Occasionally, he is unable with exhaustion to put out his kuma. (ibid.)

Shaman/Healers

Shaman/healers are similar to shamans except that they are found in large, settled communities, are often full-time specialists, receive special training, and may be organized into professional associations. In a single society, they may also specialize in certain ritual activities, such as agricultural rites, or in the treatment of specific types of illness. One well-described type of shaman/healer is the zar doctor found in North African cultures such as the Amhara of Ethiopia.

Zar doctors are the leaders of zar cults and treat mental illness, primarily in women although men may also use their services. Zar doctors diagnose, treat the illness, and then incorporate the patient into the doctor's zar cult, which provides protection for life. A zar is a particular type of spirit. Zar spirits, it is said, first appeared in the Garden of Eden. Eve had thirty children and when she tried to conceal fifteen of them from God, he punished her by declaring that all fifteen would be invisible night creatures. Zar spirits are descended from these fifteen children and may be either harmful or benevolent in their relations with humans.

Harmful spirits possess humans through magical coitus and cause illness, including mental illnesses such as fatigue, depression, seizures, and mood disorders. All humans are susceptible to zar possession. The difference between zar doctors and others is that the doctors have learned about the spirits and their victims and they can use their possession by their zar spirit to control the spirit and cure others. Doctors treat while in a trance and possessed by their zar spirit. They first diagnose the illness by interpreting the words of the possessed victim, by causing the victim to become possessed again, or by observing the possession as it occurs. Once the doctor determines the reason for the spirit's unhappiness, he or she negotiates with the spirit, which usually results in the patient making an offering through the doctor to the spirit that cures the illness. Then the patient is socialized into the zar doctor's cult, which provides life-long protection from the spirit. Cult members attend treatment sessions for other patients, which involve the burning of incense, drumming, poetry recitations, and possession.

Many zar doctors inherit the role from their mothers, or they may claim the status on the basis of having been kidnapped by a zar spirit early in life. In either case, the zar doctor must complete an apprenticeship with an established doctor and at the end receive his power directly from his teacher. Zar doctors are respected members of the community, free from some social obligations required of other people, and often wealthy. Zar doctors may specialize in treating certain types of illness or may gain reputations as being especially skilled at treating difficult cases, such as a person possessed by more than one zar spirit at one time. The zar doctors hold an annual convention, open only to them and their most dedicated cult members, at which new diagnostic and treatment techniques are presented and tested.

Mediums

A medium is a type of shaman/healer whose power comes from possession by a supernatural force such as a god or spirit. Across cultures, the most common function of mediums is divining—predicting the future or explaining the past—although they may also conduct various rituals and cure illness. For the Ganda of what is now Uganda, a medium (*mandwa*) served as the spokesperson for the god who possessed him or her. The person was selected as a medium by a god and a person was identified as a medium through his or her knowledge of events or his or her ability to predict the future. The first possession was called "being married to the god" and subsequent possessions were called "being seized by the head." A female medium was considered to be a wife of the god and had to keep separate from men and refrain from sexual activity. There was generally one medium per temple. The medium became possessed in order to divine, smoking a pipe filled with ordinary tobacco and gazing intently into a fire. While possessed and under the influence of the god, the medium spoke the words of the god, which were interpreted by the priest for the Ganda rulers.

Religious Healers

Religious healers are religious specialists who form a distinct occupational group of high status and considerable influence in their communities. While possession may be involved in achieving healer status, it is not always required, and religious healers cure not through possession but through the use of spells, rituals, and formulas to communicate with the supernatural. Healers are especially common in agricultural communities, where certain individuals may be identified as having powers they can use to cure others. The use of these powers requires knowledge and skills in ritual activities and, therefore, training, often as an apprentice.

Priests

Priests are not found in all societies but primarily in societies with large settled communities, a subsistence system based on agriculture, and centralized political leadership. In anthropological usage, *priest* is a generic term that is used for any individual who is specially trained to conduct rituals in order to communicate with the supernatural world. Thus, Catholic priests, Baptist ministers, and Jewish rabbis are all priests. The influence of priests often concerns both religious and secular matters. They may serve as advisors to political leaders or conduct rituals for many important events, such as planting and harvesting, birth, naming, marriage, and death. Priests do not usually occupy themselves with treating illness, although part of their work is to provide comfort and guidance to the sick and their families. In some religions, such as Roman Catholicism and Judaism, priests may be called on to perform exorcisms to heal someone who is believed to be possessed by evil spirits.

INFORMAL HEALERS

Informal healers are individuals who provide health care services but do not occupy a socially defined role as a healer in the community. In most cultures informal healers are women, and they provide health care mainly to family members, usually their own children. They do not have an office or a clinic where they work, but usually provide care in their homes or in the homes of relatives. Their work focuses mainly on the prevention of illness and the treatment of chronic conditions, with acute illness left to the professionals and folk healers. That most informal healers are women that work in the home has led many experts to conclude that the informal healer–patient relationship is quite similar to that between mother and child and thus represents a continuation of emotional attachment that characterizes mother-child relations in infancy and childhood. This pattern may also apply to female folk healers in some societies, and it is no accident that some female folk healers are called "Mother."

An example of the role of informal healers is provided by the Saraguro Quichua of Ecuador. As noted above, the Saraguro choose among *curandoros* (ritual healers), herbalists, midwives, pharmacists, nurses, physicians, and female relatives when seeking medical care. Work in Saraguro is allocated on the basis of one's sex, with women responsible for domestic work and caring for the children. Men work more often outside the home. As part of their domestic role, women care for sick children and other relatives. Girls assist their mothers, learning the basics of disease prevention, the identification of the early signs of illness, and appropriate treatments. Girls then practice these methods on their younger siblings. Since Saraguro informal care is learned at home and through discussions with other women, experience is considered a key marker of skill, and older women are considered more knowledgeable than younger, less experienced women. Saraguro women become informal healers after the birth of their first child. Saraguro informal healing reflects Saraguro ideas about the cause of illness. The home is considered a safe place and illness is attributed to influences outside the home, including other children, malevolent supernatural forces, and poisonous plants. The first line of defense is prevention, and children are dressed to protect against the weather and their diets are balanced with "hot" and "cold" foods to maintain a balance of the humors. Saraguro informal healers watch for such early signs of illness as sleeplessness and poor appetite and, through experience, learn to lump various symptoms together to diagnose specific diseases such as measles. Treatment combines drugs purchased from a pharmacist, massage, bathing, rest, herbal remedies, and emotional support. Perhaps it is emotional support—missing from many other types of treatment available to the Saraguro—that separates informal healing from professional and folk healing, both in Saraguro and elsewhere.

See also HEALTH CARE SYSTEMS.

Atkinson, Jane M. (1992) "Shamanisms Today." *Annual Review of Anthropology* 21: 307–330.

Balzer, Marjorie M., ed. (1990) *Shamanism: Soviet Studies of Traditional Religion in Siberia and Central Asia.*

de Laguna, Frederica. (1972) *Under Mount Saint Elias: The History and Culture of the Yakutat Tlingit.*

Eliade, Mircea. (1964) *Shamanism: Archaic Techniques of Ecstacy.*

Finerman, Ruthbeth. (1989) "The Forgotten Healers: Women as Family Healers in an Andean Indian Community." In *Women as Healers: Cross-Cultural Perspectives*, edited by Carol S. McClain, 24–41.

Harner, Michael. (1982) *The Way of the Shaman: A Guide to Power and Healing.*

Hultkranz, Åke. (1992) *Shamanic Healing and Ritual Drama: Health and Medicine in Native North American Religious Traditions.*

Jochelson, Waldemar. (1933) *The Yakut.* Anthropological Papers of the American Museum of Natural History, vol. 33 (2): 33–335.

Kendall, Laurel. (1985) *Shamans, Housewives, and Other Restless Spirits: Women in Korean Ritual Life.*

Krauss, Friedrich S. (1888) *Yakut Shamanism.*

McClain, Carol S., ed. (1989) *Women as Healers: Cross-Cultural Perspectives.*

Messing, Simon. (1957) *The Highland Plateau Amhara of Ethiopia.*

Tschopik, Harry, Jr. (1951) *The Aymara of the Chucuito, Peru: 1. Magic.* Anthropological Papers of the American Museum of Natural History 44: 133–308.

Winkelman, Michael. (1986) "Magico-Religious Practitioner Types and Socioeconomic Conditions." *Behavior Science Research* 20: 17–46.

———. (1990) "Shaman and Other 'Magico-Religious' Healers: A Cross-Cultural Study of Their Origins, Nature, and Social Transformations." *Ethos* 18: 308–352.

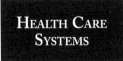

HEALTH CARE SYSTEMS

In all cultures people are concerned about their health and in all cultures there are shared beliefs and behaviors about the prevention and treatment of illness and injury. All of these beliefs and behaviors form the health care system of the culture. While health care systems can differ from culture to culture, all health care systems share a number of common elements:

1. Definitions of health and illness
2. Beliefs (theories) about the causes of illness
3. Treatment strategies
4. Healers
5. Specific methods and techniques of treatment
6. A decision-making process for using the health care system

Although in many cultures one health care system is dominant, in nearly all cultures today people have a number of different health care system options to choose among. Such cultures are said to have a pluralistic health care system. For example, in the United States, scientific medicine is dominant, but alternative systems such as homeopathy, chiropractic, natural healing, and a wide range of additional techniques are also used by as much as 30 percent of the population. This same pattern holds in many cultures around the world, and one of the main health care issues is how and why people choose one system rather than another.

In order to describe the major features of health care systems across cultures and to note the differences between them, we describe here different systems from four different cultures: the Hausa of Nigeria, an Andean Indian community, the Amhara of Ethiopia, and rural Taiwan.

HAUSA HEALTH CARE SYSTEM

The essence of Hausa views on health and illness can be found in the broad meanings for two words, *lafiya* and *magani*. Lafiya, in the narrow sense, means health. More generally, however, it refers to "the proper ordering, correct structuring, and general well-being of the social order and the individual's relations within it, as well as the state of wellness in the human body." (Wall 1988: 212) Magani means medicine, in the sense of something that cures an illness, but also has a more general meaning: it "encompasses practically the whole range of human activities, since it can include any act which results in the restoration, maintenance, or creation of order and balance. . . . In common usage magani generally refers to *substances* which are thought to possess powers that can bring these things to pass." (Wall 1988: 212–213) Thus, an important element of Hausa beliefs about the causes of illness and its treatment is the issue of maintaining or restoring balance. Another important element of good health is strength, and much of preventative medicine is meant to maintain one's strength. The linkage of strength with health is common in many cultures where people produce their own food because the inability to feed oneself and one's family, which depends on one's strength, creates considerable risk.

Hausa beliefs about the specific causes of illness are complex and derived from a mix of sources. Many Hausa are Muslims and they attribute some illnesses to Allah, not in a direct causal sense but in the more general sense of God being responsible for some human afflictions. Second, the Hausa see a balancing of "hot" and "cold" elements as vital to health and view cold as especially harmful as it both kills the blood and produces phlegm, which also kills the blood. The Hausa also attribute some illnesses to spirit possession and, while not necessarily believing in a scientific theory of disease, accept Western medicine as a treatment of last resort.

The Hausa choose among a number of different treatment strategies with the treatments mostly provided by professional healers. The most common strategy is herbal medicine, and it is used both to prevent illness in the form of tonics that maintain strength and to treat a wide range of disorders. Its importance to the Hausa is reflected in the presence of three types of herbal healers as well as the regular use of herbs as home remedies. The most important herbalist is the boka, who is a medical specialist and may achieve this status either by inheriting it or through an apprenticeship. The boka may run an herbal practice from his or her home, treat individuals at the marketplace, or travel to patients' homes. The second type of herbalist is the magori, or medicine seller. He is a traveling salesman of herbal remedies and specializes in love potions and aphrodisiacs. Unlike the boka he enjoys little prestige. The third type herbalist is the kantankar, who sells herbal remedies in the village markets. The herbs he sells are usually unprocessed plant materials that his customers then process into home cures. He draws his clients from the local population and may be a full-time or part-time herbalist. He enjoys more status than the magori but less than the boka. Herbal medicine is considered by the Hausa to be their own medical system and thus is often the treatment of choice for many illnesses. It is also used, in the Hausa's more general conception of illness, to cope with many life situations and problems. However, the traditional use of herbs has been influenced by Islam, and many herbal remedies are promoted as medicine from Allah. Thus, some herbalists see themselves as religious as well as medical specialists.

The second major type of healer is the wanzami, or barber-surgeon. Unlike the herbalists, who dispense either herbs or advice, the wanzami is a hands-on healer. In addition to giving haircuts to boys and men his healing specialty is cupping. Cupping is an ancient technique for removing "bad blood" from the body. This blood is believed to cause illness, usually indicated by fatigue. In addition, the wanzami performs circumcisions on boys, removes the uvula of newborns, and tattoos infants when they are named, as well as girls and women. Another hands-on healer is the ma'dori, or bonesetter, who sets broken bones with sticks and plaster made from dung. In rural areas he is more accessible than Western medical facilities and his casts are considered more attractive than white plaster ones.

A third type of practitioner is the ungozoma, or midwife, who assists at birth. The Hausa take pregnancy and childbirth quite seriously and in addition to using the services of the midwife engage in various food and behavior taboos and strength-building techniques to assist the mother and child before and after birth.

The final type of healer is the mallam. He is an Islamic teacher whose status comes from his ability to read Arabic (which most Hausa do not), his collection of sacred books, and his knowledge of the Quran (Koran). Mallam practice "the medicine of the Prophet." The core of this practice is the use of passages from the Quran, as follows:

> The Prophet Muhammed is believed to have recommended a few *aayat* or verses from the Quran for healing, but ever since that time the Quran has increasingly become a major source of therapy among Muslims the world over. Various verses from the Quran are prescribed as remedies for different sicknesses, pathological or otherwise. The common feature of such verses is that they contain an explicit or implicit reference to the sickness for which they are prescribed. A person suffering from continuous vomiting, for example, will be treated with the aaya: "And We said, swallow up thy water, Of Earth, Sky cease thy rain—And the water disappeared." . . . while the aaya "I have bestowed love upon thee" is prescribed for the unsuccessful lover in order to remove all obstacles between him and the beloved. (Abdalla, quoted in Wall 1988: 235)

These verses from the Quran are mostly written in Arabic and then worn as amulets or placed around the house.

The final element of Hausa health care is Western medicine, provided in clinics and hospitals and more readily available in cities than in rural villages. Western medicine is used for two main reasons: (1) for vaccinations that control epidemic diseases such as smallpox and (2) as a treatment of last resort for illnesses or injuries that fail to respond to traditional therapies. Interestingly, since Western medicine is a last resort, it is often ineffective at the late stage it is used, reinforcing the belief that traditional approaches are usually better and should be tried first.

SARAGURO HEALTH CARE SYSTEM

Like the Hausa, the Andean Indians who live in the mountain village of Saraguro in Ecuador use a pluralistic health care system, composed of elements from their traditional culture combined with elements from outside introduced more recently. Two beliefs are central to the Saraguro health care system. First, they do not differentiate neatly between being healthy and being ill. While being healthy is desired, the reality of health and illness in Saraguro is more complicated. No one is healthy all the time and health is never permanent. Some illnesses are so common that they are not considered illnesses at all. Pain and emotional stress are expected and are seen as making a prolonged condition of good health unlikely for most individuals. As for the Hausa, health is not simply a matter of the condition of one's body; it also includes being a productive worker, enjoying a happy family life, and being free from supernatural harm. And, again like the Hausa, because they too produce their own food, Saraguros equate good health with physical energy. In this regard, a heavy and steady body is considered a sign of good health. The second major belief underlying the health care system is the linking of the mind and the body, seeing both as possible causes of illness. Fright, stress, anger, and other emotional states are seen as causes of illness, and physical illness is seen as a cause of emotional distress. Thus, treatments address both mind and body.

Saraguros attribute illness to both natural and supernatural causes. Natural causes include infection, injury, aging, a poor diet, as well as an imbalance between hot and cold properties in the body. Supernatural causes center on the harmful actions of spirits and witches and include illnesses caused by the evil eye, soul loss, and fright. Children are more susceptible to supernatural illnesses than adults, and much of childhood care is devoted to keeping children away from supernatural harm. This mix of ideas about disease causation reflects the outside influences Saraguro has experienced. The humoral theory expressed in the notion of balancing hot and cold elements in the body was likely borrowed from the Spanish colonists and is common elsewhere in Latin America as well. The availability of scientific medicine in clinics and through community nurses has given some credence to infections as a cause of illness.

Saraguros have a number of choices in health care providers. Which type of healer they choose depends on a number of cost and benefit factors. Costs include the actual financial cost of the treatment, its effect on time lost from work, and other factors, such as the embarrassment it might cause the person and the emotional distress caused by unfamiliar treatments, an unfamiliar treatment facility, or using a treatment that does not fit with the indigenous theory of the illness. Since Saraguros do not separate physical and emotional disease, using Western medical treatment, which focuses on the former, can cause much distress.

The first treatment choice for many Saraguros is the senior woman in the household. This is especially the case with children and reflects the Saraguro concern about children being harmed by supernatural forces when outside the home. In addition to members of the family who act as healers, there are other traditional healers and Western medical providers. The traditional healers are the curanderos, herbalists, and midwives.

Curanderos are magico-religious specialists who attend mainly to illness attributed to spirits or supernatural forces. As with all traditional healers, they have no formal training and their status is based on a combination of experience and reputation. Partly because they are feared and not trusted—some are considered to be witches—few Saraguros use curanderos to cure illness. In addition, the availability of Western medicine and the continuing role of women family healers makes the curanderos somewhat superfluous. Herbal healing is an important treatment modality in Saraguro, and most people have some knowledge of herbal treatments. Herbalists tend to be used when home remedies fail. Midwives, like curanderos and herbalists, are also used only sparingly, mainly by first-time mothers who need advice and perhaps assistance during childbirth.

Relatively new to Saraguro are the healers associated with scientific medicine—pharmacists, nurse practitioners, and physicians. Pharmacists provide herbal and other medications without prescriptions. Thus, they also diagnose and provide medical advice, although their primary function is to provide the drugs preferred by their clients. Nurses work at the local hospital or in neighborhood medical offices. They serve as gatekeepers in involving Saraguros in the biomedical system, often by providing such preventative care as prenatal and nutritional counseling and vaccinations to children. Physicians are affiliated mainly with the hospital. They are outsiders and male, two factors that make them undesirable as healers for Saraguro women. Thus, they are used only in emergency situations when home and community interventions fail.

AMHARA HEALTH CARE SYSTEM

The Amhara, like all cultures, attribute illnesses to a variety of causes. Most significant are the zar and ganel spirits. Both cause many diseases, including fatal ones, but both can also be communicated with by humans and, therefore, can be made to cure, or help cure, illnesses. The zar spirits work as follows:

> Zars select their victims carefully, most often choosing girls and women. Typically, their choice is signaled by the onset of stomach pain, persisting headache, and arthritic complaints, although powerful zars are capable of sending any ailment. Once selected by a zar, a host can expect the subsequent attentions of other zars. Periodically, each of these will dramatize his domination over the human partner by sickening him and demanding tribute in the form of clothes, jewelry, and specially prepared food. Zars are visible only during the dreams of their human partners; in addition they frequently speak through their hosts. From these sources, it is known that the zars have human forms and live in a bisexual and culturally pluralistic society which duplicates that of traditional Abyssinia. The means by which zars cause sickness is not known to humans, however. (Young 1971: 5)

While zars are of the supernatural world, ganels are of the human world and are similar to witches or the devil in earthly form:

> The ganel's appearance is known from scriptural references and, in addition, they are infrequently seen. When visible, the ganel appears as a tall and thin black man, Nilotic except for certain details. Descriptions by laymen are generally hearsay, since madness (*ibidet*) strikes the unprotected human who looks on a ganel; if the glance is returned, the effects are mortal. So dangerous is the ganel's person that even contact with his shadow leaves the victim stammering and given over to undefinable fear and anxiety (*ayni tila*); the ganel's shadow is sufficient to render the constitutionally frail child feeble-minded (*mun*). Although ganels in nocturnal ambush sometimes strike blows resulting in epileptic seizures or apoplexy, and although their human partners may oblige them to send almost any ailment, most ganel-caused sicknesses result from

indirect contact with their malignant persons (*likift*). (Young 1971: 6–7)

Likift is a third major explanation for disease for the Amhara. It has to do with contamination and contagion and thus is more about how than why a person becomes ill. Likift is the transformation of harmless substances into dangerous ones—ones that cause a person to become ill. Especially dangerous are substances that have been touched by a ganel, including food and water, which can lead to stomach problems, fatigue, heart problems, and rashes. Contamination leading to diseases such as ringworm are caused by contact with crawling creatures such as snakes, insects, and lizards.

While the actions of zars and ganels and the contamination of likift are three primary explanations for illness, there are others of more limited scope. Some illnesses are caused by the sun (gerifta) although only under specific circumstances:

> When, however, sunlight falls upon an unclean body part—a perspiring torso, a diner's unclean mouth, a nursing breast—or upon a body emerging naked from a togo's cool confines, gerifta threatens. . . . Even the absence of special conditions, prolonged exposure to the sun of certain body areas can produce painful body complaints, such as headache, conjunctivitis, blindness, earache, tonsillitis, and toothache. Lastly, gerifta-mists are created when sunlight falls on soil recently moistened by showers and urine. . . . Although urine-mists can cause pubic sores, more frequently, gerifta-mists are inhaled, to affect the body internally. (Young 1971: 9–10)

In addition to the supernatural and the sun, the Amhara also see physical explanations for illness, including the following:

1. The idea of contagion, that one individual can get sick by coming into contact with another individual who is already ill, as well as a fetus from its mother and hu-

mans from animals. The key element in the Amhara notion of contagion is that the human or animal spreading the disease already has it.

2. Diseases and injuries result from a poor diet, too much physical exertion, and emotions such as anger, fear, and deep sorrow, which can cause serious heart problems.

3. The association of certain illnesses with physical location—malaria in the hot region near the Sudan and wind disease in the hills.

4. Some are believed to cause others; for example, epilepsy leads to mental illness or measles leads to deafness.

The final Amhara explanation for illness focuses on the ability of humans to cause others to become ill. Those who can cause illness are sorcerers, witches, and casters of the evil eye. Sorcerers cause illness and other mishaps through spells. Witches are inherently evil and enter their victims through the victim's abdomen, proceeding to eat the internal organs and driving the victim to near-madness. Casters of the evil eye cause people to become ill when they stare at them. However, the illnesses they cause are less severe than those caused by witches. In these three types of human-induced illness, envy plays a major role and the people who become ill are often ones who are rich or who have desirable physical features such as light skin color.

This system of beliefs about the causes of disease, and misfortune in general, is quite complex. In diagnosing the cause of a specific illness, the Amhara consider five questions:

1. What agent—human or supernatural—can cause this illness?

2. Is the illness caused by a deliberate or an opportunistic action?

3. Is the illness caused by physical factors; introduced into or onto the body; the

result of assaults by ganels, of sympathetic magic, or of unknown methods such as possession by a zar?

4. Which method of causation do the symptoms of the illness indicate as a cause?

5. How does the disease progress: by devouring internal organs, by irritation, or by disrupting internal balance?

Using these factors, the cause of the disease can then be determined and a treatment selected. Four types of treatment are used:

1. Aligning the body parts so that they are in their normal positions
2. Removing certain body parts, such as the tonsils or teeth
3. Removing the causal agent from the body
4. Inducing or forcing the supernatural agent to end its influence over the sick person

Treatment is provided by some twenty-one different practitioners of traditional Amhara medicine. Other treatments are provided by physicians and health workers who practice Western medicine.

The twenty-one indigenous healers fall into three general categories based on the type of treatment used. In category one are those who treat illness by aligning body parts or by removing body parts. Their specialty is physical treatment. Category two is composed of those who heal by removing the causal agent from the body. Category three is composed of those who use magic to remove the influence of the zar and ganel spirits. The specific healers are as follows:

Category One

Tagan	bonesetter
Ankar Korac	tonsil remover
Yiters Medhaniyt Awlakiy	tooth extractor
Awalaj	midwife
Agamiy	cupper
Tokwariy	tattooer

Category Two

Medhaniyt Korac	herb gatherer
Medhaniyt Seci	herb gatherer/advisor
Medhaniyt Ateci	herb gatherer/preparer/advisor
Medhaniyt Awakiy	herbal healer

Category Three

Balazar	healer possessed by a zar
Debtera-Ganel Gelac	ganel-pulling healer
Debtera-Meshav Gelac	a weak ganel-pulling healer
Atmakiy	baptizer

In addition to these diagnostic categories, causal theories, and healers, the Amhara also make extensive use of cult healing through the zar cults, which are led by zar doctors. These specialists treat disorders associated with one zar or with a few zar spirits and their cults consist mostly of women who have been cured but remain susceptible to further attacks. A healing takes place in a group setting and involves dancing to an ecstatic state, possession of the victim and the zar doctor by the zar spirit, and the zar doctor's negotiations with the spirit to convince it to leave the sick person.

TAIWANESE HEALTH CARE SYSTEM

Of the four health care systems profiled here, the one used by the rural Taiwanese town of Chaochang is the most complex. It is comprised of Western medicine, Chinese secular medicine, Chinese sacred medicine, and home care.

Western medicine was introduced early in the twentieth century during a time of Japanese rule and is widely available and used. The villages of the town have access to ten physicians, nineteen druggists who also provide medical advice, a laboratory technician, midwives, three nearby hospitals, and over-the-counter medications sold in general stores. All Western medical providers have some formal training, with the physicians trained at Taiwan's two medical schools. There is also a government public health program and office whose main activities are providing birth control advice and methods and vaccinations for children. In addition, the four factories all provide some form of on-site medical care. In terms of treatment approach, Western medicine in rural Taiwan is firmly rooted in the scientific approach, with a strong emphasis on preventative medicine.

Secular Chinese medicine as practiced in Taiwan is similar to the system on the mainland. It dates back over 2,000 years, is supported by a long and detailed literature, and is concerned with maintaining a balance between the yin and yang forces and a harmony of the five elements (wood, fire, earth, metal, and water). The treatment core of Chinese secular medicine are the drugstore-clinics, which are run by Chinese secular doctors. A doctor examines a patient, makes a diagnosis based on the ancient Chinese medical texts, and prescribes herbal treatments, which are available in both processed and raw form in the drugstore. In addition to the doctors there are bonesetters and acupuncturists who work in the Chinese secular tradition.

Chinese sacred medicine "is an amalgamation of the concepts of China's great traditions of Taoism, Confucianism, and Buddhism, combined with folk religion, translated into practice, and expressed symbolically with ritual and everyday objects." (Gould-Martin 1983: 90) The major underlying beliefs of the system include:

1. A desire for harmony in all aspects of one's life
2. A desire for good luck and avoidance of bad luck
3. A belief that a person's fate in life is set by the hour, day, month, and year of his or her birth
4. A belief that gods, ghosts, and deceased ancestors influence the lives of the living and can cause disease or good health
5. A belief that the souls of children are not firmly fixed, making children especially vulnerable to certain types of illnesses
6. A belief that magic can be used to cause harm or to reverse harm
7. A belief that at certain stages in life certain people, such as a woman who has recently given birth, are polluting and therefore may bring harm to those who come in contact with them
8. A belief that foods can be classified as either hot or cold and that these properties affect one's health

Chinese sacred healing takes place at a number of places of religious worship—Taoist temples, cult temples dedicated to deceased ancestors, and homes—and involves a hierarchy of healers. Healing at the temples involves a Taoist priest and takes place regularly throughout each month and over the course of the ceremonial cycle during the year. The rituals, music, and prayer focus on bringing harmony to one's life and controlling fate. Other rituals center on information about one's fate obtained from fortune-tellers, restoring one's soul, driving off harmful spirits, and protecting the unborn. Rituals performed in cult temples and homes are often more specific and concern the immediate needs of the family or individual. In addition to the Taoist priests, the category of sacred healer includes mediums, fortune-tellers, and specialists who treat fright disorders of children.

In addition to these three fully developed health care systems, Taiwanese also use various forms of home care that do not require the use of healers. These include special foods that restore the balance of hot and cold in the body, secluding the mother after birth to allow her to rest, and altering the diet of sick children.

These major forms of healing form both separate health care systems and one interrelated system, as follows:

Western style medicine is similar to Chinese secular medicine; Chinese secular medicine is similar to Chinese sacred medicine. The first two have published theories and pharmacopoeia, schools for training doctors and druggists, diplomas, legal regulations, associations and lobbying groups, hospitals, clinics, drugstores, technology, pharmaceutical factories, and relations with other countries through the import and export of drugs, the travel of practitioners, and the publication of journals, advertisements, and manuals.

Chinese secular and sacred medicine share the cosmology of yin, yang, and the five elements, the food and herb classifications, many theories of disease causation and cure, and many remedies.

But Chinese sacred medicine shares virtually nothing with the Western-style medicine practiced in Taiwan. It is practiced in temples or in front of household altars with the smoke of incense, candles, and burning spirit money and the sound of chants, instrumental music, and firecrackers. The practitioners are often old, blind, and lame. Their remuneration is considered a gift, not a payment. Their equipment makes no attempt to resemble the scientific and they have no official sanction or regulation. Training is through apprenticeship or revelation. The herbs prescribed are often those growing wild by the rivers or in the mountains. And the behavior of the spirits is important in most diagnoses and treatments. (Gould-Martin 1983: 89–90)

On a practical level, the interaction among the three systems typically involves Western doctors sending patients to Chinese secular medicine doctors and druggists; Chinese secular doctors sending patients to Western doctors, hospitals, and the Public Health Service; and Chinese sacred healers sending patients to Western doctors and Chinese secular druggists. In general, the Western system is the primary system, as people routinely use it for a wide range of illnesses and also for preventative medicine. While the other systems are also used commonly, they are used mainly for illnesses that do not respond well or at all to Western medicine. These include chronic diseases, chronic pain, and minor ailments and injuries. People will also use the non-Western alternatives to speed up the results of or supplement the Western treatment they are already receiving.

An individual's decision about which treatment or combination of treatments to use is based on a number of considerations. One is the type of illness, with Western medicine favored for acute, serious illnesses. A second is cost, with Western medicine often the cheapest option. Western medicine is the cheapest because it is supported by the government, while the other systems require payments by the users. However, cost is not the most important consideration and poor people often use the more-expensive Chinese systems. Another consideration is the "entertainment value" of the various medical offerings. Western medicine is boring, while visiting a druggist, where one can gossip with others in the waiting room, or attending a festival at a temple is far more meaningful socially. A final consideration is the effectiveness of the treatment and the comfort of the treatment process. This is especially important with regard to the choice of drugs. Western drugs are considered faster-acting and are easier and cheaper to obtain. But they may irritate the stomach or have other unpleasant side effects while Chinese herbal medicines are soothing, if not as fast-acting.

MAKING HEALTH CARE CHOICES

There is a key issue facing health care providers and planners in societies with pluralistic health care systems (basically all societies in the world): How and why do people make the health care decisions they do? That is, why do they choose a particular type of treatment or type of healer from the various options available to them? Across cultures in the contemporary world, one of the choices is usually Western medicine, with the other major choice being the indigenous healing system. Some experts suggest that when people opt for indigenous health care they do so because they either do not know or do not understand that the Western approach is superior or because Western medical facilities are not readily available. The four health care systems described above as well as numerous other pluralistic systems around the world suggest that this view is wrong. The decision-making process regarding health care is complex and varies from culture to culture. The Hausa lean toward Islamic healers because of the importance of Islam in Hausa society. Saraguros prefer women healers because they prefer to keep health care in the family and community. The Amhara consider the illness, its cause, and its nature in selecting a treatment approach. And the rural Taiwanese, faced with the most choices of our four example cultures, consider a mix of factors, of which cost is not the most important.

The customary decisions people make about health care point to the major role culture plays in health care. The following are among the aspects of health care that are influenced by culture:

1. Beliefs about what is a health problem
2. Behaviors meant to deal with the problem
3. Definitions of what is a symptom
4. Ideas about the disease process
5. Definitions of what constitutes treatment and who is a healer
6. What is considered to be appropriate treatment
7. The treatment setting and locale

In all cultures, people routinely consider these factors when making health care decisions.

See also ALTERNATIVE AND COMPLEMENTARY MEDICINE; BIOMEDICINE; CHINESE MEDICINE.

Eisenberg, D. M., et al. (1993) "Unconventional Medicine in the United States: Prevalence, Costs, and Patterns of Use." *New England Journal of Medicine* 328: 246–252.

Finerman, Ruthbeth. (1989) "The Forgotten Healers: Women as Family Healers in an Andean Indian Community." In *Women as Healers: Cross-Cultural Perspectives*, edited by Carol S. McClain, 24–41.

———. (1989) "Tracing Home-Based Health Care Change in an Andean Indian Community." *Medical Anthropology Quarterly* 3: 162–174.

Gould-Martin, Emily. (1983) *Women Asking Women: An Ethnography of Health Care in Rural Taiwan.*

Nichter, Mark. (1992) *Anthropological Approaches to Ethnomedicine.*

Wall, Lewis. (1988) *Hausa Medicine: Illness and Well-Being in a West African Culture.*

Young, Allan L. (1971) *Medical Beliefs and Practices of the Begemder Amhara.*

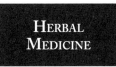

HERBAL MEDICINE

The use of plant matter in the prevention or treatment of illness or injury is a cultural universal. In all cultures and as far back in human history as we know, with the exception of some Inuit groups in the Far North who lack regular access to plants, people have used medicines made from plants to cure everything from the effects of the evil eye to headaches to broken bones. The plants, often gathered, prepared, and administered by health specialists in villages and communities, are crushed into powders or made into teas, tinctures, and poultices. Herbal medicine is a large part of major medical systems such as Ayurvedic, Chinese, and homeopathic medicine and although we often think of herbal medicine as a treatment approach outside modern, scientific medicine, between 60 and 70 percent of all drugs are derived from plant material.

In Western medicine, until the nineteenth century most drugs were composed of whole plant materials and taken orally or made into compresses or healing baths. In 1803, a German pharmacist succeeded in separating one of the active elements of a plant—morphine from opium—and suddenly the focus in medicine shifted from using the whole plant in healing to using an isolated, active component. While this was a dramatic change in Western medicine, knowledge of the healing properties of thousands of plant components had already been known for hundreds or even thousands of years in many traditional cultures around the world. Part of the reason for this shift in Western medicine was that many plants have a number of different active chemical properties and it was believed that by separating them out, medicines would be more effective and specific. But the overwhelming number of side effects (toxicity) that occur from such drugs point to the negative side of isolating one part of the plant. Advocates of herbal medicine argue that there is a natural balance of substances in a whole plant that is destroyed when the individual elements are isolated. Isolating one element and administering it in high doses may make it more effective but also potentially harmful.

Which is not to say that herbal remedies are never toxic. Some plants are harmful, even fatal, to humans. One can imagine the poor patients involved in the trial and error of discovery of some herbal remedies. It was an inexact process—the patient never knew with certainty what was being administered and doses were often determined by the healer's intuition. But many cures that were passed off as "old wives' tales" turned out to provide the basis for modern drugs. One such drug is digoxin, a modern heart disease medicine. In eighteenth-century England, Dr. William Withering's heart patients started thriving, seemingly out of the blue. He discovered that they were being treated by a village curer with the herb foxglove. The active ingredient, later isolated and administered in high doses, was digoxin.

HERBAL MEDICINE IN WESTERN CULTURES

Although herbal medicine plays a role in scientific medicine, in many Western cultures it also stands alone as a medical system, used both for the prevention and treatment of illness and injury. Adherents of herbal medicine view it as a holistic approach that reflects the fact that human beings are part of nature and should trust nature. Although components of plants may be used, the emphasis is on the use of whole plants, or major parts such as the leaves, stalks, or bark. Such use rests on the belief that the effect of the sum of a plant's parts is greater than the effect of any single part and that, therefore, medicines using the entire plant will be more effective. For this reason, the scientific approach of isolating pharmacologically active chemical components is rejected as being less effective and as causing harmful chemical side effects. Herbalists also recognize that some plants or parts are harmful to humans and this knowledge guides which plants are used and how they are used.

As is the practice in both major non-Western medical systems and traditional cultures, herbal medicines in Western cultures are prepared and used in a number of ways: tinctures, baths, inhalants, ointments, moist dressings, dry compresses, and consumed as teas and vegetables and in juices and salads. They are used in prevention (cleanse the blood, prevent infection, reduce stress, stimulate the heart) and in the treatment of both symptoms and specific disorders. The selection, gathering, and preparation of herbs is an important component of an herbalist's practice. Here are one internationally known herbalist's directions for picking and drying herbs:

> Flowering stems and leaves should be picked as soon as the dew has evaporated. Flowers such as hawthorne should be gathered while they are still like young maidens, before they have bloomed into maturity. This is very important: the flowers of the common broom, one of our best diuretics, can cause gastric disturbances if they have been picked while they are turning into pods. . . .
>
> Many plants are best gathered in the summer solstice, around midsummer day, as our forefathers knew. The weather should be neither too damp nor too dry. Roots must first have all soil removed, then be quickly washed and brushed before drying. The actual drying of the plants is of prime importance, for on this depends the extent to which plants retain their effectiveness. It is all a question of touch. Plants should neither be too dry nor too fresh and never completely dehydrated. The initial drying should be done in the shade, never in the sun, in a well-ventilated but never a draughty spot, away from insects, and the plants should be spread out on a sheet, and turned at frequent intervals. After this, they can be "finished," an operation for which a sieve is ideal, since it allows air to circulate freely. The most usual method, however, is to hang the plants in little bundles, heads down, inside the house. . . . The dry herbs should be stored out of the light, for light draws the color and some of the goodness out of them. (Messegue 1973: 108)

Western herbal medicine ranges from what is often considered backwoods folk medicine to self-healing to mainstream acceptance. One famous French healer, Maurice Messegue, has gone to court many times to defend his practice of his family's traditional occupation. Messegue's successes, particularly where orthodox approaches have failed, gained him a reputation that included treating European heads of state. He has tried to legitimize the use of unorthodox healing, giving himself the title phylotherapist.

The modern herbalist usually takes a medical history from the patient. He or she may take a diagnosis from a medical doctor and then do an independent assessment by examining certain parts of the body. Dowsing, the use of a pendulum suspended over the body to identify areas in need of healing is also still used by some herbalists. It is believed that diagnosis can be aided by the quality and speed of the vibration created.

Some herbalists trained in Chinese or Ayurvedic medicine may use pulse diagnosis, and intuition is an important element in the health assessment. Some herbalists "dowse" the remedies, while remaining in physical contact with the patient, to determine an appropriate dosage of a particular remedy.

As elsewhere, herbal medicine in the West is used both to prevent illness and maintain well-being and to treat specific problems. Two examples from the practice of Rosemary Gladstar Slick, an herbal healer and teacher, indicate the uses of herbs in prevention and healing. To maintain well-being during the cold winter months, Slick suggests cold water baths; appropriate clothing; regular exercise; a diet rich in specific plants such as rosehips, root crops, peppers, and citrus fruits that provide ample amounts of vitamins and minerals; and herbal teas to maintain the respiratory and immune systems. For specific health problems that occur commonly in winter such as influenza, sore throats, and colds specific herbal remedies are suggested. The treatment regimen for a head cold is as follows:

> A good head cold, as far as I'm concerned, is one of the worst miseries. Treat it early to avoid the awful symptoms.
> A. Avoid all mucous forming foods: bread, dairy products, sweets.
> B. Take Golden Seal Capsules; 2 capsules every 2 hours.
> C. Take Immunity Tincture; ½ tsp in warm water every hour.
> D. Horseradish; fresh grated horseradish is one of the best specific remedies for

head colds. Store bought horseradish is not as strong as that you grate yourself. When you make it yourself, it's so strong it makes your eyes water. It's almost painful to eat but it will clear your sinuses. Eat on toast, with soup, or on rice.

E. Herbal Decongesting Steams. Place a drop or two of pure essential oil(s) into a large pot of boiling water. Remove from heat. Place a large towel over your head and the pot and breathe in deeply for 10 minutes. Do this 2–3 times daily until sinus cold is gone. Select one or two of the following oils: Eucalyptus, Sage, Pine.

F. Golden Seal and/or Salt Snorts. See under ear infections. (Slick n.d.(2): 7)

In addition to being used to treat specific illnesses and maintain general health, herbs are also often used to maintain particular body systems, such as the immune system, circulatory system, and nervous system. For example, Slick recommends a category of herbs called Herbal Nervines that should be taken to maintain the nervous system and thereby prevent or minimize problems such as headaches, insomnia, depression, and pain. There are four types of herbal nervines. Nerve tonics such as chamomile and hops strengthen the nervous system. Sedatives such as catnip and lemon balm soothe and relax the nervous system. Demulcents such as comfrey root and flaxseed heal inflamed nerves. And stimulants such as peppermint and ginseng activate the nervous system.

Herbal remedies are now sold over the counter in supermarkets and drugstores as well as natural food stores. Administering these medicines to oneself, harmless as some of them may be, is not recommended. Over-the-counter herbal preparations are not subject to the same scrutiny as are prescription drugs. The Dietary Supplement and Health Education Act of 1994 includes herbal preparations in a list of supplements that do not need to be tested for safety or efficacy or to meet any kind of independent standards. An herbalist has the experience needed with both plant preparations and illnesses to administer the medicines properly. Herbalists usually mix remedies themselves from herbal extracts, custom mixing them to meet the needs of their patients.

In the United States, licensing for herbal healers varies from state to state. Some license only naturopathic doctors to prescribe herbal remedies. Some practitioners call themselves "botanical consultants" and are not licensed medically. The resistance that many medical doctors had when the resurgence of interest in herbal remedies arose in the 1960s and 1970s has been replaced with cooperation in many cases, particularly when scientific medicine has not been successful and herbal medicine has. Herbalists report referrals from medical doctors whose attempts at healing have been unsuccessful. In England, since 1986 herbalists may write prescriptions.

Practitioners in the United States order herbs from a number of distributors that are regulated by government agencies like the Food and Drug Administration. Master herbalist Mark William McDermott of Connecticut says that it is important to remember that herbs are foods. What heals is their nutritional value and the strength that they give to the body naturally.

In the United States, Native Americans continue to practice traditional herbal healing. Sometimes they work with local physicians in government health centers and hospitals. They believe that nature is sacred and give offerings whenever a plant is taken—acknowledging the gift they are receiving. Though the technique of identifying and preparing herbs is passed down from elder to younger, usually the healer must feel a calling or intuitive relationship to the plants. Illnesses and accidents are often seen, as in Chinese traditional medicine, as a deviation from the natural path of health. Thus, other healing powers are often invoked to complement the actual plants. In addition, remedies are used by ordinary people at home.

Descendants of the first white settlers of North America have continued the tradition of using herbs, particularly in rural areas of the United States. In the mountains of Appalachia, goldenrod is used for coughs and colds. Boneset is for fever and flu, pokeroot for rheumatism, catnip tea for babies, and horehound for kidneys. Sassafras gives energy. One American researcher of folklore queried listeners of a radio show in the 1970s about herbal remedies. He asked them to send in home remedies made from plants or natural sources. He received replies from all fifty states, an indication of the broad appeal of herbal remedies. During the 1960s, a high school project researching the folk traditions of Appalachia resulted in a series of *Foxfire* books. They provide recipes and home remedies like taking blackberry juice for diarrhea and placing a spiderweb across a wound to speed its healing. Coughs and sore throats are cured with honey and vinegar. The students also added some nonherbal folk wisdom—curing cramps could supposedly be accomplished by simply turning one's shoes upside down before going to bed.

In the early 1950s, a Vermont doctor named DeForest Clinton Jarvis experimented with natural remedies. In his *Folk Medicine,* published in 1958, he claimed that the body's need for vitamins and minerals could be met by eating common plants such as dandelion, anise, catnip, and peppermint. He recognized the value of kelp, a seaweed, and caster oil for moles, warts, and skin ulcers. Some other treatments include using sap from a pine tree for boils and a plaster of ground dog bones for fractures.

HERBALISM IN MAJOR, NON-WESTERN MEDICAL SYSTEMS

In major, non-Western medical systems herbs are used to restore the body's vital energy so that the body's own healing capabilities can be activated. It is a holistic approach similar to the concept of balancing chi in Chinese medicine. In Ayurvedic, or ancient Indian, medicine it is called the balancing of the doshas. Solutions may be sought in the physical, emotional, or spiritual realm, and restoration of harmony and balance is the goal. Messegue's guiding principle—"Treat the patient, rather than the disease"—applies to the uses of herbs in most medical systems. Studies indicate that animals instinctively eat healing herbs if wounded, and somehow know enough to stay away from toxic ones. Some experts argue that humans have the same intuitive abilities.

Herbal healing has ancient roots: fifteen Sumerian prescriptions were inscribed in cuneiform characters over 4,000 years ago in what is now southern Iraq. Most of the ingredients came from trees and plants, but some came from animals as well, and they were mixed into solutions with water, wine, milk, and beer. Five hundred years later a scroll sixty-six feet long, written in Egyptian hieratic script, included more than 800 medical recipes, along with incantations and spells.

In the first century A.D., a Roman named Pedanius Dioscorides wrote a five-volume work called *De Universa Medicina,* which includes thousands of plant, animal, and mineral ingredients. The ancient Greek, Hippocrates, whose oath all modern U.S. physicians take, was an herbal practitioner.

Pen Ts'ao Kung-mu is a fifty-two-volume encyclopedia, compiled in sixteenth-century China, that lists natural plant and animal substances that had been used for centuries for healing. Its roots are believed to be with a legendary god of farming, Shen Nung, in 3000 B.C. Healing with herbs constitutes about 85 percent of the traditional Chinese medicine used in China. The Chinese use the concept of opposites in their healing with herbs. Everything in the universe is classified as either yin (cold, female, expansive) or yang (hot, male, contracting). This includes plants and herbs, which are administered in hopes of balancing the vital energy, or chi, which is composed of yin and yang energies. Some healing plants from Asia, like ginseng, are used for many types of illnesses and have diffused to other parts of the world.

In Indian Ayurvedic medicine, balance is also the aim of herbal healing, but Indian healers use the concept of balancing the doshas—the three metabolic principles that exist in the body. The doshas reflect qualities such as cold, hot, sticky, dry, moist, heavy, light. Foods and herbs are classified according to the system and are used to balance out the doshas.

HERBALISM IN TRADITIONAL HEALING

As noted above, herbal medicine is a cultural universal and remains a major element of many traditional healing systems. People in traditional cultures around the world use tens of thousands of different plants to maintain health and cure illness. A survey of the use of plants for medical purposes by Native Americans shows that some 2,397 plants were used for 17,634 medicinal purposes. Of these plants, twenty-three families include species that account for 55 percent of the medicinal plants. These are Aceraceae, Apiaceae, Araceae, Araliaceae, Asclepiadaceae, Asteracae, Berberidaceae, Caprifoliaceae, Corylaceae, Cupressaceae, Ericaceae, Fagaceae, Lamiaceae, Liliaceae, Pinaceae, Polygonaceae, Polypodiaceae, Pyrolaceae, Ranunculaceae, Rosaceae, Salicaceae, Saxifragaceae, and Solanaceae.

An interesting feature of this list of plant families is that while they include 55 percent of plants used medicinally, they include only 37 percent of plant species in North America. This differential in availability versus use is related to the question of why traditional peoples use certain plants in healing and how they learn that they are effective. As the above percentages suggest, availability alone does not insure that a plant will be used in healing. Two other factors that

people consider when using a plant for healing are the qualities of the plant and whether or not it has observable effects thought to cause healing. Across cultures, a plant's taste, smell, color, size, shape, and texture are all considered and, in some cultures, people also consider certain qualities of the plant as they relate to ideas about disease and healing. For example, in cultures where disease is attributed to an imbalance of hot and cold qualities in the body, plants will be used because they are either hot or cold in order to restore a balance. The physical effects of the use of a plant are also considered by people in many cultures when they judge a plant's healing effectiveness. For example, in many cultures people believe that whatever agent is causing an illness must be forced to leave the body. Thus plants that cause sweating, salivating, or vomiting are considered healing because they can help flush the disease out of the body.

A question related to what plants people choose is how they determine that a plant actually has healing qualities. Evidently, throughout human history people have used trial and error to make this determination. Because the harmful effects of a poisonous plant can appear quite suddenly and dramatically, only a few trials are needed to eliminate those plants that are harmful. In making this decision, people must also decide what parts of a plant are beneficial and which are harmful or of no use. For example, apple flesh is seen in American culture as medicinally useful, while the seeds, leaves, wood, and bark are not eaten.

Variation in the use of plants across cultures for healing has to do not with whether herbal medicine is used or not but rather with issues such as how important it is, the types of healers involved, and what it is used for. Among the Zulu of South Africa, some 225 plants are used, along with animal matter and inert matter, for medicines to ward off evil and thereby prevent illness or misfortune. The Zulu recognize six categories of these medicines:

amaKhubalo	to fortify oneself against evil
imiKhando	to destroy the power of others
imBhuelo	to cause disease to others
izinTelezi	to ward off evil
izimPundu	to confuse an evil doer
izinGqunda	to lessen the harm of evil

The Zulu distinguish among medicines made from herbs and roots—*amaKhambji* (green medicines)—and those made from other substances (black and white medicines).

For the Amhara of Ethiopia, herbal medicine is a component of their highly complex indigenous medical system. Herbs are used to treat anxiety, bleeding, sores, scabies, stomach pain, tapeworm, smallpox, leprosy, infected cuts, rashes, headaches, coughing, and spirit possession. Herbs are believed to work by removing the cause of the illness from the body and thus are usually ingested and used as diuretics or emetics. The effectiveness of any herb is based on a combination of the strength of its active ingredient and whether the techniques used to gather, process, and administer it maintain its healing power. The Amhara recognize twenty-seven types of medical practitioners, five of them herbalists, who are categorized on the basis of the types and completeness of techniques used:

medhaniyt seci	gatherer of herbs who supplies them to patients
medhaniyt ateci	one who administers processed herbs as an infusion
medhaniyt awakiy	a medical expert who provides the full range of herbal treatments
medhaniyt korac	professional medicine gatherer
kitab kitabiy	maker of herbal amulets

Which type of healer a person selects is based on the ailment to be treated, the reputation of a specific healer, and the ability of the patient to pay.

As suggested by the use of herbs among the Zulu and Amhara, in many traditional cultures herbal medicine is used to ward off or reverse the work of evil spirits who cause illness. For example, among the Ashanti of West Africa, healers use herbs in a number of ways to deal with evil spirits. The Ashanti believe that "everything works by spirit on spirit." Thus, in curing an illness, the healer uses a specific herb for a specific disease not because of the medicinal properties of the herb but because the herb has a more powerful spirit than the spirit that caused the illness. The Ashanti also use herbs to divine the causes of illnesses and learn their cure. A priest or herbalist uses an herb mixed in water as a dip for some other object, which is then touched to the patient's shoulder in order to communicate with the patient's spirit, which communicates to the practitioner what has made it angry and what offering is needed to reverse the illness.

See also ALTERNATIVE AND COMPLEMENTARY MEDICINE; CHINESE MEDICINE; DIET AND NUTRITION; HEALTH CARE SYSTEMS.

Ackman, Lonnelle. (1977) *Nature's Healing Arts: From Folk Medicine to Modern Drugs.*

Bryant, Alfred T. (1966) *Zulu Medicine and Medicine-Men.*

Christensen, James B. (1952) *Double Descent among the Fanti.*

DeWaal, M. (1980) *Medicinal Herbs in the Bible.*

Etkin, Nina L. (1990) "Ethnopharmacology: Biological and Behavioral Perspectives in the Study of Indigenous Medicines." In *Medical Anthropology: A Handbook of Theory and Method*, edited by Thomas M. Johnson and Carolyn F. Sargent, 149–158.

Hill, Ann, ed. (1979) *A Visual Encyclopedia of Unconventional Medicine: A Health Manual for the Whole Person.*

Mairesse, Michelle. (1981) *Health Secrets of Medicinal Herbs.*

Messegue, Maurice. (1973) *Of Men and Plants.*

Moerman, Daniel. (1986) *Medicinal Plants of Native America.* 2 vols.

Rattray, R. S. (1927) *Religion and Art in Ashanti.*

Santillo, Humbart. (1984) *Natural Healing with Herbs.*

Slick, Rosemary Gladstar. (n.d.) *Herbs for the Nervous System.*

———. (n.d.) *Herbs for Winter Health.*

Theiss, Barbara, and Peter Theiss. (1989) *The Family Herbal.*

Weil, Andrew. (1983) *Health and Healing: Understanding Conventional and Alternative Medicine.*

Weiss, Gaea, and Shandor Weiss. (1992) *Growing & Using the Healing Herbs.*

Woodham, Anne. (1994) *HEA Guide to Complementary Medicine and Therapies.*

Young, Allan L. (1971) *Medical Beliefs and Practices of the Begemder Amhara.*

HOLISTIC HEALTH AND HEALING

Holism emphasizes the organic or functional relationship between parts and wholes. A holistic concept of health, then, sees health as the result of the proper functioning and integration of all components of the human being, with body, mind, and spirit working together as a harmonious unit. In addition, there is a synergistic dividend: when all of the parts are functioning optimally, a feeling of wholeness, or wellness results. Deviation from this state of harmonious balance creates opportunities for accident, illness, and disease.

A second important element of holistic health is the relationship of the human being to nature. Holistic cures are almost exclusively natural cures, because the breakdown of vital energy through analysis or processing of a natural substance is believed to render a cure less effective in most holistic approaches. In most cases, holistic healing is the application of the wholesomeness of nature to a body that is out of balance or, in disease, the stimulation of the body's inherent healing ability, thus restoring it to wholeness and balance.

In Chinese and Indian medical systems, as well as in the beliefs underlying Western naturopathy, homeopathic medicine, and anthroposophical medicine, health is conceptualized as a state of balance acted upon by natural, psychological, and spiritual forces. When one of these forces pushes the person out of the state of well-being, whether on a physical, emotional, or spiritual level, disease may result. Such a force may be the result of an accident or an injury, lack of balance in work or family responsibilities that creates stress and tension in the body, repressed emotional or spiritual disease, and so on. These forces are seen as compromising the immune system, the body's own natural defense against infection and disease.

Most holistic therapies attempt to restore this lost balance of health by stimulating the body's own natural healing abilities. Instead of attacking and destroying the agent of disease or suppressing the symptoms, the typical approach in scientific medicine, restoring the body's integrity and ability to fight disease itself is primary.

Key to this approach is the belief that health or wholeness or wellness is the result of the sum of the workings of all the parts. There is an invisible "state" where health resides, called the balancing morphogenic field by healer Barbara Brennan and the quantum body by Deepak Chopra and described by the union of opposites in Chinese medicine, the yin and yang. This state is rarely continuously maintained by anyone and hard to achieve with conventional medicine alone. The holistic approach is often contrasted with that of scientific medicine in which surgery, drugs, and other invasive methods are used to attack an invading toxic agent and destroy it. While these methods restore functioning to the body, proponents of a holistic approach argue that they do not necessarily produce overall well being or health.

HOLISTIC APPROACHES

The holistic approach is the basis or a component of many approaches to healing that are classified as alternative or complementary.

For example, many people are exposed to influenza viruses during any given winter, and some develop influenza. In treating the flu, various holistic approaches may differ in their specific methods, but all focus on the entire human being and restoring balance to the system, as indicated by the following examples.

A homeopathic physician examines the patient and takes a detailed history of diet and lifestyle to develop a profile of the patient. Even emotional and psychological traits are examined. The homeopathic remedies, which were developed over many years by homeopathy's founder, Samuel Hahnemann, are specific to a profile of symptoms, rather than specific to one disease, like the flu. The remedies are tremendously distilled, naturally occurring substances that actually cause those same symptoms in a healthy person. The theory is that the imprint of the substance will stimulate the body's immune system into fighting off the cause of the imbalance.

A Chinese physician might prescribe herbal remedies, foods that counteract the flu, or acupuncture to revive the ailing life force of the patient. In the system of energy meridians used by the Chinese, certain points help stimulate the life force, or chi, back into balance, creating the conditions for healing many complaints. These points, which exist throughout the body, are stimulated using very thin needles or burning herbs.

A naturopath might recommend certain vitamins to boost the immune system, and a change of diet or fast to strengthen the system. Herbs might also be recommended, and hot baths to sweat out the illness. Rest would be an important recommendation. If the flu was recurrent, the naturopath might look for more systemic problems, like food allergies, that might be a contributing factor to ill health.

An anthroposophical physician might ask a patient to consider why they are vulnerable to illness at this time in their lives. Is there an emotional or spiritual matter of consequence that is seeking resolution? Does the patient need to be "stopped" by illness in order to solve this problem? Assistance in solving these questions is given, as well as homeopathic diagnosis and remedies if appropriate.

If stress and over-stimulation is making a person vulnerable to the flu, a mind/body healer might suggest meditation and biofeedback to calm and center the individual. Affirmations like "My immune system is strong and vital" might be suggested, as well as visualizations like the white blood cells surrounding the virus and consuming it.

A holistic nutritionist might recommend the elimination of dairy products (which are mucous-producing), more fruits and vegetables, or even a fast to rest the digestive system.

A Reiki or Therapeutic Touch practitioner would lay hands on the client in an attempt to relax and rejuvenate the person. The belief is that divine energy courses through the hands of the practitioner and is directed through intuition and experience to where it is needed by the patient.

A faith healer would pray to the gods or God for the healing of the individual, and in some cases would also lay hands on the recipient.

A polarity therapist would use the hands and knowledge of the body's energy field to rebalance the body's energy. This rebalancing strengthens the body's ability to ward off illness. Dietary recommendations might also be made.

An aromatherapist might use aromatic oils known to be antiseptic and to strengthen the system in a steam bath, or recommend that the patient inhale them nightly.

The beliefs underlying these and other holistic approaches run counter to one of the basic assumptions of Western philosophy—that the body and mind are separate and the body is not a source of wisdom or knowledge. The body-centered holistic therapies take the opposite view; they see the body as a source of knowledge of health for the individual and seek to cultivate it. For this reason, body-centered and other holistic mediums are often not accepted in Western medicine.

See also ACUPUNCTURE; ALTERNATIVE AND COMPLEMENTARY MEDICINE; ANTHROPOSOPHICAL MEDICINE; AROMATHERAPY; AYURVEDIC MEDICINE; CHINESE MEDICINE; FAITH HEALING; HOMEOPATHIC MEDICINE.

Brennan, Barbara Ann. (1988) *Hands of Light: A Guide to Healing through the Human Energy Field.*

Chopra, Deepak. (1991) *Perfect Health: The Complete Mind/Body Guide.*

Gottlieb, Bill, ed. (1995) *New Choices in Natural Healing.*

Hill, Ann, ed. (1979) *A Visual Encyclopedia of Unconventional Medicine: A Health Manual for the Whole Person.*

Hulke, Malcolm, ed. (1979) *The Encyclopedia of Alternative Medicine and Self-Help.*

Olsen, Kristin G. (1989) *The Encyclopedia of Alternative Health Care.*

Weil, Andrew. (1983) *Health and Healing: Understanding Conventional and Alternative Medicine.*

HOMEOPATHIC MEDICINE

The development of homeopathic medicine or homeopathy, which is translated from the Greek as "same suffering," but more accurately means "like cures like," coincides with the rise of what is now called allopathic, orthodox, scientific, or Western medicine, or simply biomedicine. In the early days of Western medicine in the United States and Europe, there were some questionable practices in use. Between 1780 and 1850, heroic medicine was the standard medical treatment. Venesection, or bloodletting, and the administration of high doses of anesthetics and purgatives like calomel were the standard practices of the day. George Washington died after complaining of a sore throat and losing almost two quarts of blood to venesection. Medicine was not the respected profession that it is today, and journalists of the time continually poked fun at the medical profession through editorials and cartoons, which claimed that it killed more people than it healed. Though orthodox medicine sought to eliminate the inexactness of folk remedies and herbalism, the natural cures remained popular and their use continued. Uneducated practitioners like Samuel Thompson maintained that natural remedies were superior to heroic medicine. He had success with herbs and heat-inducing treatments, much to the chagrin of the "scientific" doctors.

Into this mix, in the late eighteenth century, came Samuel Hahnemann, a trained German physician who was dissatisfied with the results of conventional medicine. His approach was similar to Thompson's in that he stressed noninvasive techniques and prescribed exercise, good diet, and clean air. He was similar to the scientific physicians in that he was interested in studying the precise effects of drugs on the human body. As with the rest of medicine, pharmacology was not held in high esteem because of the lack of standard preparation. Hahnemann sought to remedy this.

His first order of business was to determine the actual effects of drugs by taking them himself and noting the symptoms they caused. He started with a remedy for fever, cinchona, also called Jesuit's bark. His symptoms were a quickening of his pulse, coldness of the extremities, and fever. When he stopped using the drug, the symptoms disappeared. This experiment became the basis of homeopathic medicine—the law of similars. It states that disease (in this case fever) could be cured using drugs that caused the same symptoms in a healthy person. In short, "like cures like."

Hahnemann continued his investigation into other drugs, using a variety of people and medications. These experiments, which used healthy people, were called "provings." Experimental provings continued for the next 150 years of homeopathic medicine. In 1810, he published his most important work, *The Organon of Homeopathic Medicine.* Hahnemann's provings became the basis for a catalog of remedies called *Materia Medica Pura*, printed in 1811.

Hahnemann's explanation of how the law of similars works is that the drug creates an artificial form of the same illness that stimulated the body's defense system or what he called "vital powers" into action. The homeopathic dose engaged the spiritual aspect of the person into causing material change in the form of healing. This explanation suggests homeopathy's holistic approach. The homeopathic physician operates from the belief that the body is constantly striving for balance or health. The "vital force," which can be compared to the concepts of chi and prana in the philosophical-medical systems of China and India, respectively, is the guiding intelligence that keeps the body "on track." Homeopathy is similar to herbalism, another holistic approach, in that it stimulates the body's own healing properties. The body is seen as a group of interdependent parts, and the person is treated as a whole. As we discuss below, the patient's overall condition, including the emotional and spiritual

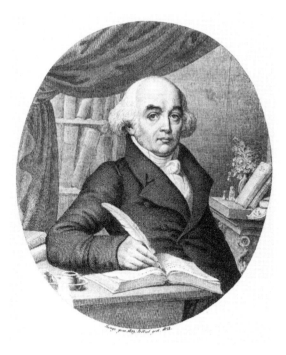

German physician Samuel Hahnemann (1755-1843), founder of homeopathic medicine, in about 1805.

as well as the physical, is considered in a homeopath's diagnosis.

Homeopathy rose in popularity during the early nineteenth century. Its reputation solidified after it appeared to cure many more people during the cholera epidemic of the 1830s than did heroic medicine. A thousand doctors and laymen created a homeopathic society, and a college was formed in Cleveland in 1850. Most homeopaths were trained physicians who "converted." Hahnemann actually coined the term "allopath" after declaring that orthodox physicians prescribed according to neither the law of similars nor the law of contraries (prescribing drugs contrary to the symptoms), but according to "allos," meaning "other basis of prescription." In 1890 there were 14,000 homeopaths in the United States, compared to 100,000 conventional physicians. There were 22 homeopathic medical schools and over 100 hospitals that dispensed homeopathic medicine.

But the spiritual explanation of the effectiveness of homeopathy became a part of its downfall as orthodox doctors feared homeopathy's competition and began to ridicule its premises. In addition to the law of similars, Hahnemann had developed the law of infinitesimals, which states that the smaller the dose, the more effective the treatment in stimulating the body's vital forces. The doses became so small as to be undetectable by chemical analysis. The following is a description of the preparation of homeopathic remedies.

Using the law of potentization, a remedy is prepared by successive dilutions and shaking (succussion):

- A tincture is prepared by soaking the plant (most homeopathic remedies come from plant sources, some from mineral sources) in a mixture of alcohol and water for a prescribed amount of time.
- One part of the tincture is diluted in 99 parts of alcohol and water and shaken vigorously for a prescribed amount of time. This becomes a "1" potency.
- One part of this mixture is mixed and succussed with 99 parts of alcohol and water, resulting in a "2" potency.

The process continues, with some plants reaching up to 1,000 parts. There are two ranges of potency—the one to ten or "X" potency and the one to one hundred or "C" potency. A few "M" potencies are diluted 1 to 1,000 parts. Home remedies are made up to a 30 times dilution.

The remedy may be made into easily taken globules by dropping the remedy onto lactose globules, or the tincture may be mixed with other ingredients to create lotions or ointments. In the case of an insoluble medicinal substance, one part of the substance is ground together with 99 parts of an inert substance like lactose. Two globules equals one or two grains of remedy and can be repeated by a patient three to four times with two to six hours between doses. The dose is cut in half for children. The standard pharmaceutical texts are *The American Homeopathic Pharmacopoeia* (1928) and J. H. Clark's *Dictionary of Materia Medica.*

The lesser dilutions are known as the low potencies, and the greater dilutions as high potencies. Homeopaths believe that the effect of shaking the remedy releases the vital force and the subtle energies of the remedy, so that each successive shaking increases the potency. This quote from a newspaper report in 1954 describes one possibility: "The power of the solution does not depend solely on the degree of dilution but on a special progressive method in its preparation; the energy latent in the drug is apparently liberated and increased by a forceful shaking of the liquid at each stage of the process." (Panos and Heimlick 1980: 13) The doses are so small there is virtually no toxicity and, therefore, no noxious side effects.

In addition to the potentized remedies, biochemics, or tissue salts, are also prescribed. Described as low-potency mineral preparations, they were developed in the nineteenth century and are used to help restore inner balance.

Aside from the issue of actual successes in healing, the law of infinitesimals provided ammunition in the orthodox physician's fight against homeopathy. From 1840 to 1870 a series of punitive measures were taken by orthodox physicians to limit the practice of homeopathy. It started in 1842, with physician, poet, and medical educator Oliver Wendell Holmes's lecture "Homeopathy, and the Kindred Delusions." He compared the successes of homeopathy to superstition and faith healing and doubted that all of the people cured by homeopathy were sick to begin with. He said that although no harm might come from the mild homeopathic remedies, the real harm came from the truly sick not seeking the cures of orthodox "scientific" medicine. He therefore placed homeopathy in the ranks of quackery.

Part of the effect of the popularity of homeopathy was to strengthen orthodox medicine, and improvements in medical education and research were made as a result. Physicians organized the American Medical Association and by the 1870s had purged homeopaths from their ranks. Though this was reversed somewhat in the 1880s and 1890s, the result was polarization. Although homeopathy continued, so did the battle with orthodox medicine. So many advances and improvements were made in orthodox medicine that homeopathy lost ground in the 1920s. Though it never died out completely, and has experienced a resurgence with the increased interest in holistic health since 1960, it never gained a firm institutional footing again. Today, there are no national standards for practicing homeopathic medicine. Some physicians adopt it as a specialty and may attend a homeopathic school or simply take courses or seminars and do self-study. In Massachusetts, any physician can dispense homeopathic medicine—in fact any type of healing professional may do so. Some other states have licensing for homeopathic medicine. In Europe homeopathy is more widespread and accepted.

Disease is not seen as an "entity" in itself by homeopaths. Instead of identifying the invading germs and destroying them with powerful drugs, homeopathy aims to strengthen the body's own natural defenses. Patients are treated according to symptoms, but symptoms are to be supported rather than stopped. It is opposite from the orthodox view that symptoms are manifestations of the disease. Symptoms are seen as important parts of the body's defense: coughs clear the mucus that blocks the respiratory tract; mucous surrounds and carries off irritating material; and fever heats up the body to kill off viruses.

HOMEOPATHIC TREATMENT

Homeopathic diagnosis is a process of identifying, categorizing, and analyzing symptoms. It begins with careful case-taking. The physician may spend an hour or more with a new patient, seeking information on the mental, emotional, and physical conditions of the patient. Success depends on the closest match of the patient's symptoms with that of the remedy, so great attention is paid. "A close doctor-patient relationship is essential to homeopathy. We treat the patient, not the disease, which means getting to know every patient as an individual— knowing that person's feelings, thoughts and family situation. You can describe this approach as either 'holistic' or a return to the old-fashioned family doctor." (Panos and Heimlick 1980: 31) X rays and laboratory tests may be used, but less frequently than in scientific medicine because the belief is that the symptoms indicate an alteration of the vital force before any change is seen in blood or tissues. Treating on the basis of the symptoms may head off a disease.

A sample case-taking is as follows:

Mr. R., aged 42

Complaint
This man, who was an engineer and worked with synthetic oils, came complaining of a rash on his hands and feet for 4 months, following domestic upset. He had also been off work for 9 months, his palms and soles were covered with small itchy blisters which burst and wept moisture. He had been using steroid creams and taking diazepam.

Past history
Nil

Family history
Wife under psychiatric care—she had been running up debts.
One daughter.

Social history
Smokes 40 per day. Drinks some beer. Plays tennis and badminton.

Homeopathic history

Generals
Heat: cold.
Appetite: good.
Desires: pickles, salt, sweet, some fat, cheese, eggs.
Sleep: good.
Other systems: nil.

Mentals
Worries.
Irritable—slow to reach a temper.
A bit self-conscious, upset in anticipation.
Tidy and exact.
Likes to be busy, frustrated at being off work.
Can be a bit emotional.

A tall grey-haired man.

A chilly patient, with liking for tasty, salty foods, tidy in his habits, but irritable and frustrated.

Nux Vomica 30c was prescribed.

Within 10 days his feet were improved and his palms less moist and not so itchy. He was keen to get back to work. Within a month his hands were almost clear and he had started a clerical job. (Boyd 1981: 42–3).

Generals represent an overall picture of the symptoms affecting the entire body and, thus, the first suggestion of the remedy. Since, from the beginning, homeopathy stressed the significance of mental and emotional state in determining health or illness, *Mentals* ties remedies to psychological symptoms. Physical characteristics, food cravings, and sleep patterns have been observed by homeopathic researchers to bear a relationship to certain remedies as well.

The modalities of a symptom are factors that aggravate or improve each symptom. The patient's wife's mental illness is called a contributing cause. All of this information is analyzed, and a homeopathic medicine chosen that best suits the illness.

In this case, nux vomica was chosen. Here is the description of the remedy from *Materia Medica*:

Persons of anxious, zealous, fiery temperament, offended at the harmless word or malicious and IRRITABLE, with anger and violence or desire to kill. They hate contradiction, are troubled by little things, must attend to details, fastidious. Cannot sleep as business affairs crowd upon them. May fall asleep after 3 a.m., and wake with bad taste and headache. They worry over others, and may be sullen and quiet and averse to doing things. It is a remedy for indiscretion of eating or drinking or overdoing things, work, stress.

Generals

Chilly persons, worse in dry or windy weather, from draughts and dislikes stuffy atmosphere.

Burning heat with red face in fever but cannot move or uncover without feeling chilly.

Sensitive to smells, noise, pain. . . .

Gastrointestinal

Desire for tasty food, fat, rich food which upsets. . . . (Boyd 1981: 23)

Remedies are usually given one at a time so that symptoms are not confused. They should be kept away from strong light, which can decrease potency, and only one remedy should be opened at a time to prevent cross-potentization. Coffee interferes with the working of most remedies, and patients are asked to remove it from their diet.

No food or drink should be taken for an hour before or after high-potency remedies. Globules and tablets are dissolved on or under the tongue in a clean mouth free of food, toothpaste, mouthwash, etc., and rinsed with clean water so the medicine can be absorbed. Some remedies must be taken at certain times during the day. There are 500 remedies in daily use, each with a multitude of symptoms.

For homeopaths, illnesses are divided into two types, acute and chronic. Acute diseases are not deep-seated and easily treated. If they continually recur, it is surmised that they are symptomatic of an underlying chronic illness. Chronic diseases are seen to be a result of genetic inheritance or of suppression of symptoms by using strong allopathic drugs. For example, many homeopaths believe that using steroids to suppress eczema may cause asthma. This concept of disease resulting from symptom suppression is called miasm, and Hahnemann believed that chronic diseases caused by miasm could be transmitted generationally.

Causal factors are also very important to homeopathic doctors in the treatment of chronic diseases. After the remedy is prescribed, changes in the patient's condition are observed closely. In the classic reaction, aggravation, the symptoms temporarily get worse. Mental symptoms then tend to improve and are followed by physical improvements. In other cases the patient improves for a while, but then the condition worsens slightly. If the symptoms have not changed, the remedy is repeated. Another possible reaction is that the symptoms change. A new prescription is then given, based on the new symptoms. This may happen especially with, for example, a respiratory condition, where symptoms tend to change very quickly. A common error in homeopathy is over-prescribing, which can cause confusion and a worsening of the condition.

Homeopathy is also used for primary care, first aid, infections, respiratory disease, gastrointestinal illness, headaches, rheumatism, skin conditions, and genitourinary distress. Psychosomatic states and anxiety are also often treated. A homeopathic first aid regimen includes the following:

- For wounds involving only skin and no deeper structures, calendula lotion is applied after cleansing. For lacerated wounds contaminated with dirt and debris, arnica is given and the wound cleaned and covered with calendula.
- For bites that cause stinging and puffiness aphis is used. Arnica alleviates soreness afterward. Calendula used externally decreases the risk of infection. For horsefly bites, hypericum is recommended and ledlum is used for mosquito bites.
- Bruising remedies are arnica taken internally and arnica ointment if muscle or soft tissue is bruised, but not if skin is broken. Ledlum is for blows to the eye causing pain, discoloration, and swelling. Ruta lessens pain to bruised bones.
- For burns, after cleansing the area with cool water and keeping the patient hydrated, a biochemic named kali mur is given for first and second degree burns. Arnica is given at 200c. Cantharis relieves the pain and hypericum lotion can be used externally.
- For sprains and strains, arnica is given and an ice pack applied to the area. Bryonia helps painful joints. Rhus tox is used for hot, swollen, painful joints and ruta for aching pains made worse by movement.

See also ANTHROPOSOPHICAL MEDICINE.

Anderson, David, Dale Buegel, and Dennis Chernin. (1978) *Homeopathic Remedies for Physicians, Laymen and Therapists.*

Boyd, Hamish. (1981) *Introduction to Homeopathic Medicine.*

Cummings, Stephen, and Dana Ullman. (1984) *Everybody's Guide to Homeopathic Medicines: Taking Care of Yourself and Your Family with Safe and Effective Remedies.*

Hamlyn, E. C. (1979) *The Healing Art of Homeopathy: The Organon of Samuel Hahnemann.*

Hill, Ann, ed. (1979) *A Visual Encyclopedia of Unconventional Medicine: A Health Manual for the Whole Person.*

Kaufman, Martin. (1971) *Homeopathy in America: The Rise and Fall of a Medical Heresy.*

Panos, Maesimund B., and Jane Heimlick. (1980) *Homeopathic Medicine at Home: Natural Remedies for Everyday Ailments and Minor Injuries.*

Rose, Barry. (1992) *The Family Health Guide to Homeopathy.*

Woodham, Anne. (1994) *HEA Guide to Complementary Medicine and Therapies.*

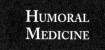

HUMORAL MEDICINE

In many medical systems, both Western and non-Western, health is seen as a state of being that exists when the body, mind, and spirit are in harmony with all of the internal and external forces that interact with it. When the body is negatively affected by outside agents like extremes in temperature, accidents, or overwork, or by internal agents such as family disharmony or guilt arising from unethical behavior, the result is disease. Some cultures also posit a supernatural element—offending the gods by, for example, not orienting one's house toward the graves of one's ancestors can bring on injury or disease as well.

Within this framework, the goal of healing is to restore balance to the system. Not surprisingly, the simple elements of food and temperature were the first agents to be used in trying to restore it. These two factors are intricately connected in humoral medicine in different cultures. Though there is wide variation in how these elements were and are still applied, the idea of applying the opposite element to counteract a situation—hot to heal a "cold" disease, and vice versa—and doing so with food, forms the basis of humoral healing.

HUMORAL MEDICINE IN GREEK THOUGHT

The word *humor* comes from the Greek, meaning "wet" or "damp," and itself has little to do with either food or temperature. It refers to the four bodily fluids that were believed by the Greeks to circulate through the body and regulate health. The key to health was maintaining the proper proportions of one to the other in the body's system.

The four humors, as set forth by early Greeks like Hippocrates and Galen, are blood, phlegm, black bile, and yellow bile. The humors are associated with four qualities: hot, cold, moist, and dry. Blood is considered hot and wet, yellow bile hot and dry, phlegm cold and wet, and black bile cold and dry. It is not entirely clear what the black and yellow bile refer to: black bile could be coagulated blood, yellow bile the serum that forms on the top of healing wounds. Lymph, which circulates in the lymphatic system, is another possibility for one of the humors. The important thing is that the Greeks believed that these circulated throughout the human system, and that an overabundance of one or the other would offset their interrelationship, causing disease. An imbalance in the humors caused a temperature or "moistness" imbalance.

The humors were also associated with the four earthly elements: earth, air, water, and fire. In the same way that the humors must maintain proper relationship for a healthy body, it was believed that elements maintained balance and order in the world at large. The system was believed to be dynamic: constantly changing. Not only do the elements interrelate in this system, they are part of an energy system that keeps the earth, and body, vital. In the same way that one season of the year gives way to another, life energy moves in specific cycles, from one into another. Spring builds up life and growth after the barren winter, in summer it reaches its height, and then it slowly disperses in the fall. Earth goes to water, which goes to fire and then to air.

When the natural balance of the body is off, it means that one of the humors has gained precedence and that the ratio between the humors is disturbed. The system becomes too hot, too cold, too wet, or too dry, resulting in the loss of vitality or health. (Though not humoral, this conception of health as a balance of different forces at work in the body also appears in Indian Ayurvedic medicine.)

Greek humoral medicine healed by forcing the elimination of the putrefied material that was believed to have been created by the abnormal mixture of the humors. They did this by focusing on the blood, one of the humors. This may be the origin of the practice of bloodletting, which continued into the early twentieth century. Cupping, scarification, venesection, and leeching (using leeches to suck blood out of sick patients) were the methods used.

In addition to bleeding, purging the body using laxatives and regulating the diet were the main methods used to reestablish balance in the system. The Greek physician Galen (A.D. 130–200) postulated a relationship between food and the increase of humors. "Foods of a warmer nature tend to produce bile, while those of a colder nature produce an excess of phlegm. An excess of bile produced 'warm diseases' and an excess of phlegm resulted in 'cold diseases.'" (Magner 1992: 92) Prescribing warming foods to heal a cold disease and vice versa were part of his treatment.

HOT AND COLD FOODS

Many cultures designate certain foods as either hot/warming or cold/cooling. An examination of the cultural variations of this concept shows that, while widespread, there is much variation in such systems. Some do not have the same

physiological basis as the Greeks vis à vis the four humors. Some only use the hot/cold dichotomy, and not the wet/dry.

Environmental differences account for some variations. Concepts of humoral medicine may have been brought to these cultures through conquest, or they may have evolved independently. In Latin America, Australia, and Africa, especially, indigenous cultures assign hot or cold properties to various substances and designate them as dangerous or as healing.

There is some physiological basis for the distinction of hot and cold as it applies to food.

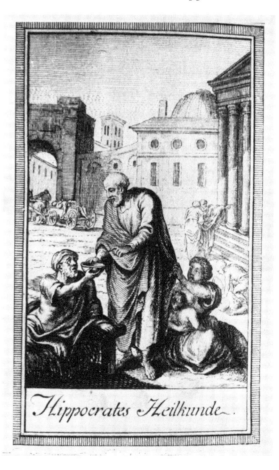

The Greek physician Hippocrates (c. 460–377 B.C.), considered the father of medicine, practices his healing arts in a public marketplace.

Modern nutritionist Annemarie Colbin believes the body requires both warming and cooling foods to accommodate the body's metabolic needs and explains it in the following way. The metabolic structure of digestion and elimination corresponds to a building-up and breaking-down cycle. The body takes in nutrition and converts it into energy that is used to build and strengthen cells for all of our various bodily functions. It breaks down what is not usable and disperses it or eliminates it. Traditionally "hot" foods, generally animal protein, aid the building process. Traditionally "cold" foods aid the elimination process. They include vegetables, fruits, herbal teas, and soups, which include higher quantities of vitamins, minerals, fiber, and water than animal protein.

Humoral Medicine in Non-Western Cultures

Aside from this possible physiological explanation for the division of hot and cold foods, there are culturally specific philosophical ones. While humoral medicine has its roots in the Greek description of the body's "humors," it is also associated with ascribing healing properties to the balancing of opposites, particularly temperature. While Chinese culture may not be strictly humoral, the division between hot and cold foods and the balancing of them illustrates the concept. They add a third category of "clean" foods, which help rid the body of poisons, and is associated more with cold.

The Chinese division of all aspects of existence into two opposing forces—yin, representing the cold, female, or receptive energy, and yang, representing the hot, male, or forceful energy—helps illustrate the dynamic tension between opposites that is at the heart of the humoral idea. In Chinese culture, the play of opposites appears in diet as an extension of Chinese philosophy.

The proper union of yin and yang forces creates divine harmony and balance of the life energy, or chi, whether in the body or in the universe. When there is a lack of harmony the opposite energy to that which is in deficit is applied, whether in the administering of food or herbal medicine or in the balancing of the energy using acupuncture.

The Chinese also relate foods and herbs to the five elements—wood, metal, fire, water, air—and each of these elements, which flow into one another, have some combination of qualities of hot/cold and moist/dry.

The Chinese believe that losing blood means losing heat; therefore, postpartum women who had lost blood during labor are given a "hot" diet. A soup containing hot ingredients—meat or chicken, oils, etc.—called a tonic or "patching medicine," is given to build strength. This remedy might be given to anyone who has suffered loss of blood. Similarly, the Tamil of India classify pregnancy as a hot condition, and so hot foods are prohibited for the pregnant woman. It is believed to cause boils and other skin conditions for the new child. But after birth, the postpartum woman is fed "hot" chicken broth and garlic to restore balance.

Ailments such as arthritis, colic, and diarrhea are considered "cold" in Chinese medicine, while headaches and heart trouble are considered "hot." Meat, fried foods, spices, and tropical fruits are some "hot" foods that counteract "cold" illnesses, while vegetables, soupy rice, and pears are "cold" and used to cure fever. In the event of exposure to an extreme temperature, it is believed that the cold or heat becomes trapped inside the body, requiring an opposing remedy.

Remedies using hot and cold foods to treat illness in Chinese medicine are common in rural Taiwanese villages as indicated by the following report: "When I grew faint with the heat I was told to drink some bamboo-shoot soup because it was 'cold' (*lieng*). When my landlady served some eggs she announced that they were not 'hot' (*zuag*) because they had been boiled in teas, which was 'cold'." (Ahearn 1975: 91) Likewise among the Chinantecs, medicinal plants are selected by their relative "hot" or "cold" properties to aid pregnancy and childbirth. The origin of the phrase "feed a cold—starve a fever" may have its origin in humoral medicine.

In some cultures the stage of life of a person has a particular quality of heat or coolness, in others it can be a way of determining a personality type. Relationship to the earth and the seasons of the year enter into judgments of heat and coolness.

Among the Chewong of Malaysia, coolness is the supreme state and it represents health, fertility, and everlasting life. Coolness is somewhere between hot and cold. Everything human is "hot" and heat is the source of illness, disease, and death. "Abod" represents the feeling of heat, and it is the opposite of "tokad," or cold. Both states are extreme and to be avoided in favor of the desired coolness, called "sedig." It is a middle ground that may be compared to the idea of balance or harmony. A bath of tepid water is sedig; the forrest is sedig. A person who wishes to contact the superhuman beings that are their culture's gods must be in a state of sedig.

The Chewong believe that the heat in the human body is a direct result of the consumption of red meat. The superhuman beings eat only fruit. Meat and fish are called "ai," vegetables and fruits are known as "ratn." Those who eat ai are considered "hot" and predisposed to disease; those who eat ratn are likely to be cool and closer to the gods. Spices, salt, chilies, and oil must not be mixed with ratn foods or they become hot. A sick person is more likely to be treated with coolness through the application of dew or smoke (smoke being the "cool" aspect of fire) than with heat. The dew will be brought and a bath made to restore moisture to an ill person. Dew represents moisture and coolness, which signifies life.

At certain times of life this dichotomy is reversed. A newborn must be bathed in warm water and cannot leave the warmth of the house. Its head must always be covered. But a corpse must always be washed in cool water.

The Maenge of New Guinea use hot and cold plants in their medicine and share the Chewong view that excessive heat is the source of illness. The source of the heat may be a plant, like a fragrant red flower called rolana; a roasting animal like a pig, the smell of which is believed to cause illness; a natural phenomenon like an earthquake or a volcano; a supernatural force; or an emotional reaction. Women are believed to induce disease because they are considered to be "hot," and men are believed to be more vulnerable to evil during sexual intercourse.

Moistness and dryness enter into the Maenge concept of health, as well as the Greek idea of the condition of the blood being the source of health:

> When a person is in good condition, his blood is liquid (veta) though stagnant, it is clean (leke), it is red (tente), its temperature is not too high, and it is equally distributed throughout the body. When a person is sick his blood becomes dry (manani) and as a result heats the body . . . "the blood becomes dry and cooks the body." (Howell 1984: 168)

Bloodletting is also used among the Maenge.

Treatment of a "hot" illness by the Maenge differs radically from those previously mentioned, in that treatment is homeopathic, meaning "like cures like." Hot diseases are treated with heat. Therefore, ginger, a hot plant, is given to treat hot illnesses. Hot plants include astringent plants, bitter plants, and peppers, those with an irritant effect on the skin, those with a strong smell, or those that are otherwise associated with the quality of heat. The leaves of hot plants like *Cinnamomun* and *Zingiber* are cooked and pressed on the body or ingested. Other materials considered hot that may be used in curing include such insects as scorpions and centi-pedes, lime, pork fat, and the bones of dead warriors. These remedies are also used as preventatives: someone entering warfare rubs his legs with a mixture of the above.

Cold plants have rich foliage and abundant sap, and they do not rob the soil of nutrients. *Ficus pungens,* a type of fig tree, is considered cold; fresh water is cold, while sea water is hot.

When certain hot remedies are combined with the "cold" qualities of fresh water, the bal-ance of hot and cold is believed to produce an aphrodisiac effect. One such "charm" used by men involves wrapping a cordyline leaf with some fresh water in the leaf of a hot plant and placing it over the fire for two days. Before the meeting with his love interest, the man has eaten only warm foods and refrained from water. He then rubs his legs with the leaf, and supposedly cannot fail to win his beloved. If he loses interest in her, the leaf is "cooled off" by placing it in the river.

For the Tamil, fasting and bathing are part of the hot/cold dichotomy. Fasting is believed to create a state of heat and spiritual strength. Ado-lescence is a period of heat, and during puberty rites cooling measures are taken.

In Latin America, the use of the hot/cold dichotomy as the basis of medical belief is found in Mexico, Guatemala, Colombia, and Chile. It may have existed prior to the Spanish conquest, as it has been noted in Inca medical practices, although there is debate in anthropological circles about whether it existed in North America prior to the Spanish conquest.

Again, there is not always agreement regard-ing the classification of hot and cold food, and the determination is based on the *effect* of cer-tain foods on a hot or cold illness. In other words, a substance (not just food) that cures a hot illness will be considered cold, and vice versa. The temperature or quality *(calidad)* of the substance is believed to cause or cure the ill-ness. Some examples of illnesses attributed to cold and hot in one Mexican community are as follows:

- **Chest cramp.** Cold air enters the chest when a person is overheated.
- **Earache.** A cold draft of air enters the ear canal.
- **Headache.** The cool mist or night air, called aigre that enters the head.
- **Paralysis.** A part of the body is "struck" by aigre. Stiffness, considered a partial, temporary paralysis, is ascribed to the same cause.
- **Pain due to sprains.** Such "cold pains" are the result of cold entering the damaged part.
- **Stomach cramp.** When the body is warm, and not adequately covered, cold can en-ter from the air or from a body of water.
- **Rheumatism.** Cold from some outside source lodges in the afflicted bones.
- **Teething.** The pain of teething is a "cold pain," originating in the coldness of the white new teeth that are growing in.
- **Tuberculosis.** Cold enters the body from water or carbonated beverages, especially when the body is overheated from work or travel.
- **Algodoncillo.** Heat rises from the center of the body to the mouth, causing the gums, tongue, and lips to turn white.
- **Disipela.** Overexposure to the sun can cause the sun's heat to collect in the skin, resulting in an outbreak of red spots on the hands, arms, or less commonly the feet.
- **Dysentery.** Since it is accompanied by bloody stool, and since blood is intensely hot, dysentery is classed as a hot disease and may be caused by consuming too much hot food.
- **Sore eyes.** A person may overstrain his eyes, causing them to "work hard" and

thus to heat up, or alternatively, cold wet feet can cause the body heat to rise to the head, overheating the eyes.

- **Fogazo.** Heat rising from the center of the body causes the mouth and tongue to break out in tiny red spots. In contrast to algodoncillo, this is not a serious disease.
- **Kidney ailments.** Any pain in the kidneys is a hot pain; most kidney ailments are accompanied by itching feet or ankles, a reddening of the palms of the hands, and fever.
- **Postemilla.** An abscessed tooth results from heat concentrating in the root of the tooth, evidenced by the fact that when the abscess bursts it releases blood.
- **Sore throat.** Wet feet cause sore throat by driving the body heat up into the throat.
- **Warts and rashes.** Whatever the cause, these ailments are the result of heat. This is a conclusion from the fact that warts and rashes are irritating, and irritation is always ascribed to heat and never to cold.

Some diseases are considered either hot or cold, based on the particular form of the condition, as in diarrhea and toothache. Cold seems to be associated with overheating, which allows the cold in and which affects motor and sensory function. Hot illnesses seem to be generated from within the body itself. Sensations of pain are considered hot. Fear of heat, as a result of overexposure to the sun and poisoning from hot plants, is commonplace, but fear of the cold is equally threatening.

Again vegetables and fruits are classified as cold, while chili peppers, meat, water fowl, and oils are considered hot. Dairy foods and chicken are considered cold in this system, while cereal grains, liquor, and aromatic beverages are considered hot. The method of cooking can change the calidad of a food. Easily digested food is considered "warm."

In Guatemala, children are believed to be especially vulnerable to temperature fluctuations. In one case, a child who died after being given penicillin was believed to have died from the "coldness" of the medicine. Vitamins are considered to be "hot," and are therefore to be avoided when one has a "hot" illness. Conflicts have arisen when Western-trained physicians have prescribed medicines for Guatemalans that have a similar calidad to the illness. Heat is believed to result from strenuous labor and emotional or sexual excitement.

For the Kallaway-Andean people, the parts of the body are believed to be organically united with the natural environment, and the circulation of air, blood, and fat are considered a mirror of the waterways. Air is the principle that touches all and unites all. The movement of blood controls the health of the body, and its relationship to other body fluids: it can be classified as hot, cold, wet, or dry. When it is in proper condition it moves the various fluids around the body, distributing necessary nutrients; when it is not moving correctly it causes disease.

Hot sicknesses are considered to be associated with high fevers and inflammation, and hot herbs stimulate and irritate. Cold sicknesses include respiratory and mobility problems. Dry sicknesses relate to thirst and dry herbs like glutinous plants are used for drying wounds or setting bones. Health is seen as a neutral or "gray" area between the extremes of heat and cold.

See also AYURVEDIC MEDICINE; CHINESE MEDICINE; DIET AND NUTRITION.

Ahern, Emily M. (1975) "Sacred and Secular Medicine in a Taiwan Village: A Study of Cosmological Disorders." In *Medicine in Chinese Cultures: Comparative Studies of Health Care in Chinese and Other Societies*, edited by Arthur Kleinman et al., 91–113.

Barrett, Robert J., and Rodney H. Lucas. (1994) "Hot and Cold in Transformation: Is Iban Medicine Humoral?" *Social Science Medicine* 38: 383–393.

Bastien, Joseph. (1989) "Differences between Kallaway-Andean and Greek-European Humoral Theory." *Social Science Medicine* 28: 45–51.

Chopra, Deepak. (1991) *Perfect Health: The Complete Mind/Body Guide.*

Colbin, Annemarie. (1986) *Food and Healing.*

Howell, Signe. (1984) *Society and Cosmos: Chewong of Peninsular Malaya.*

Logan, Michael. (1977) "Humoral Medicine in Guatemala and Peasant Acceptance of Modern Medicine." In *Culture, Disease and Healing,* edited by David Landay, 487–495.

Magner, Lois N. (1992) *A History of Medicine.*

Panoff, Françoise. (1970) "Maenge Remedies and Conceptions of Disease." *Ethnology* 9: 68–84.

Reynolds, Holly B. (1978) *To Keep the Tali Strong: Women's Rituals in Tamilnad, India.*

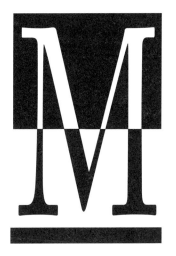

The work of Soviet biologist Alexander Gurwitsh is cited as support for the theory: "Every cell in the body is stimulated by the resonating interaction of the rhythmical flow of electromagnetic currents from the cosmos and the environment." (Hanneman 1995: 9) Measurements of electromagnetic cell energy can be compared to ultraviolet radiation—and some researchers in this area believe that there are contact points within the human body that act as receptors to the "outer" radiation.

The key to health is believed to be the smooth flow of this energy. The idea that healthy cells produce energy and contain contact points to receive it is fledgling at best, but resonates with more ancient approaches to health. In the Chinese philosophy of Taoism, the universe is believed to be composed of and held together by forces of energy called yin and yang. Yang represents expansive, active, male energy, and yin receptive, calm, female energy. All life is believed to be created by the interaction of these two forces. They are in opposition to each other, yet create each other. The symbol of yin and yang is a circle divided by a curved line, with one side shaded and one not, and a small circle representing the opposing quality inside each half. This small circle represents the idea that the seed of one is a part of the opposite. Darkness gives way to light, male gives way to female, and vice versa. There is constant exchange of one into the other. When this relationship is harmonious, it is the basis for health and well-being in Chinese philosophy. The energy that results from this interaction is called chi, and it is the quality of the chi that is examined by Chinese doctors when diagnosing health and illness.

Chi, or energy or "natural power," is carried on invisible lines through the body called meridians. They can be understood as long stretches of a magnetic field's currents. In Chinese medicine, points along the meridians called acupuncture points are stimulated to rebalance the chi.

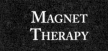

MAGNET THERAPY

Magnet therapy is based on the idea that the human being is a "biocosmic creature." The argument is that, as a part of nature, human beings are integrally connected to all other animate and inanimate forms of nature in an energy relationship. This energy is believed to interact with the very cells of living organisms and, according to the principles of science, transform them.

Cells are equipped with "receivers," according to this theory, that pick up the energy, but energy is also created by the activity of the cells. An example of a cell creating energy is the process of digestion of food, by which food is transformed into biochemical energy for use by the body. This all-encompassing energy system therefore resides within and outside the body. The cells in the body take in energy from the larger system and send out energy from their own functions. This is called the macrocosm/microcosm theory: the biochemical reactions within the body mirror those occurring in the larger world.

These acupuncture points can be compared to the receptors discussed above.

Dysfunction in this energy system is believed to cause illness. The energy that keeps cells of the various organs of the body running smoothly has not been adequately received—or sent out—and the energy pathway becomes blocked.

In Chinese medicine, acupuncture needles or moxa (a burning herb) is applied to the points on the meridian to restore the energy flow and stimulate healing. In magnet therapy, magnets are placed strategically to enhance the current of energy to the organs or parts of the body in need of that energy for healing.

The fragile energy balance of the body is believed to be constantly threatened by inside and outside forces. Magnet therapy is a holistic medium because it stimulates the body's innate ability to heal itself by restoring its overall balance and integrity.

From a standpoint of physical science, magnets consist of electrons circling around atoms of iron molecules. It is the electron activity that is key. Dr. Linus Pauling discovered the magnetic properties of hemoglobin in the blood. Copper, which occurs naturally in the body, is also conducive to magnetism.

To treat using magnets, knowledge of acupuncture points is needed, as well as the best time to treat individual organs. Each organ is believed to have an internal clock, a rhythm that reflects an ebb and flow of activity.

Magnet therapy was used during the Middle Ages. It was clumsy and unwieldy, with magnets sewn into clothing. Today, small magnets of high magnetic resonance are available. Pea-sized magnets are made in Japan that can be adhered to the body with adhesive. The magnet is applied to the source of the pain, to the acupuncture point that relates to the diseased part of the body, or it is applied to an extremity. It stays on the body for a period of between five minutes and two hours. This is done on a number of suc-cessive days, with five being the recommended number for full efficiency.

The body is divided into sections. For problems on the right side of the body, one magnet's north pole is placed under the right hand, and another magnet's south pole under the right foot. The opposite is true for problems on the left side.

Magnet therapy should not be used by those who have pacemakers, during pregnancy, or near mealtime. Magnets should not be attached to the heart area, and care is recommended when treating the head or eye area.

Cleansing the body using magnetized water is the first step in many treatments. To prepare magnetized water, two Yama magnets are immersed in water, south side facing up. After about ten hours, the water will be magnetized. Four equal portions should be drunk each day, totaling one liter. This should continue for several months.

Homeopathic remedies are often used in concert with magnet therapy. The subtle effects of the remedies are strengthened by the magnet therapy. Illnesses treated by magnet therapy include headaches, high blood pressure, insomnia, muscular pain, sexual dysfunction, cystitis, back problems, bronchitis, and burns. Magnet therapy is especially popular in Japan for muscular pain reduction and wound and burn pain.

The positive and negative sides of the magnet have very different effects. The south pole is believed to positively affect all living systems, including germs and bacteria. Therefore, only the north poles of magnets are used to cure infections.

See also ACUPUNCTURE; BODYWORK; HOLISTIC HEALTH AND HEALING.

Hanneman, Holger. (1995) *Magnet Therapy: Rebalancing Your Body's Energy Flow for Self-Healing.*

MEDITATION Meditation, a peaceful state of mind achieved by performing various focusing techniques or rituals, is present in most ancient Asian religions as a method of expanding consciousness and making contact with the spiritual world or one's own spirituality. Within the Judeo-Christian tradition, practices such as chanting and singing and repetitive prayer are used in a similar way.

In the Asian meditative traditions, God is experienced as within us as well as outside of us. In Western traditions, God is generally experienced as outside of us, as someone we pray *to*, but the process of letting go of our daily thoughts and emotions to allow for divine contact comes from the same impulse—to merge with God or a higher energy.

Commonalties among most Asian meditative practices include the following:

1. A calm environment, with silence or simple rhythmic sound
2. An attempt to quiet daily thoughts and emotion and quell "busyness"
3. An acceptance that by stopping the flow of rational thought and normal mental activity, a state of passive awareness can be achieved
4. The belief that by achieving this passive awareness, doors to higher consciousness can be opened

One form of Hindu meditation from India and Tibet is known as kundalini meditation. It teaches that we all have divine energy, or kundalini, suppressed in our bodies. This energy, coiled at the base of the spine, is believed to be a tremendous power, and it is released through the practice of meditation. It is usually experienced as radiant warmth and light and can sometimes overcome a practitioner.

Traditionally, a student who wished to learn this meditation—or most Asian forms of meditation—would renounce the world and, under the guidance of a teacher called a Master, engage in strict and lengthy meditation practices. He (most students, until recently, were men) would leave his family, and any aspirations for a career or family would be left behind. He would become a monk, devoted to the goal of union with God that comes with the unblocking of the kundalini.

Modern practitioners of meditation, especially in the West, may not renounce the world, but by practicing meditative techniques daily, they may achieve some aspect of this experience. It is generally not as profound or life-consuming—or it may be, depending on the person's goals and the length of time they engage in the practice. Meditative techniques are used in the West as complements to psychological and medical treatments, as relaxation is one of the most demonstrated effects of the practice (relaxation has been proven to aid the body/mind in healing). Others may meditate to reduce stress and feel more relaxed and energized.

TECHNIQUES OF MEDITATION

Whatever the goals, there are similar techniques used in both spiritually based Asian traditional meditation and Western adaptations and approaches. They are:

1. Mantra or sound
2. Focus on breathing
3. Moving meditation
4. Visual meditation
5. Guided meditation

The various methods used are points of mental focus so that the falling away of everyday thoughts and emotions can occur. The mind may stray from the focus, but it is continually returned. Eventually what is left is the point alone: the sound, the breath, the image, the motion, and then *that* begins to slowly dissolve. When the mind is empty and there is no grasping onto any thought or sensation, a person experiences a flood of relaxation, often accompanied by a sense of warmth and light. There is generally a feeling of well-being and increased energy. With repeated practice, states of higher and more expanded consciousness may be achieved.

To allow the conscious mind to release its hold, a person generally closes his or her eyes or focuses them on a fixed point and is either seated or lying down. The traditional Asian posture is called the lotus position, with the legs crossed and hands resting in the lap, or with palms facing upward while resting on the knees. The spine is held very straight with the top of the head pulled upward toward the sky. The chin is in. This can be an uncomfortable pose at first, but the spine is straight to allow for an unimpeded flow of the life force, and the legs are crossed to contain it in a closed system. Often, the tips of the index finger and thumb are pressed together in each hand to further complete the "circuit."

Once the posture is assumed, the point of focus is brought in and the practitioner begins to allow his thoughts to disappear.

In vocal meditation, a sound is repeated over and over as a way of blocking conscious thought and moving from the rational mind to passive awareness. In traditional meditation, a mantra, the Sanskrit word for "thought form" is used. A mantra is a word or phrase, usually having a religious significance, that is given to the student. Traditionally, the belief is that a particular mantra resonates in a special way for that student and is therefore not to be shared with anyone else. The word's resonance is often to a particular deity and is believed to assist in the person's connection to the life force. One of the most commonly used mantras is "Om," which is believed to be the universal sound from which all other mantras spring.

Transcendental Meditation (TM), a method developed for modern life, is derived from such an ancient Indian technique. It was developed by Maharishi Mahesh Yogi, who brought it to the United States in the 1960s. TM is taught by the International Meditation Society and can be mastered in four days. One does not have to believe in any spiritual or religious doctrine, but the concept of the secrecy of the mantra is maintained. The mantra is given to the student in a special spiritual ceremony called the puja.

In her research on meditation, clinical psychologist Dr. Patricia Carrington found some TM meditators who had shared their mantras found that they had all received the same one and that TM mantras are often assigned on the basis of age. TM teachers reported that there are 16 mantras regularly used. In Clinically Standardized Meditation (CSM), developed by Dr. Carrington, students are allowed to choose their own mantra.

Breathing meditation also has its roots in Indian philosophy and religion. Pranayama is the Sanskrit name for the life force, and it is also the name for the yoga of breathing. In pranayama, a devotee sits in the lotus position and, using one of the many forms, fixes his or her awareness on the sensation of breathing. Eventually the breathing becomes automatic, as the body/mind relax. There are many types of pranayama, including the alternate breath, in which the practitioner inhales in a particular way, holding one nostril closed, then opening it for the exhale. Use of the throat in ujaya breathing imitates the relaxing sound of ocean waves. Another technique is the cleansing breath, during which the lips are pursed on the exhale for a forceful expulsion of the breath. Practitioners experience a sense of wholeness and peace from the practice.

A Harvard Medical School cardiologist researched meditation techniques to determine their use as tools to combat heart disease. Herbert Benson developed a breathing meditation

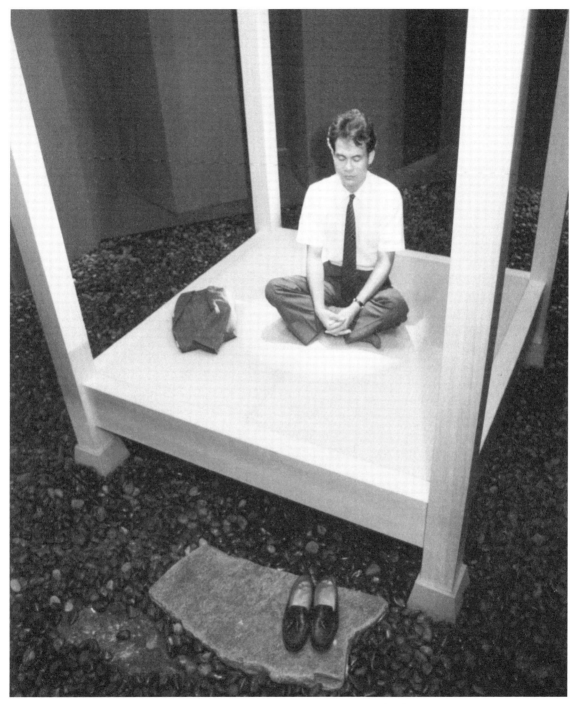

A worker in Japan achieves harmony in a Zen meditation room.
Meditation, the peaceful state of mind achieved by performing focusing techniques or rituals, is present in most
ancient Asian religions. Such relaxation can aid body and mind healing.

technique that he called "Benson's Method." Using the focus on simple breathing as his starting point, he added the repetition of the word "one" to his instructions to his students, thereby mixing breathing and vocal meditation.

Other forms of breathing meditation include the Japanese-based Zazen, a strict and rigorous discipline from Chinese Zen Buddhism. Students are not allowed to move during the meditation, and they are forced to ignore any and all distractions, including insects, numbness, or any painful sensation within or outside of the body. They sit in the lotus position, their eyes open and focused on a spot a few feet in front of them. Often an unanswerable riddle, called a koan, is offered by their teacher. "What is the sound of one hand clapping," goes one popular koan. Again, there is a mixture of the two techniques, with the goal of derailing conscious thinking so that the divine energy can enter the body/mind.

An example of a moving meditation is the ecstatic dancing of the whirling dervishes of the mystic sect of Islam, the Sufi order. In this repetitive group twirling, dancers are lifted out of ordinary consciousness. Another type of moving meditation, from Chinese Taoism, is called t'ai chi ch'uan. In this meditation, a series of slow and meditative martial arts postures are strung together into a form that is repeated over and over. Relaxing into the movement, with practice, allows release of the life force, or chi.

Not all moving meditation uses the whole body. A simple moving meditation described by Carrington is as follows:

> Sit with a pillow on your lap so that your hands are resting comfortably on the pillow and cup your hands together in a "prayerlike" position with fingers lightly touching. Then gently open your palms while still keeping their lower edges resting against the pillow and in contact. Now once again bring your palms together so that all fingers touch lightly, returning to the position. . . . This meditation consists of opening and closing

your palms over and over again, gently and easily. . . . Use as little energy as possible for this exercise and let your motions be easy and rhythmic. (1977: 81)

Traditional visual meditation includes use of a mandala, or spiritual painting:

> In Sanskrit, the word mandala literally means the "centerpoint." And, in fact, spiritual meditation is largely based on holding your attention on one point over a period of time, while also expanding your consciousness to include the whole that surrounds the centerpoint. . . . These paintings offer a calm, clear path to finding one's visual center, and to expanding one's mind in all directions around the centerpoint. (Selby 1992: 68)

In another, more simple visual meditation, a natural object is placed at eye level a few feet away from the meditator. A candle is often chosen, but a plant, a flower, or any other pleasing object can be used. While sitting comfortably, the meditator rests her eyes on the subject, but instead of consciously focusing, she lets the object slowly enter the awareness. Periodically, the attention is taken away from the object to a more distant place in the room. It is then returned. Each time the meditator becomes more absorbed in the object, until conscious attention falls away. In Tratak meditation, from Hinduism, one stares unblinkingly at a flame until the eyes tear.

Guided meditations involve the gentle, calm voice of someone telling a detailed story, praying, or repeating inspirational messages. A guided meditation may involve asking meditators to imagine that they are in a relaxing place, like the beach or the woods. There may be a very detailed description of the place or the journey to the place, which allows the meditator to relax deeply in this imaginary state. He may be led to some point of catharsis or given directions to increase self-love and love of others. These meditations may be directed toward a goal, promoting self-esteem or some other positive psychological state.

Meditation has helped many people reduce or stop addictive behaviors. It has been proven to improve academic performance in college students, increase job satisfaction, and reduce anxiety. Some research supports personality changes such as increased self-esteem, creativity, and ability to achieve intimacy and self-actualization. Benson refers to "the principle of the maximum mind" in meditators, a kind of mental agility marked by the ability to see ourselves and the world in new ways.

Benson also found that meditation lowered metabolism—decreasing breathing rate, heart rate, and blood pressure. He measured brainwaves and found that deep meditation produced alpha waves that indicate relaxed alertness. Meditation can benefit those suffering from high blood pressure, chronic pain, tension headaches, Raynaud's disease, asthma, insomnia, and other stress-related problems.

Many books are available on the subject of meditation, with descriptions of how to begin meditating. Some individuals may learn from a book, but others may need a teacher. Each discipline or method has its own training programs. Daily practice is usually recommended or required, with length of time varying from twenty minutes to an hour for most Western approaches.

The benefits of meditation do not come immediately, although one may feel relaxed after only one session. Changes in attitude, personality, or health may take months or years. It is recommended that meditators stay away from stimulants like caffeine, especially prior to meditating. The hours before sunrise are said to be advantageous times to meditate.

See also Mind/Body Healing; Yoga.

Arguelles, Jose. (1992) *Mandala*.

Carrington, Patricia. (1977) *Freedom in Meditation*.

Elliot, C. (1969) *Japanese Buddhism*.

Selby, John. (1992) *Kundalini Awakening: A Gentle Guide to Chakra Activation and Spiritual Growth*.

Watts, Alan. (1957) *The Way of Zen*.

Yogananda, P. (1946) *Autobiography of a Yogi*.

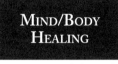

MIND/BODY HEALING

Mind/body healing rests on the belief that there is a causal relationship between an individual's emotions and thoughts and their physical health. The causal relationship works both ways. If a person is unhappy or angry, they may become ill, or if they are ill, they may become unhappy or angry. Although there has been a recent resurgence of interest in the mind-body-disease relationship in Western medicine, the mind/body relationship is a common assumption in many traditional healing systems and in many contemporary alternative healing approaches. In many traditional societies, no clear distinction is made between the mind and the body and the two are often seen as interacting and influencing one another on a regular basis. For example, meditation as practiced in Buddhist communities in Central Thailand requires personal study of one's own mind and body:

> Nama-rupa lumps the five heaps of conditioned reality into nama or "mind," referring to feelings, perceptions, mental formations, and consciousness, and rupa, referring to form, corporeality, or body. Thus to meditate on mind and body can lead to knowledge of all the khanda and thus wisdom, according to some meditation schools. To many meditators this is the message of the satipatthana, which advises mindfulness of the body, and the nama group of feeling, perception, mental formations, and consciousness. (Van Esterik 1978: 77)

In cultures where illness is attributed to supernatural causes, body and mind are often linked because both are believed to be equally susceptible to supernatural influence. For example, for the Garo of India: "Every ill of body or mind is attributed to the wrath of numerous malignant demons, to appease whom sacrifices are offered." (Hunter 1879: 155)

In biomedicine the mind/body relationship is not ignored entirely and there is much research on the relationship between emotions and illnesses such as heart disease and cancer. Many experts believe that emotional stress can reduce the disease-fighting capabilities of the immune system.

In alternative health care, the emphasis is on using one's mind to heal, help heal, or maintain health in one's body. The argument is that one does not need a practitioner to use mind/body medicine, although there are many kinds of practitioners who can teach people to use it. The basic approach is to align one's mind in the belief that health and well-being will follow and to learn the words and symbols that resonate with one's consciousness to "train" one's body to heal itself. The power of the mind to "persuade" the body of its point of view is the basis of mind/body healing. For some people, the best evidence of the potential of mind/body healing is the placebo effect. The placebo effect is a phenomenon that researchers use when testing new medical treatments, and especially when testing the effectiveness of new drugs. For some significant proportion of people, the sheer suggestion that a drug will have a powerful effect is enough to cause the effect, regardless of whether that drug is actually administered or a sugar pill is given instead. Thus, tests of drug effectiveness require comparison with the effects of a placebo. While some people taking the placebo will benefit, an effective drug will benefit a significantly larger number of people. For adherents of mind/body healing, the fact that some people taking the placebo show improvement is evidence of the importance of the mind in healing the body. For example, in one dramatic case, subjects were told that a drug they were given would have the *opposite* effect of its known purpose, and many of the subjects experienced the symptoms the researchers suggested. Another explanation for the placebo effect suggests that when people believe someone else is taking care of them, they will feel better.

A less well-known but well-documented case of mind/body healing involved a man with a terminal illness. Reported by Dr. Bruno Klopfer in the *Journal of Projective Techniques* in 1957, it involved a man with metastatic cancer and tumors that had spread throughout his body. The patient had tried every available form of medicine and his condition had hopelessly deteriorated to the point where he was bedridden and gasping for air. His doctors agreed that he had only a few days to live. Then the man heard about an experimental drug called Krebiozen, which was in the process of being tested. He insisted on being included in the experimental trials. His doctors, feeling he had nothing to lose and would soon be dead anyway, out of compassion agreed to give him the experimental drug. To their amazement, the man's tumors soon began to shrink dramatically and he was discharged from the hospital. Two months later, the man read news accounts of the research on Krebiozen that reported serious doubts with the drug. Within a matter of days, the man's tumors had returned and were again threatening his life. His doctor cleverly convinced him that a new and more potent shipment had been received and proceeded to give him injections of plain water. His tumors once again began to shrink dramatically. He remained healthy for several more months until another news report declared that "nationwide AMA tests show Krebiozen to be worthless as a cancer treatment." The man died within two days.

Not everyone is so sensitive to or believes in mind/body connections. But some healers believe that every person has some and that the connections can be improved. Techniques like meditating, visualization, inner dialogs with the subconscious mind, and hypnosis can "instruct" the immune system to improve its job of fighting foreign and toxic materials and promote healing. They can also slow the heartbeat and respiration, reduce high blood pressure, and relax the nervous system. Mind/body medicine is primarily used as a complementary form of therapy in conjunction with other forms of conventional or alternative treatments.

The idea that thoughts and emotions can influence health is not new. As noted above, it is common in traditional societies and is also found in some ancient civilizations. Ancient Indian medicine called negative or violent thoughts "mental ama" and considered them a legitimate cause of disease. Hippocrates and other ancient Greeks commented on the influence of one's mental state on health. In Chinese culture, the idea of balance, which includes a healthy state of mind, is believed to be critical to health.

In the West, naturopathic, homeopathic, chiropractic, and anthroposophic schools of medicine stress the analysis of the emotional state of patients before recommending treatments. Indeed, any form of holistic medicine considers the mind as interrelated to the functioning of the body.

Scientific Studies

The increasing pace of life and the awareness that chronic stress has a negative physiological effect on the body led to explorations of alternative healing in the 1960s and 1970s. With the reintroduction of holistic methods of healing that incorporate relaxation and integration of the body, mind, and spirit, interest in research on the mind/body connection began. In the late 1970s Herbert Benson and his colleagues at the Harvard Medical School began to research "the relaxation response." Combining knowledge of meditative techniques from other cultures and applying Western scientific principles, he developed a form of meditation that would predictably induce this response.

Medically significant results of the positive effects of meditation on hypertension and heart disease were found. Studies have included those that showed the effect of the release of stress hormones into the bloodstream. Changes in the body include increased tendency for blood to clot, a surge in the pressure on the coronary artery, increased blood pressure, and other demands on the heart. Subsequent studies in mind/body medicine have included the effect of relaxation on reducing chronic pain and other conditions.

The nervous system and the circulatory system are the two primary physical sites of the mind/body connection. In addition to the beneficial effects of relaxation on health, interest began in the study of the possibility of using the mind to strengthen the immune system, the system that fights off the numerous germs, viruses, cell dysfunctions like cancer, and other negative stimuli that the body comes into contact with.

The study of the effect of the brain on immune response is called psychoneuroimmunology. In the early 1980s Suzanne and David Felten discovered nerve fibers that physically link the nervous system and the immune system. That was the first physical evidence that feelings affect the physiology of the immune system. The brain, in the form of our thoughts, secretes chemicals and releases them into the bloodstream and receives feedback, in some form, from all of the organs of the body. According to David Felton:

> The higher centers of the brain can generate signals that very clearly influence hormonal outflow. In certain psychiatric disorders there are changes in some of the hormones. And when you're frightened, there's a huge outpouring of adrenaline and noradrenaline from the sympathetic nervous system and the adrenal gland. What we

haven't contemplated before is that some of these signals that leave the brain when we feel certain emotions may well have an impact on the immune system. (Moyers 1993: 215)

Some researchers are studying whether the stress that accompanies certain experiences, such as taking an exam, getting a divorce, or going into a nursing home, is attended by changes in immune response. They have found that one factor contributing to a diminished response is whether or not an individual is in control of the situation; another is whether or not the individual feels lonely.

Given this relationship between emotional state and immune response, researchers are now trying to discover if the brain can be "trained" to teach the immune system how to work better. One technique being tested is biofeedback, in which special instruments that measure the body's vital signs amplify those signs that represent relaxation, in order to train the person to recognize and replicate it themselves. Electromyographic (EMG) feedback involves sensors attached to the skin and registers muscle tension. Other types of feedback include thermal feedback, which senses the temperature of the skin, and electrodermal feedback, which registers perspiration and finger pulse for cardiovascular symptoms. Biofeedback can also monitor breathing patterns.

In one study using biofeedback, the possibility of diabetics replacing additional insulin with relaxation when stress would otherwise require a higher dosage is being studied, as well as treating chronic lower back pain and muscle-related pain. Another study is using guided imagery, a system of using symbols to imagine the desired physical changes happening to the body, in the treatment of asthma and cancer. Studies indicate that some people who repeatedly imagine a healing scenario can positively affect their immune system. For example, a person might imagine their healthy white blood cells as white

knights on horses subduing some source of infection. A cancer patient might see their white blood cells like the computer game Pac Man, gobbling up cancer cells.

A final and major interest in mind/body is the study of so-called Type A and Type C personalities and their links to heart disease and cancer. The Type A personality is characterized by anger, lack of emotional control, competitiveness, and achievement, and one aspect of the personality type—hostility—is clearly related to increased risk of heart disease, although the exact nature of the relationship is not clear. The Type C personality, characterized by extreme emotional control, has been linked to an increased risk for cancer, although the link is not as firm as the Type A heart disease link.

ANECDOTAL EVIDENCE

While research on mind/body medicine continues, many people, with and without medical training, believe intuitively in the process and hold that restoring harmony to the system will create the conditions for the body to heal itself. They recommend emotional healing and reconciliation with the past, using visualization and affirmations.

Affirmations are positive statements about oneself or an outcome that one desires, that, repeated over and over, are thought to train the body to heal itself. For example, "I affirm in my mind that I have the power to heal myself" is an affirmaton, developed by one of the most popular proponents of this method, Louise Hay. The essence of her approach is summarized as follows:

- We are each responsible for all of our experiences.
- Each thought we think is creating our future.
- The point of power is always in the present moment.

- Everyone suffers from self-hatred and guilt.
- The bottom line for everyone is "I'm not good enough."
- It's only a thought, and a thought can be changed.
- Resentment, criticism, and guilt are the most damaging patterns.
- Releasing resentment will dissolve even cancer.
- When we really love ourselves, everything in our life works.
- We must release the past and forgive everyone.
- We must be willing to begin to learn to love ourselves.
- Self-approval and self-acceptance in the now are the keys to positive changes.
- We create every so-called illness in our body. (Hay 1984: xiii)

Hay's audiotape *Love Your Body* addresses every part of the body with a loving affirmation of its beauty and worth, and a corresponding emotional connection. "I love my bladder. I am at peace with my thoughts and emotions. I am at peace with those around me. No person, place or thing has any power over me, for I am the only thinker in my mind. I choose the thoughts that keep me serene. I willingly and lovingly release old concepts and ideas. They flow out of me easily and joyously. I love and appreciate my beautiful bladder."

Some proponents of mind/body medicine believe that the very content of our thoughts can translate into a physical change. Barbara Hoberman Levine says:

> Emotions and your overall sense of illness or well-being are felt and expressed in your body. . . . Sometimes you ignore physical sensations, but *subconsciously, every thought tells your body how to react.* Every thought promotes health or illness. Once an idea has gained a foothold in your physical world,

other thoughts, words and images may affect its existence. Words are not the sole cause of dis-ease. But they certainly are a link in a chain of causative factors that also includes environment, lifestyle, and heredity. Words create the climate that allows disease to flourish. Language affects the quality of life. (1991: 65)

Levine believes that "seedthoughts," or core emotional beliefs, are the beginning of ill health. With counseling and self-appraisal, these beliefs can be rooted out as part of the overall process of healing. Mental affirmations help turn the thoughts around. For example:

- *Seedthought and Symptom:* I am burning up. The rash was so red hot it burned my skin.
- *Core Belief:* Burning up was indicative to me of my stored anger burning me as it was released through my skin.
- *Mental Antidote:* I transform the warmth within to love and peace. I am cool and at ease.

Levine also believes that illness can be an opportunity to illuminate the areas in the emotional and psychological life that need to be addressed for spiritual growth.

INTEGRATION WITH SCIENTIFIC MEDICINE

The medical profession has been most sympathetic to mind/body medicine in the treatment of terminal illness, such as cancer, when used in conjunction with conventional treatment, believing that an improved attitude and emotional healing cannot hurt. A modern marriage between ancient Indian medicine and modern techniques has resulted from the work of Deepak Chopra and is called Maharishi Ayurveda. Mind/body medicine is its core concept:

> Maharishi Ayurveda looks at the meeting point between mind and body. Clearly the

two do meet. Every time there is an event in the mind, there is a corresponding event in the body. If a child is afraid of the dark, his fear takes physical shape in the form of adrenaline shooting through his bloodstream. Ayurveda says that this interconnectedness is accomplished at a place sandwiched between the mind and body, where thought turns into matter. (Chopra 1991: 25)

This place is explained in his theory of "Quantum Healing." He posits the existence of an inner world, where intelligence, thoughts, and beliefs are formed and *can be changed*. He compares it to the "software" that drives the human being—with abilities much greater than just the brain.

> It is a network of intelligence, the collected know-how of not just the brain but the body's other 50 trillion cells; it responds immediately to our slightest thought and emotion, giving rise to the constant flow and change that is basic to our nature; it is not localized in space-time, but is far more general, extending in all directions like a field. (Chopra 1991: 107)

This inner world is called the quantum body, and Chopra believes that we experience it as a level of awareness. In it, perfect health resides. The more we access this quantum body, the more our body will begin to restore itself to health. His techniques—which include transcendental meditation; a purification regime called panchakarma to rid the body of toxins (or ama); pulse diagnosis; a massage technique called marma therapy; and sound, music, and aroma therapies—ultimately encourage a healthy lifestyle, but also provide contact with this quantum body:

In a serious or life-threatening illness, there can be many layers of imbalance concealing the depths where healing exists. Each layer is like a mask hiding the self from itself—one could spend a lifetime never suspecting that the quantum mechanical body exists. Perfect health is a reality at this deepest level, and it waits to be brought to the surface of life. (Chopra 1991: 111–112)

See also ALTERNATIVE AND COMPLEMENTARY MEDICINE; ANTHROPOSOPHICAL MEDICINE; HOMEOPATHIC MEDICINE; MEDITATION; NATURAL HEALING; YOGA.

Chopra, Deepak. (1991) *Perfect Health: The Complete Mind/Body Guide*.

Collinge, William. (1996) *The American Holistic Health Association's Complete Guide to Alternative Medicine*.

Hay, Louise. (1984) *You Can Heal Your Life*.

Hunter, William W. (1879) *Statistical Account of the District of the Garo Hills*.

Leventhal, Howard, and Linda Patrick-Miller. (1993) "Emotion and Illness: The Mind Is in the Body." In *Handbook of Emotions*, edited by Michael Lewis and Jeanette M. Haviland, 365–379.

Levine, Barbara. (1991) *Your Body Believes Every Word You Say: The Language of the Body/Mind Connection*.

Moyers, Bill. (1993) *Healing and the Mind*.

Van Esterik, John L. (1978) *Cultural Interpretation of Canonical Paradox: Lay Meditation in a Central Thai Village*.

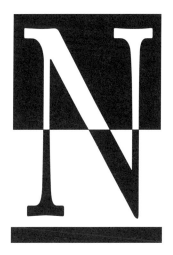

- Flower Remedy/Essence Therapy—the use of the color, smell, shape, and medicinal qualities of flowers to relieve stress and prevent and cure illness
- Food Therapy—the use of diet and nutrition to maintain health and prevent disease
- HERBAL MEDICINE—using plant matter—usually in processed form—to prevent and cure illness
- HOMEOPATHIC MEDICINE—the healing system based on the concept that like cures like
- Hydrotherapy—the use of water through baths, showers, compresses, and inhalation to maintain health and treat illness
- Imagery—the use of positive mental images to reduce pain, fatigue, and anxiety and to speed healing
- Juice Therapy—drinking fruit juices to maintain health and help the body fight disease
- MASSAGE—using touching, rubbing, and manipulation to relieve pain, improve circulation, and relax the body and mind (*see* BODYWORK)
- REFLEXOLOGY—applying pressure to specific spots on the feet to stimulate the body's healing energy
- Relaxation and Meditation—clearing one's mind to relieve stress
- Sound Therapy—listening to pleasing and soothing sounds to relax
- Vitamin and Mineral Therapy—taking vitamins and minerals to supplement those obtained through the diet to maintain health
- YOGA—the ancient Asian/Indian techniques for relaxing and toning the body and mind

ORIGINS AND DEVELOPMENT

The origins of naturopathic medicine can be found in the natural healing methods that have been employed for centuries, especially herbal

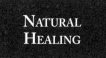

NATURAL HEALING

Natural healing, also called naturopathic medicine, nature cure, or natural medicine, has been called "a great cornucopia." A healing approach based on a return to nature, it incorporates a variety of means to restore balance with nature, from whence we receive our vitality. It works principally through the regulation of diet and lifestyle, herbal remedies, manual manipulation, bathing, and detoxification to achieve a balanced and harmonious lifestyle that allows the inherent healing power of nature to work through the body.

The dozens of specific methods used in natural healing fall into sixteen general categories. These are listed below, with separate articles in this volume for those appearing in ALL CAPITAL LETTERS.

- Acupressure—applying pressure to specific points on the body to stimulate the body's healing energy
- AROMATHERAPY—using pleasant smells for relaxation and stimulation
- AYURVEDIC MEDICINE—the ancient Asian/Indian medical system

medicine, healing with food, and massage. All cultures have recognized the healing properties of foods and herbs, and, along with the power of touch, these methods were among the earliest forms of healing. Humoral medicine, which incorporates the healing properties of hot and cold, especially in food, to rectify imbalances in the system, was also widely used. As medicine in Western countries became more focused on eliminating specific symptoms rather than supporting the body's inherent healing system, respect for natural cures waned.

Natural cures regained popularity in modern times as a specialty form of medicine when the healing baths of an Austrian priest named Sebastian Kneipp attracted the notice of a German named Benedict Lust in the late 1800s. Lust was suffering from tuberculosis at the time, and he cured himself by using Kneipp's method of alternating hot and cold hydrotherapy treatments. Lust believed in the curative powers of the natural world, including fresh air, healthy foods, massage, and exercise, and went on to incorporate them, with hydrotherapy, into his "new" medicine.

Hydrotherapy is a system that exploits the healing property of water, which was believed to stimulate circulation and the lymphatic system, dissolve germs, and draw out toxins from the body. The origins of our current "health spas" lie in water cures, which used the movement of water and the altering of temperature of the water to produce therapeutic effects.

Healing herbs were added to baths as another form of treatment. Valerian and chamomile were commonly added to water to cure nervous conditions. Seaweed, peat, salt, Epsom salts, soda, and sulfur were believed to cure arthritis, rheumatism, paralysis, and poor circulation. The effect of alternating cold and hot water, applied to the body with towels, was to stimulate the circulatory system to act like a pump. Inflammation was reduced when these were ap-

plied to congested areas, and improvement in circulation was observed. Neutral temperature baths promote relaxation and were used to treat insomnia and tension. Pine, oats, bran, soda, and herbs such as elderflowers, peppermint, and horsetail enhanced the effects of these baths.

Lust came to the United States a believer in the power of nature to cure. Nutritional therapy, manual manipulation therapies like chiropractic, the emerging science of psychology, herbal medicine, and homeopathy all became a part of Lust's system. He studied to become a physician and then started a school of naturopathic medicine, in which he taught all of the above. He said, "There is really but one healing force in existence that is Nature herself, which means the inherent restorative power of the organism to overcome disease." (Collinge 1996: 99) Lust's New York City school graduated its first class in 1902; Dr. James Foster founded a similar school in Idaho at about the same time.

Lust viewed his medicine as "orthodox," posing the question "Is it more amenable to combat disease by irritating drugs, vaccines and serums employed by superstitious moderns, or by the bland intrinsic congenial forces of Natural therapeutics?" (Collinge 1996: 99) The three major components he used were the elimination of such "evil" habits as drinking alcohol, coffee, or tea, using drugs, overdoing it socially or sexually, and eating meat; the implementation of restorative habits like proper breathing, moderation in lifestyle habits, exercise, and a balanced mental attitude; and the introduction of new techniques like fasting, hydrotherapy, and forms of manual manipulation like chiropractic and osteopathy.

Since Lust first "packaged" these therapies for modern consumption, natural medicine has waxed and waned in popularity in the West. Many of the types of natural therapies that he employed never left the medicines of the Eastern world. Both Chinese and Indian medicine employ food, herbs, exercise, and massage as the principle methods of healing. Chinese acupuncture, which employs the use of energy highways in the body that are stimulated at various points for healing, may have originated with the observation of the results of acupressure massage. In fact, many modern naturopaths incorporate Chinese medicine and Ayurvedic medicine from India in their practices.

Since there are so many different forms of healing to choose from, naturopathy can vary widely from practitioner to practitioner. They are eclectic and seek to match a cure to a condition. Some naturopaths may specialize and become more focused on one aspect of treatment than another. The commonality among naturopaths is the emphasis on prevention and curing of disease by maintaining balance in the system.

Naturopathy rose in popularity between the turn of the century and the 1940s, in concert with homeopathy and other more traditional and less strictly scientific medicines. The political pressure of conventional medical doctors was successfully brought to bear on these medicines and resulted in a decline in these systems of healing. Licensing became law, and allopathic doctors became the only "real" doctors. The term "allopathic" was coined by Samuel Hahnemann, the originator of homeopathy, and was eventually adopted to describe modern medicine as having no philosophical basis. It focused on alleviated symptoms, rather than on healing the whole person, as is the case in most traditional systems of healing. Homeopathy was more popular—and more successful, particularly in treating the cholera epidemic of the late 1930s—than allopathic medicine, but was trounced in favor of allopathic medicine.

Naturopathic medicine has resurfaced as a popular form of healing since the 1960s, when the back-to-nature movement and awareness of ecology came to the forefront of the thinking of many. As people analyzed their diets and lifestyles, the harmful effects of laboratory-created medicines, adverse environmental effects like pollution and pesticides, and the stress of modern living, they recognized that these conditions may have a serious effect on health and well-being. The number of naturopaths rose.

NATUROPATHIC PRACTICE

A visit to a naturopath usually involves a long initial meeting, during which the patient's diet, work, and lifestyle habits are explored. Special attention is paid to the diet, as digestion is a cornerstone of naturopathic diagnosis. Food intolerances and allergies often interfere with nutrition being properly absorbed by the system and can also result in the build-up of toxins that are left within the digestive system from improperly digested foods. Clearing the pathway for food to be properly digested and eliminated is an important focus. Stress-related conditions at work or at home may be discussed, as well as the amount of exercise taken. After this initial interview, an examination may follow, which may include pulse diagnosis and examination of the tongue.

Though the naturopath is "light" on diagnostic tests and does not usually use expensive invasive laboratory analysis, a few tests are used, especially to determine the condition of the digestion. A urine test to detect putrefaction in the digestive system may be ordered, and hair analysis may be used to determine the level of various minerals and vitamins being delivered to the organs by the blood.

Once an assessment is made, the practitioner may recommend a detoxification program. Detoxification is one of the key methods of healing most conditions. Toxins—harmful substances that build up in the body—are believed to affect the proper functioning of the body's organs as well as inhibit the optimal working of the immune system. Pollution, food intolerances that result in improper digestion, and chronic stress, which releases excess lactic acid into the system, are examples of toxins. Toxins, along with poor nutrition, lack of fresh air and exercise, and exhaustion from stress combine to wear down the body's natural ability to heal itself.

The removal of toxins from the body requires the elimination of all drugs, alcohol, coffee, meat products, and disturbing emotional or sexual habits, and the addition of a new, more nutritious diet. Hydrotherapy, light and air baths, osteopathy, or chiropractic may contribute to the process. A cleansing diet or fast may be recommended.

Since the spine covers the spinal chord, chiropractic and osteopathic techniques are brought in to restore the proper flow of blood through the nervous system and aid in the elimination of toxins. Chiropractic and osteopathy are methods of bone and joint manipulation that restore the proper alignment of the spine. Again, the removal of toxins from the system is a key concept to reestablishing the body's ability to heal itself. Through detoxification, the natural force of healing is given the proper environment to come forward and restore the system.

Once the pathways of the circulatory and digestive systems are clear, relaxation techniques that reduce tension and enhance the breathing may be recommended. Exercise and meditation may be recommended to bring more oxygen into the body and preserve a feeling of well-being. Herbal remedies may be prescribed. Naturopaths use herbal systems from around the world in their healing. Some traditions of naturopathy do not use herbs to effect specific results, but to strengthen the system overall. Others employ herbal medicine or work together with allopaths who prescribe pharmaceutical drugs. Naturopaths may not prescribe prescription drugs, but many view their healing as complementary to allopathic medicine and refer their clients to allopaths and to other holistic practitioners for particular ailments.

After the initial session, follow-up meetings of about a half-hour in length are common, until the condition subsides.

An example of the difference in approaches to healing between allopathic medicine and naturopathic can be seen by the approach to healing infections. In the event of infection, an allopath will prescribe medicine to suppress unpleasant symptoms—in a cold, for example, antihistamines may be used to stop the flow of mucous, which is causing congestion. A naturopath would see that the symptoms of infection—an increase in white blood cells resulting in mucus or pus—are an indication that the body is engaged in fighting the infection. Instead of suppressing the symptoms, which naturopaths believe can result in conditioning the body *not* to respond and result in a weakening of the immune system, naturopaths would support the body's work. Vitamins would be prescribed to strengthen the white blood cells in their work of eliminating the virus, herbal remedies known to help with the particular conditions would be ordered, and so on.

The following treatment for a large diabetic ulcer on the leg is recorded in *The American Holistic Health Association's Complete Guide to Alternative Medicine:*

> The practitioner gave her zinc, beta carotene, and a topical goldenseal cream to apply to the ulcer. He also recommended the use of hydrotherapy each night before bed to aid in the circulation problem. This involves first soaking the feet in warm water, then putting on a pair of cold wet socks, covered by a pair of dry wool socks, and going straight to bed.
>
> After she followed this regime for three weeks the ulcer on Sandra's leg had disappeared. She continues the hydrotherapy treatment four times a week on a preventative basis. . . . The cold moisture has the effect of provoking the body's protective response of increasing peripheral circulation, especially in the feet and legs. Usually they

become so warm during the night that the socks dry out and the person has to remove both pairs. The method is used commonly in diabetes and other problems associated with poor circulation in the extremities, including the hands. (Collinge 1996: 112)

NATUROPATHY TODAY

Naturopathic education includes training in the biomedical sciences such as biochemistry, pathology, microbiology, immunology, laboratory diagnosis, and radiology as well as the holistic therapies described above. Naturopaths view themselves as primary care providers, with an eye to preventative medicine. They are especially attuned to recognizing the early signs of chronic degenerative diseases like cancer. Since they view degenerative diseases as an overall function of the wearing down of the system through negative environmental, emotional, and dietary stresses, they believe that their system of maintaining the proper balance of forces for health in the body is the best defense against these conditions.

The Office of Alternative Medicine at the National Institutes of Health is engaged in studying the effects of diet and vitamins on a number of conditions. For years naturopaths prescribed vitamins C and E to strengthen the immune system, and research has found a strong link between the use of these vitamins and the prevention of cancerous tumors in laboratory animals. It is becoming apparent to most health care practitioners that stress is a major factor in the onset of disease, even if it does not cause it, and stress management programs are now offered by many health maintenance organizations and promoted by most physicians.

Research into the effect of toxic material on the body has resulted in an increased attention to pollution, a concern that has been held by naturopaths for years. Pollution is seen as contributing to chemical sensitivity disorders, which some people believe are increasing in number and severity.

The Council on Naturopathic Medical Education has accredited three colleges for training naturopaths: Bastyr University of Natural Health Sciences in Seattle, Washington; the National College of Naturopathic Medicine in Portland, Oregon; and the Canadian College of Naturopathic Medicine in Toronto, Ontario. Another in Scottsdale, Arizona, has accreditation pending. Some states have adopted a national exam called the Naturopathic Physician Licensing Exam. About 10 states have specific licensing laws and others have right-to-practice laws that allow naturopaths to practice.

The American Association of Naturopathic Physicians (AANP) has 750 members and lobbies on behalf of research and regulations for practice. It publishes the *Journal of Naturopathic Medicine,* which publishes original research and clinical practice articles. There are twenty-four state associations of naturopaths.

See also AROMATHERAPY; AYURVEDIC MEDICINE; BODYWORK; HERBAL MEDICINE; HOMEOPATHIC MEDICINE; REFLEXOLOGY; YOGA.

Collinge, William. (1996) *The American Holistic Health Association's Complete Guide to Alternative Medicine.*

Gottlieb, Bill, ed. (1995) *New Choices in Natural Healing.*

Hill, Ann, ed. (1979) *A Visual Encyclopedia of Unconventional Medicine: A Health Manual for the Whole Person.*

Murray, Michael, and Joseph Pizzorno. (1991) *Encyclopedia of Natural Medicine.*

Woodham, Anne. (1994) *HEA Guide to Complementary Medicine and Therapies.*

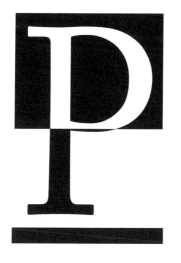

onset of an illness or with an injury, seems to occur and be expressed in all cultures. Chronic pain, which may be either physical or emotional in origin, seems to be expressed and perhaps actually experienced only in some cultures. Perhaps the only general statement that we can make about pain across cultures is that it is usually interpreted as a sign that something is wrong with one's body.

In non-Western cultures, as in Western cultures, pain is seen as a sign of physical illness, but in accord with the supernatural explanations for illness in many of these cultures, pain is also seen as supernatural in origin and subject to supernatural cures. For example, among the Khasi of India:

> If . . . any member be afflicted with illness or pain, the spirit is understood to be restless and in want of something; the breaking of eggs is resorted to, and [the pain] may indicate that it is necessary to sacrifice a fowl or goats, and that the bones of the defunct be taken up and buried in another spot. (Godwin 1872: 131)

The pattern is much the same for the Iban of Indonesia:

> When a person complains of pain in the body the familiar will often suggest that some mischievous devil has put something into him to cause the pain. The *manang* [healer] will thereupon manipulate the part and pretend by some sleight of hand to draw something out of it, a stick, or a stone, or whatever it may chance to be, which, no doubt, he has previously concealed about his person, and he will hand it about and exhibit it as the cause of the pain in the body, which he has thus been able to remove without so much as leaving a mark on the skin. (Roth 1892: 116)

Among the Toradja of Indonesia, beliefs about the cause of pain are somewhat more specific, although the treatment is much the same as in other cultures:

PAIN

Pain is a cultural universal, as in all cultures people experience pain, often associated with illness, injury, and in many cultures, as discussed below, with the death of a close relative or friend or as a component of religious observance. However, despite the fact that probably all people experience pain at some time in their lives, very little is known about pain across cultures. In part, this is because the actual experiencing of pain is a highly personal and individual matter and, especially in the context of illness, seems not to follow any pattern either within or across cultures. It is also because pain transcends language—there are often no words to describe the exact experience of pain—and therefore the experience is not easily described to others. Sometimes, pain is described by certain qualities such as sharp, throbbing, dull, deep, or aching and other times it is described through comparison with other sources of pain, such as the pain of passing a kidney stone's being compared to that of childbirth. Experts classify pain as either acute or chronic. Acute pain, often associated with the

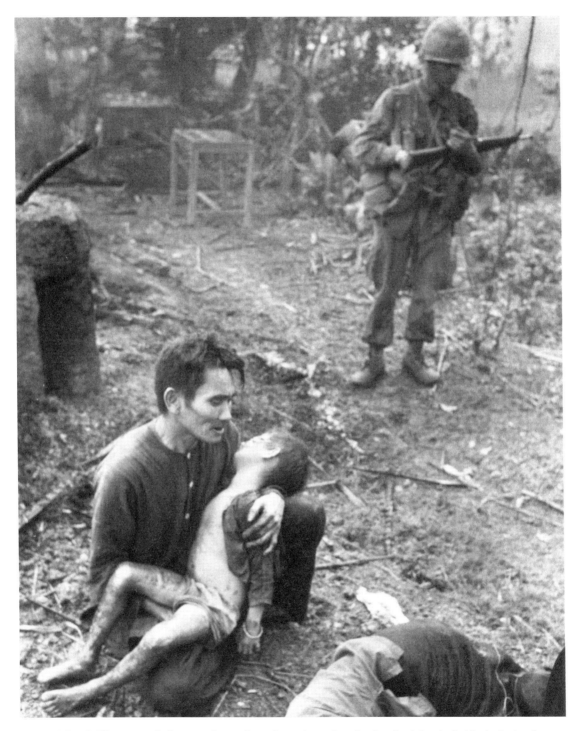

A South Vietnamese father experiences the universal emotional pain of grief as he holds the body of his dead son, killed during a U.S. attack on the Viet Cong in the village of Bon Son.

The morbid matter that is pulled out of the body has the shape of an object connected with the kind of pain in the treated part of the body. Usually onions, pieces of curcuma, or ginger root are brought to light, for the burning sensation that the patient has felt reminds one of these things. Often it is sharp pieces of bamboo that are brought to light; they must have caused the sharp pain that the patient felt. Once we saw a piece of iron pulled out of the stiff neck of a person; this iron had made the neck stiff. (Adriani and Kruyt 1951: 253)

Similarly, the Aranda of Australia are quite specific in their beliefs about the causes of pain and what to do about them:

As a result, the medicine man will perhaps pronounce that the sick man is suffering from a charmed bone inserted by a magical individual, such as Kurdaitcha; or perhaps, worse still, the verdict is that one of the Iruntarinia has placed in his body an Ulinka or short barbed stick attached to an invisible string, the pulling on which by the malicious spirit causes great pain. If the latter be the case it requires the greatest skill of the renowned medicine man to effect a cure. (Spencer and Gillen 1927: 399)

In some cultures pain is not just seen as supernatural in origin but is also believed to be a form of punishment meted out by supernatural beings such as gods or spirits. For example, the Cagaba of Colombia believe that sickness and death are supernatural punishments, and that pain is a sign that death is lurking. Thus, when a Cagaba complains of pain, he is told "Be careful or you will die." The warning means "Take care, observe the law of the Mother so that you may not be punished by death."

Across cultures, emotional pain is a common reaction to the death of a close one and in some cultures that emotional pain is expressed through the self-infliction of physical pain. For example, grief among the Amhara of Ethiopia is expressed, in part, as follows:

. . . hands are thrown into the air in a gesture of loss and abandonment in grief, and the mourners leap into the air, dancing about in semi-formal style, as if suffering such intense pain that they cannot stand on one place. Some roll on the ground, some hit themselves with rocks. (Messing 1957: 484)

Use of pain to express grief was customary among the Blackfoot of the North American plains:

When the Blackfeet went into mourning, they denied and tortured themselves to excite the pity of the Great Spirit, to display to the tribe their indifference to pain and to show their high regard for the departed. During this period which often lasted for several months, they withdrew daily at sunrise and sunset to the summit of a hill, where they wept and gashed themselves with arrow points and knives, until a relative, a man, or a woman, according to the sex of the mourner, went to urge their return to camp. They sometimes cut off a finger, generally the first joint of the small finger. (McClintock 1968: 150)

An especially poignant account of the experience of pain in mourning is provided for the Ona of the Tierra del Fuego:

I observed old Saipoten during this procedure; he had permitted me to sit down in his hut. He was occupied with this for 90 minutes, during which time he never turned his eyes away from his wound, did not utter a sound, and, with a sad expression on his face, shed a few tears. He drew seven lines of blood. Finally, he raised his head again and stared in front of him, deep in thought. He kept both legs drawn in, bent at the knee, so that every visitor or occupant of the hut could see his work of self-torture on his lower right leg. But no one would have fixed his eyes on it out of curiosity; people let their glance pass over it only fleetingly and avoided everything that could disturb the old man in his feelings. Saipoten spent the time from eight o'clock in the morning until four in the afternoon in his hut, demonstrating his grief. Then he stood up and went outside for a short time. Finally he took a little food. He remained very silent the whole day, however, occupied only with his own sorrows over the loss of his child.

This playing with the self-produced flow of blood is customary only among men, is not practiced by the women. They content themselves with a few hasty, irregular scratches up and down and over their breasts and legs. They inflict these scratches on themselves during their mourning song; what matters to them above all is a conscious feeling of pain. (Gusinde 1931: 799)

In some cultures, pain is part of religious practice and is used by adherents to prove the strength of their belief and to draw closer to the supernatural world. The use of pain in religious rituals was common among the indigenous people of the Americas. In South America, for example, people whipped themselves

to purify oneself and to drive out spirits. . . . The Merida Indians celebrate a festival at which the dancers beat themselves with whips while swinging rattles. The Arawak in Guinea whip their guests with plaited whips three feet long, until blood flows. In the same way, the Mundurucu on the Tapajoz and the Caua and Cubeo on the Rio Ayari whip themselves with pieces of fabric at the nahore dance. (Bolinder 1925: 245)

Adriani, N., and Albert C. Kruyt. (1951) *The Bare'e-Speaking Toradja of Central Celebes (the East Toradja)*. Translated from the Dutch by Jenni K. Moulton.

Bolinder, Gustaf. (1925) *The Indians of the Tropical Snow-Capped Mountains: Investigations in Northernmost South America*. Translated from the German by Frieda Schutze.

Godwin, Austin. (1872) "On the Stone Monuments of the Khasi Hill Tribes, and on Some of the Peculiar Rites and Customs of the People." *Journal of the Anthropological Institute of Great Britain and Ireland* 1: 122–143.

Good, Mary-Jo Del Vecchio, et al., eds. (1992) *Pain as Human Experience: An Anthropological Perspective*.

Gusinde, Martin. (1931) *The Fireland Indians. Vol. I. The Selk'nam: On the Life and Thought of a Hunting People of the Great Island of Tierra del Fuego*. Translated from the German by Frieda Schutze.

McClintock, Walter. (1968) *The Old North Trail; or Life, Legends and Religion of the Blackfeet Indians*.

Messing, Simon. (1957) *The Highland Plateau Amhara of Ethiopia*.

Reichel-Dolmatoff, Gerardo. (1951) *The Kogi: A Tribe of the Sierra Nevada de Santa Marta, Colombia*. Vol. 2. Translated from the Spanish by Sydney Muirden.

Roth, H. Ling, ed. (1892) *The Natives of Borneo*.

Spencer, Walter B., and Francis J. Gillen. (1927) *The Arunta: A Study of a Stone Age People*.

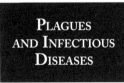

PLAGUES AND INFECTIOUS DISEASES For the purposes of this entry, a plague is defined very broadly to include diseases that affect humans and/or economically important animals by causing debilitating symptoms and much death. Additionally, it is assumed that plagues result from communicable infectious diseases, that is, diseases that spread directly from one human to another or indirectly among humans by animal or insect carriers such as rodents or mosquitoes. From the viewpoint of culture and society, plague becomes an important consideration when it disrupts the normal functioning of society. This disruption—which typically results from the loss of human power due to incapacitation or death—may take a number of forms: (1) the extreme form of societal extinction, as the population can no longer reproduce itself; (2) the somewhat less extreme form of cultural death, as some people survive, but the culture and its institutions are so weakened that key elements of the cultural system disappear and the survivors are absorbed into another society; (3) societal dislocation, as the people relocate to a new region that they believe to be free of disease; and (4) the society continues to survive but various institutional changes take place such as permanent reliance on outsiders for medical and other assistance, the development of new economic activities, and changes in leadership. The study of plagues and the spread of infectious diseases over time and across cultures is extremely difficult, as not until the twentieth century in most parts of the world have reliable medical records been kept that document the spread and effects of plagues. In addition, it is difficult to identify accurately the actual diseases involved in plagues of the past, making it hard to study the spread of different diseases across societies.

Despite these obstacles, it is possible to see that over the 4 million years of human existence, disease—including infectious disease and plague—has evolved through three clear transitions.

The first transition occurred about 8000 B.C. and followed the development of agriculture and permanent settlements. Prior to this time all humans had lived in nomadic hunting/gathering bands that were too small and too mobile to develop epidemics of infectious diseases, although people certainly got sick. The first transition brought with it a decline in health as people now had more contact with human waste and domesticated animals, both of which harbored bacteria, parasites, and viruses that caused infectious diseases in humans. And when cities housing tens of thousands of people developed about 3000 B.C. and then more rapidly in the

early centuries A.D. alongside frequent trade and travel routes between Europe and Asia, and with exploration and colonization of the Americas and Africa, epidemics of infectious diseases emerged. Two factors seem especially important over time and across cultures in the development of these plagues, such as the Black Death of the 1300s which took some 25 million lives in Europe (about 25 percent of the population). First, there must be a population that is large and dense enough to allow infectious disease to spread from one person to another or throughout the population. Second, there must be contact between different populations so that infectious diseases that one group is resistant to can spread to other groups which are not so resistant.

The second major transition in disease happened in economically developed nations beginning in the middle of the 1800s but occurred mainly in the twentieth century. This transition is marked by a decline in infectious diseases and an increase in other diseases due to poor nutrition and age such as cancer and heart disease. The key factor in causing a decline in infectious disease was the twentieth-century discovery of the germ theory of disease and the resulting development of new methods of sanitation, new medical procedures, and antibiotics to control certain kinds of infectious disease.

The third transition is occurring in the 1990s and is marked by the emergence of new and old infectious diseases that are resistant to treatment by antibiotics. Although many of these diseases are called "new" it is likely that few are new to human beings, but, rather, they are now being transmitted more readily to different populations. Those that cause the most alarm are ones that move from the less developed world (Africa, parts of Asia, and Latin America) to the Western world, although the effects in terms of number of deaths and disruption are more devastating in less developed societies. These diseases are discussed below under the heading "Infectious Diseases in the 1990s."

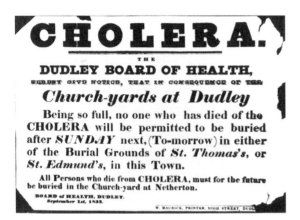

An epidemic of cholera in 1832 caused so many deaths that victims had to be sent to a nearby town for burial.

Throughout human history and across cultures, records of plagues repeat the names, over and over again, of a relatively small number of diseases—smallpox, cholera, typhoid, measles, bubonic fever, tuberculosis, influenza, dysentery, venereal diseases, whooping cough, mumps, scarlet fever, and diphtheria. While no doubt some of these diseases are misnamed in historical accounts, it is clear that the first five alone have accounted for hundreds of millions of deaths in epidemics and pandemics throughout human history and have been a major factor in the destruction of indigenous populations in the past 500 years. The devastating effects of plagues are suggested by the experience of China and Native Americans. In China, nearly 300 epidemics occurred between 243 B.C. and A.D. 1911. An epidemic combined with famine in A.D. 312 left north and central China a "great wasteland," in 423 two out of three died in northern China, in 762 over half the population of Shantung died, in 1127 over half the population of Honan died, in 1358 over 200,000 died, in 1562 seven out of ten died in Fukien, in 1641 an epidemic left "corpses lying side by side throughout," and so on into the twentieth century. In North America, smallpox was likely introduced to the nonresistant Native Americans during Ponce de Leon's expedition to Florida in 1513. It then spread rapidly north and west through the Indian groups and some experts suggest that by 1524 about 75 percent of Native North Americans had died from the disease. While this may be an overestimate, there is no doubt that epidemics and pandemics of infectious diseases such as smallpox and measles reduced the Native American population from several million to about 250,000 over the next three centuries.

PLAGUES AND INDIGENOUS PEOPLES

As the above example from North America suggests, there is no doubt that plagues have been an important factor in the European colonization of the world and the destruction of indigenous cultures. It is likely that Cortes could not have conquered the Aztecs or Pizarro the Inca were it not that both empires were already weakened by epidemics of diseases introduced by the European explorers. For many indigenous peoples, their first contact with Europeans was disease and as often as not, disease that killed them and many other members of their community. As with the first smallpox pandemic in North America, the disease was first introduced through contact among explorers or traders and a small group of Indians who met them. The disease spread though the local Indian community and then through trade contacts to other cultures. It is estimated that the Native American population was decimated by as many as 93 major epidemics and pandemics from 1520 to 1900, including seventeen of measles, ten influenza, four bubonic plague, five diphtheria, four typhoid, three cholera, and four scarlet fever. The cause, nature, and effects of these epidemics on native groups across the continent is indicated by the following accounts and descriptions. The first account, concerning a smallpox epidemic among the Blackfoot of the northern Plains in 1837, raises an issue that continues to be controversial—

was the spread of disease from Europeans to Native Americans a "natural" result of cultural contact or were at least some Europeans involved in actively spreading infectious diseases to destroy Native American resistance?

> Much of the friendliness which followed was due also to the influence of Alexander Culbertson, agent for the American Fur Company. So long as he was present, there were no hostile incidents, despite the harrowing experience of a deadly small-pox epidemic in 1837. The disease had broken out on the company's steamer when it was about to deliver a load of goods to the fort. About 500 lodges of Piegan and Blood Indians camped there, awaiting the arrival of the boat. When they were informed by Major Culbertson that the boat must be held up they were displeased and threatened to take it by force. Unable to restrain them, despite warnings of the consequences, the boat was allowed to land its supply. For the next two months no Indian came to trade and Culbertson went out to locate them. He met a ghastly scene of death; thousands had perished. The disease had spread to Canada and over two-thirds (6000) of the Blood and Blackfoot had died.
>
> Chittendon gives a very different slant to this epidemic. He places the responsibility squarely upon the shoulders of the American Fur Co. officials who permitted a Blackfoot Indian to board the steamer at St. Peters at the mouth of the Little Missouri, and then go to his people without finding out whether he had the disease. In this way the disease was spread among the Blackfoot. (Lewis 1973: 25)

The following example concerns the Pawnee of the eastern Plains and shows how diseases spread from group to group.

> In the midst of the difficulties attending the removal, the Pawnee were afflicted again by the smallpox. An epidemic broke out in 1838 and did not subside until a year and a half later. It is said to have been communicated to the Pawnee by some Dakota women captured by them in the spring of 1838. Great numbers of children perished in the epidemic, while the mortality rate among the adults was perceptibly lower. Nevertheless the total deaths must have considerably exceeded five hundred. . . . (Lesser 1933: 7)

The next shows how diseases were directly transmitted from colonizers to the native peoples.

> There were at least three effects—two immediate and one long-range—which resulted from these unsuccessful Tarahumara [of Mexico] rebellions. One of the immediate effects was, according to Pascual (1651: 205), "a plague that struck the Tarahumara so hard that in many rancherias not one remained alive." The epidemic was most likely introduced by Spanish soldiers. (Champion 1963: 193)

The final example for North America concerns the Hopi of Arizona, whose culture has survived many plagues with many traditional cultural features intact:

> The effects of pestilence have likewise been greatly over-emphasized in the past, for there is abundant historical evidence to show that the Hopi, for instance, have stubbornly clung to their villages in spite of epidemics that have several times threatened them with extinction. In 1780 Governor Anza found their territory in such a wretched condition from "hunger and pestilence" that he reported [the] Hopi tribe to be "in the last stages of its extermination." Still, he could persuade only a few families to forsake their homes, and most of the chiefs begged Anza "not to force any of their people to abandon their pueblos, as most of them desired to end their lives there. . . ." Again and again in more recent times have the Hopi been ravaged by smallpox and other diseases, but there is not a single instance on record of their having abandoned a pueblo on that account. Indeed, when Leo Crane was superintendent of the Hopi Reservation, he complained that it was impossible to check

the smallpox epidemic of 1898 because the Hopi rejected help and preferred "to die unassisted by aliens." (Titiev 1971: 98)

Plagues affected not just North American Indian cultures but virtually all cultures European colonizers came into contact with. In South America, the effects were much the same as in the north of the hemisphere. The Ona of the Tierra del Fuego disappeared, in part, because of the depravations of disease against which their traditional methods of healing were helpless: It has only been in the most recent times that a few medicine men have joined together in connection with an outbreak of an epidemic, since warding off sickness is one of their most important tasks. In earlier centuries the Selk'nam were quite free of general epidemics. Such a one first occurred during the lifetime of Kwaiyus, who presumably lived three generations ago. In recent decades these phenomena were repeated on the occasion of the advance of the Europeans. Usually, however, the *xon*, perplexed and helpless, had to surrender before the force of an epidemic. As an excuse for their powerlessness they told the frightened ones around them, without any hesitation: "This *kwake* comes from the Koliot. It is so strong that we cannot go against it; it cannot be seized by us!" (Gusinde 1931: 1046)

Outside the New World, native peoples in Oceania were affected just as harshly:

Before the coming of the white man the Fiji Islands, like other South Seas groups, had a limited variety of disease germs. Yaws, ankylostomiasis, leprosy, and elephantiasis were present, probably also tuberculosis. It is doubtful whether or not there was dysentery. Malaria, venereal disease, and infectious fevers such as measles, influenza, and whooping cough were absent. As in other parts of the Pacific new varieties of disease germs, brought by the white man, were fatal to the natives who had no resistance or immunity against them. The most disastrous epidemic recorded in Fiji was that of measles in 1875, one year after annexation of the islands by Great Britain. It is estimated that the epidemic wiped out one-third of the entire population of Fiji, and aged Lauans who survived it still tell how they helped to bury the dead of their villages. The people of Maunaithake, Fulanga, say that a row of skeletons on the beach some distance southeast of the village bears witness to this great tragedy, during which the living could not find time to bury the dead.

In 1881 the native population had fallen to 114,748, in 1891 to 105,800, and in 1905 to a low point of just under 87,000, mainly because of dysentery, whooping cough and a second epidemic of measles. (Thompson 1940: 132)

Finally, we move to India where the Khasi, like many tribal peoples in South Asia, suffered the ravages of various European-introduced diseases.

Cholera made its appearance in the Hills in May 1869, traveling from the direction of Jaintiapur, on the borders of Sylhet. It only showed its presence by a few sporadic cases from time to time until the 11th of July, when the disease broke out in an epidemic form among the police and in the jail. The police and the prisoners were at once moved into camp, and communication restricted as much as possible. These precautions probably had the effect of preventing the spread of the disease at Shillong. The epidemic lasted a week; it attacked twenty-four persons, of whom fifteen died. From Shillong the disease traveled southwards, the people deserting their villages as the plague broke out. In the pre-eminently filthy villages on the Cherra Punji plateau the epidemic appears to have found a fitting home, for it stayed among them for a period of nine weeks and a half. The civil surgeon reports the deaths at Cherra Punji and the surrounding villages to have amounted to about 175 out of a total of 232 cases. During the year 1876–77 whooping-cough and small-pox were prevalent in an epidemic form. In the Jaintia Hills small-pox is stated to have caused 47 deaths, chiefly during the months of June, July, and August. (Hunter 1897b: 253–254)

In addition to causing much death and disrupting regular social, economic, and political life, the arrival of epidemics following European contact also influenced the religious system, which was often incapable of explaining such widespread suffering and disease or providing a cure. One way of coping with such cultural disorientation was through the development of religious ideas that explained plagues. An example of this is found among the Central Thai, who, until the arrival of scientific medicine in the twentieth century, suffered from epidemics of cholera and smallpox and whose livestock were often devastated by plagues of animal diseases such as rinderpest. The Central Thai attributed human epidemics and continue to attribute animal epidemics to a supernatural being, the Epidemic Ghost. The Epidemic Ghost causes all epidemic diseases and only epidemic diseases, other spirits cause nonepidemic diseases. The Central Thai believe that the Epidemic Ghost comes from somewhere else:

> Thus, Monk Doctor Marvin told me that Epidemic Ghost derives from a dead Muslim or Lao—explaining that those ethnic groups like to eat fresh raw meat. The Laos in fact do like raw meat prepared in certain ways. Nai Sin, on the other hand, believes that this S [spirit] derives from a Muslim who, before death, specialized in slaughtering buffaloes and chickens, and who now, as a ghost, continued to indulge killing those animals. (Textor 1973: 392)

As protection against the Epidemic Ghost, the Central Thai would obtain predictions about the coming year, enlist the aid of other spirits as protection, and spread salt and sand ritually around their home to keep the Ghost from entering. For the protection of animals, a sacrifice of an animal such as a chicken to satisfy the desires of the Ghost is thought to be protective.

INFECTIOUS DISEASES IN THE 1990s

In the 1990s infectious diseases have again become a major concern. This concern comes from four sources. First, the appearance of new, often deadly infectious diseases. Second, the appearance of new, antibiotic-resistant strains of bacterial infectious diseases. Third, more global travel, more frequent travel, faster travel, and travel to formerly isolated locations that has increased the threat of the spread of previously localized infectious diseases to other regions of the world. And, fourth, the continuing urbanization of the world's population, which produces greater and greater concentrations of people in one locale. Thus, the conditions that caused plagues in the past—contact between different populations; large, compact populations; and communicable diseases for which there are no cures—continue to exist in the modern world.

As in the past, the threat remains serious because people in other regions may not have any natural immunity to the infectious agent and the result might be widespread epidemics and high death rates. Infectious agents include viruses, bacteria, and fungi and they can lead to either new infections such as HIV, which often results in AIDS, or existing ones, such as incidents of tuberculosis, which is spreading in antibiotic-resistant forms, or the outbreak of plague in Surat, India. The agents causing the most concern are those like the Ebola, Marburg, Hantavirus, and Crimean-Congo viruses that are classified as hemorrhagic fever viruses. These viruses are spread through body fluids, not by casual contact, and cause flulike symptoms that progress to rashes, bleeding, kidney and liver damage, and eventually death in the majority of infected individuals. There is no effective treatment nor a vaccine for these viruses. While more frequent and rapid travel is the major means by which infectious disease may move from one region to other regions, other social, political, and

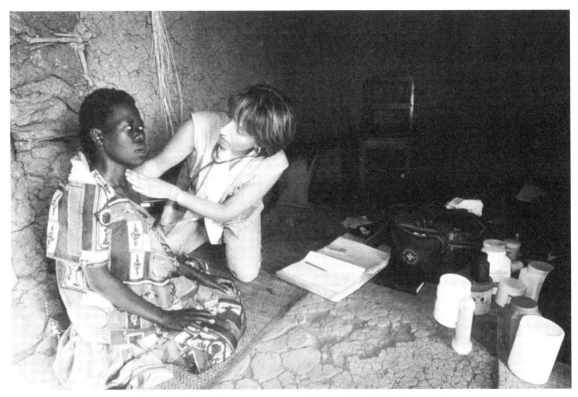

A French physician examines a Ugandan woman diagnosed with the human immunodeficiency virus (HIV). Twenty-five percent of the populations of Uganda and the other African nations of Botswana and Mozambique may be HIV-positive.

economic factors contribute to the appearance and threat posed by these diseases, including the destruction of ecosystems, the displacement of indigenous populations, poverty, environmental pollution, and economic inequalities, which limit treatment and prevention programs in less developed nations. Medical organizations such as the U.S. Centers for Disease Control and Prevention (CDC) and the World Health Organization (WHO) are developing global communication networks to monitor the appearance of infectious diseases and warn medical personnel and governments of their appearance. One major problem facing public health officials is the time and difficulty involved in identifying the disease agent in laboratories in developed nations

such as the United States and France, and the political and social problems that might result when exact information about the disease and how to best treat it is unavailable.

AIDS

Acquired Immunodeficiency Syndrome (AIDS) is a clinical medical syndrome caused by infection in the presence of the human immunodeficiency virus (HIV). HIV is transmitted from infected individuals to other individuals in blood, semen, and vaginal secretions. The origin of HIV is not yet fully known nor understood. HIV alone does not cause AIDS, although individuals with HIV are likely to eventually develop AIDS. HIV has a long incubation period and is often present in an individual for ten years or more before symptoms of disease appear. Medical personnel consider AIDS to be present when an individual's immune system is no longer able to protect the individual from opportunistic infections that would cause no harm to an individual with a healthy immune system. These infections include forms of pneumonia and cancer rarely seen in persons with intact immune systems. While various treatments have been developed that prolong the life of those with AIDS, it is still assumed that AIDS is a terminal disease. There is also no prevention for HIV other than abstaining from behaviors that make the transmission of the virus likely. Prevention programs that have proved most effective—like the one developed by the government of Thailand—include sex education, condom and intravenous needle distribution, and controls on behaviors or social institutions such as prostitution that are avenues for the transmission of HIV. However, in many nations there is often considerable resistance to AIDS prevention programs, often led by those who oppose government intervention in sexual behavior and religious leaders who are opposed to any form of birth control.

AIDS and HIV are worldwide phenomena, although in Western nations attention has been focused on the high incidence among male homosexuals, intravenous drug users, and individuals who received blood transfusions before 1975. More recently, attention has broadened to AIDS and HIV as global phenomena and to variations in their distribution both across and within nations. In the United States, for example, HIV and AIDS are more common in the African-American and Latino population than in the white population. The widespread belief that AIDS was especially prevalent among Haitians has now been shown to be false. In Subsaharan Africa, which has more HIV cases than the rest of the world combined, HIV and AIDS affect both men and women, with labor migration by men, polygynous marriage, and prostitution seeming to play major roles in its spread. In African nations such as Botswana, Uganda, and Mozambique where 25 percent of the people may be HIV-positive, a common pattern of transmittal is for husbands to become infected during sexual intercourse with prostitutes while working away from home, then pass it to their wives through intercourse, who in turn transmit the virus to their unborn children during pregnancy.

The WHO reports that in 1995 there were an estimated 18,500,000 cases of HIV around the world with the following regional distribution:

Subsaharan Africa	11,000,000
North Africa/Middle East	150,000
South/Southeast Asia	3,500,000
East Asia/Pacific	75,000
Latin America	2,000,000
North America	1,100,000
Western Europe	600,000
Eastern Europe/Central Asia	50,000

The U.S. Centers for Disease Control and Prevention estimates that by the year 2000 there will be 30 million adults and 10 million children around the world infected with HIV. As regards AIDS, the WHO reports 1,433,367 cases through mid-1995. Of these, 580,129 are in the Americas, 418,051 in Africa, 141,275 in Europe, and 293,912 in Asia and the Pacific. Experts believe that Asia, with two-thirds of the global population, will by the year 2000 have the majority of people in the world infected with HIV or AIDS. In Asian nations that already have major AIDS epidemics—Cambodia, Myanmar, Thailand, and parts of Vietnam—the pattern of spread is much the same as in Africa: from prostitutes to their clients to the clients' wives to the women's unborn children.

While AIDS has been mainly addressed as a medical problem, it is also an enormous social problem and raises many basic issues in every society where significant numbers of people are infected. Such issues include the acceptance of alternative lifestyles, the role of government and schools in preventing a problem such as AIDS, definitions of the family, and how government funds should be spent.

————————

Armelagos, George J., Kathleen C. Barnes, and James Lin. (1996) "Disease in Human Evolution: The Re-Emergence of Infectious Disease in the Third Epidemiological Transition." *Anthro Notes* 18: 1–7.

Centers for Disease Control and Prevention. (1991) "The HIV/AIDS Epidemic: The First Ten Years." *Morbidity and Mortality Weekly Report* 40: 357–369.

Champion, Jean R. (1963) *A Study in Cultural Persistence: The Tarahumaras of Northern Mexico.*

Garrett, Laurie. (1994) *The Coming Plague: Newly Emerging Diseases in a World out of Balance.*

Gusinde, Martin. (1931) *The Fireland Indians. Vol. 1. Selk'nam: On the Life and Thought of a Hunting People of the Great Island of Tierra del Fuego.* Translated from the German by Frieda Schutze.

Hunter, William W. (1897a) *Statistical Account of Assam. Vol. 2.*

———. (1897b) *Statistical Account of the Khasi and Jantia Hills.*

Lesser, Alexander. (1933) *The Pawnee Ghost Dance Hand Game.*

Levinson, David, and Karen Christensen. (1996) *The Global Village Companion: An A–Z Guide to Understanding Current World Affairs.*

Lewis, Oscar. (1973) *The Effects of White Contact on Blackfoot Culture with Special Reference to the Role of the Fur Trade.*

MacNeil, William H. (1976) *Plagues and People.*

Roizman, Bernard, and James M. Hughes. (1995) *Infectious Disease in an Age of Change.*

Stiffarm, Lenore A., and Phil Lane, Jr. (1992) "The Demography of Native North America: A Question of Native American Survival." In *The State of Native America*, edited by M. Annette James, 23–54.

Textor, Robert B. (1973) *Roster of the Gods: An Ethnography of the Supernatural in a Thai Village.*

Thompson, Laura. (1940) *Southern Lau, Fiji: An Ethnography.*

Titiev, Mischa. (1971) *Old Oraibi: A Study of the Hopi Indians of Third Mesa.*

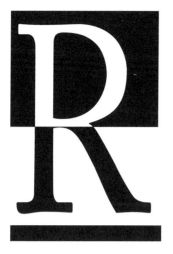

Reflexology is a form of holistic medicine used to cure various disorders and reduce stress through massage and manipulation of the feet. The beginning of reflexology can be traced to 1915, when Dr. William H. Fitzgerald, an ear, nose, and throat specialist, introduced a radical concept into medicine. His idea was similar to the ancient Chinese system of acupuncture energy meridians, which are believed to course through the body, carrying chi, or life energy. When the chi is blocked, disease follows, and unblocking the flow of energy can be accomplished by pressing on points along the meridian lines, which then "reflex" back to the diseased area, restoring balance and health.

When Fitzgerald introduced his system, he called it "zone therapy." He identified ten vertical lines that run the length of the body, dividing it into ten zones. Organs and structures within each zone are believed to be on the same "energy highway." By stimulating another part of the zone, unblocked energy would be released, healing the diseased region. One of his first demonstrations of this effect was in showing the util-

ity of zone therapy as an anesthetic. He stimulated points on a woman's hand (hands and feet, arms and legs are included in the zones) that corresponded to her face and then stuck a pin into her face. She felt no pain.

A physiotherapist named Eunice Ingham later theorized that the foot is a collecting area for the end points for all of the zones and that massaging the foot could help promote healing in any other body part. Reflexology was born.

Reflexologists do not generally diagnose illness. Reflexology is considered to be an adjunct or complement to conventional medical treatment, so patients generally come with a diagnosis. It is a holistic therapy that seeks to stimulate the body's own ability to heal itself. Intuitive and experienced reflexologists may be able to make accurate diagnoses, but most do not.

Tomb paintings from ancient Egypt depict the manipulation of the hands and feet. Practices similar to reflexology are used by some African and Native American peoples. It is a relatively simple procedure to learn and can be used on all ages of people. Babies and children are usually stroked more lightly than adults.

In addition to cleansing the body of toxins and impurities, adherents claim that it improves circulation, balances the system, and revitalizes energy. Because of all of the above, it may be viewed as a method of preventative health care. Many people seek out reflexology to relieve stress, and for overall relaxation, in the same way that people get full-body massages. There are, for example, treatments for eyestrain, neck and shoulder strain, and for building energy reserves, etc.

Over the years, maps and charts of the human body have been drawn by reflexologists, which depict the zones and the location on the foot of every point that reflexes to a corresponding organ or body part.

For reflexologists, the foot is the mirror of the body. For example, the points that reflex the waist line of the torso cross the center of the sole of the foot in the same way. The shoulder and neck line go horizontally above the ball of the foot, and the diaphragm line is halfway between the shoulder and waist points. The pelvic line is between the waist line points and the heel of the foot.

The head area is reflexed by massaging the toes; the chest and lung points are around the ball of the foot, and below, covering the center of the soles of the feet, are the reflex points for the internal organs. The pelvic area is below them. The inside curve of the foot corresponds to the curves of the spine, and the ankle area reflexes to the reproductive organs. If the foot was enlarged to the size of a human torso and set next to it, it would visually correspond to the organs next to it. Using the ends of the zone lines in therapy—in the feet or hands—is a practical decision. The points themselves are spread throughout the body, yet in the conveniently sized appendages of the hands and feet, they can be easily manipulated. There is a wealth of nerve endings in the foot and patients who may not like the other parts of their bodies touched usually have less problem with foot massage.

In addition, kneading the foot is believed to break up inorganic waste like uric acid and calcium crystals that tends to collect in the feet. It is also believed to improve circulation. There are very specific locations on the foot for the specific body parts and organs. In the toes alone, for example, are points for the brain, the sinuses, the ears, the eyes, the temple, the pineal and pituitary gland, the hypothalamus, and the neck.

When there is an injury to the foot, the hands may be used. The foot corresponds physically to the hands in the following way: the sole of the foot corresponds to the palm of the hand, the big toe to the thumb, the small toes to the fingers, the ankle to the wrist, and so on.

REFLEXOLOGY PRACTICE

The reflexologist makes initial contact by holding, shaking, and pressing into the feet for a few minutes. This is called "greeting the feet." The feet are always bare, and a cream or lotion may be used to make the skin more supple. One foot is completely worked before the other is started.

Basic reflexology techniques include thumb and finger walking, in which the bent thumb or finger inches its way along the foot with steady pressure. Leverage is created using the other four fingers. Finger walking is done on the large, fleshy areas of the feet. Troughing is done on the top of the foot, by sliding the thumb lengthwise through the ridges between the bones of the foot. Vibrating is also done on the top of the foot, by running the fingertips in a vibratory manner from the base of the toes to the ankles. In the fist slide, the underside of the foot is massaged by the backs of the fingers, pressed as a fist into the sole of the foot and slid down the surface of the sole. These are just some of the techniques that are used by the practitioner to reach all of the points that are necessary for a particular treatment. The foot may also be twisted, slapped, punched (lightly), karate-chopped, or touched lightly, as in "breeze strokes." The points on the foot that reflex to a damaged or diseased area of the body will feel tender when pressure is applied.

Relaxation techniques may be added to enhance the treatment. For example, the reflexologist may use visualization to help the client relax and get the full benefit of the treatment. A sample of a visualization for high blood pressure is as follows: ". . . imagine a shining golden liquid passing through [your] entire circulatory system, calming it and slowing it. Pay special attention to the golden liquid as it passes through the head and the heart, concentrating on it pooling in these areas and soothing them before it continues on its way. . . ." (Norman 1988: 150) For low blood pressure, ". . . imagine a shining green liquid is filling [you] with energy and vigour. Pay special attention to the heart and the solar plexus area as the liquid flows through the passageways there. . . ." (150)

Clients generally experience a tremendous feeling of relaxation and sometimes fall asleep.

This has no adverse effect upon the treatment. Most people report feeling revitalized and balanced when the treatment is over. Treatments can last for fifteen minutes to over an hour, depending on what is needed.

An example of treatment for a specific ailment is as follows:

FOR INDIGESTION

Each session should last 15 minutes before heavy meals.

Relax both feet with relaxation techniques, and end by a thumb press on the solar plexus point in both feet. Relax each foot separately.

Thumb walk up the five zones of one foot and work the points suggested below.

Thumb walk up the five zones of the other foot and work the points suggested below.

Integrate relaxation techniques throughout the session. (Norman 1988: 228)

The chart below is a partial list of reflex areas, the techniques used to cure diseases in these areas, and the rationale for the technique (229).

See also ACUPUNCTURE; AYURVEDIC MEDICINE; CHINESE MEDICINE.

Hill, Ann, ed. (1979) *A Visual Encyclopedia of Unconventional Medicine: A Health Manual for the Whole Person.*

Norman, Laura. (1988) *Feet First: A Guide to Foot Reflexology.*

Woodham, Anne. (1994) *HEA Guide to Complementary Medicine and Therapies.*

Reflex Area	Technique	Rationale
Chest	Thumb walk	Deepen breathing
Neck	Toe rotation	Relax neck muscles
Throat and esophagus	Thumb walk	Relax smooth muscles
Mouth area	Finger walk	Encourage digestive enzyme production and release; strengthen gums and teeth
Spine (thoracic and lumbar)	Thumb walk and rotate onto thumb	Stimulate spinal nerves to aid digestion
Sigmoid colon	Thumb walk along	Relax the area and allow free movement of waste products
Descending colon/ transverse colon	Thumb walk up	Encourage absorption of nutrients and water; promote regular peristaltic movement of waste
Stomach	Thumb walk across	Release gastric juices; aid stomach movement
Pancreas	Thumb walk across	Promote release of digestive enzymes; move food along intestinal tract; aid digestion
Liver	Thumb walk and rotate onto thumb	Stimulate production of bile; detoxification of blood
Gallbladder	Rotate onto thumb	Encourage proper bile release
Ileocecal valve	Hook and back-up	Encourage absorption of nutrients and water
Ascending colon	Thumb walk up	Promote regular peristaltic movement of waste
Small intestines/duodenum	Thumb walk diagonally across	Encourage release of digestive enzymes; improve intestinal movement; break down food and move it through intestinal tract

REIKI Reiki, also called the Usui System of Natural Healing, is a form of hands-on healing that originated in Japan in the nineteenth century with a Christian monk. Dr. Mikao Usui began a spiritual journey to discover the "formula" for the physical healings attributed to spiritual leaders like Jesus Christ and Gautama Buddha. Usui traveled to Japan and the United States, where he studied world religions, including Buddhism, Christianity, and Hinduism

In an early Sanskrit Sutra he found some symbols and phrases that he believed had been used by Gautama Buddha to heal 3,500 years ago. He then fasted and meditated, hoping for a vision that would unite the many things he had learned into a usable system. Usui is said to have had an ecstatic experience of oneness with all things. He then received visions of a number of symbols. When he left his fasting and meditation he met people who needed healing. When he placed his hands on them, they were healed. He called the healing energy "Reiki."

Reiki is also called the Usui Universal Life Energy Art of Healing. This healing energy is believed to be channeled through the hands of those who have been initiated using the symbols and system that Usui developed. His protégé, Chijiro Hayashi, said:

> The things most important to us, that he remembered, were these symbols and ceremonies because this is the way Reiki is brought to us, and the way we continue the teaching. But the most important thing to him was the remembrance of HOW TO RETURN TO THAT PLACE OF ONENESS WITH PURE LIGHT ENERGY. From that remembered place, all the lives he touched were changed. (Baginski and Sharamon 1988: 55)

Hayashi started a Reiki clinic in Tokyo, which operated until 1940. During this time, Hayashi, who was taught the system by Usui, trained the first Reiki practitioners. A woman who trained in the clinic, Hawayo Takata, brought Reiki to the United States. She taught practitioners who subsequently formed the Reiki Alliance, which offers first, second, and master's degrees. The alliance publishes *The Official Reiki Handbook* and a quarterly magazine called *The Radiance Technique Journal*.

During the first degree course, a student learns the basic hand positions. Though there is a sequence laid out—beginning with the head and working down the entire body, Reiki masters also encourage students to rely on their inner feelings to direct their hands to the areas in need. The hands are held gently on the body, applying little or no pressure. The treatment can also be done with the hands placed up to two inches away from the body and be effective because it is a transfer of energy.

The patient remains fully clothed and is lying down. Each hand position is held three to five minutes. All of the major positions are held and the head, the ears, the eyes, the neck, the shoulders, arms and legs, feet, and hands are covered. Problem areas can be treated for longer periods. The entire treatment lasts about one hour.

Direct treatment begins with treatment on four successive days. It is believed that this clears the body of toxins and stimulates it. After that there may be a weekly treatment, or as needed.

A first degree practitioner is initiated by a teacher called a master who uses a ritual to open up an inner channel of healing within the student. The ritual is called an attunement, and during it, the master works with particular healing symbols. It is believed that this initiation allows the energy to flow through the body and hands of a practitioner into another person's body. The more one practices Reiki, the stronger the flow becomes. Some people have strong emotional, physical, and spiritual changes after they have had the initiation, and their bodies may take some time to readjust.

In second degree Reiki, a practitioner learns to intensify the power of the treatments, using a mental method of healing. Students also receive a second initiation. In addition, it is believed that it is possible to carry out long-distance or absentee healing. The theory is that our thoughts are vibratory patterns of energy similar to radio waves, for example, and can be picked up by others.

In absentee healing, a time and a peaceful environment is arranged for. The practitioner may hold a photograph of the person to be healed and invoke his or her name while visualizing the absent healing symbol. Four successive treatments are given initially, as in direct treatment. Absentee treatment may be carried out without the conscious awareness of the patient, but never against their will.

A short treatment is given when a patient cannot, for whatever reason, lie down. It is done in a chair with hands moving from the top of the head down to the base of the spine. One hand is on the front of the body and one on the back.

In self-treatment, a person treats him- or herself using the same principles of direct treatment. The hands are placed on those areas that can be reached, and the other areas are treated using the absentee treatment method. It is especially effective when done at night and promotes a peaceful and relaxing sleep.

Believers say that Reiki can be used on plants and animals as well as inanimate objects. "Although Reiki is generally used for situations where there is a deficiency or lack of harmony, it can also be used to enrich things with additional life energy, such as food, medicine, plasters, bandages, clothes, and shoes, as well as pieces of jewelry and gems that mean a lot to you."

Reiki can be combined with traditional medical treatment, or with other forms of body work like reflexology and massage. Sometimes it is combined with homeopathy, aromatherapy, Ayurveda, or meditation. It is seen as a complement to almost any kind of therapy.

According to Hawayo Takata's biography, she cured styes, tumors or cysts, infertility, and respiratory and heart problems. One story goes that she was at a funeral and revived the person who had died. There has been no controlled scientific experiments measuring the effectiveness of Reiki. Most people experience deep relaxation and some claim to have had specific illnesses and injuries cured.

Takata believed that most illness was a result of poorly functioning organs, with low vitality. Reiki would improve their functioning, and thus relieve the symptoms. She believed that the solar plexus was the energy center of the body and recommended that treatments start either at the solar plexus or the head. She felt that the full body should be Reikied whenever possible. Takata died in 1980.

See also BODYWORK; ENERGETIC OR MAGNETIC HEALING.

Baginski, Bodo J., and Shalila Sharamon. (1988) *Reiki Universal Life Energy: Self-Treatment and the Home Professional Practice.*

Brown, Fran. (1992) *Living Reiki—Takata's Teachings.*

Haberly, Helen. (1990) *Reiki—Hawayo Takata's Story.*

Ray, Barbara Weber. (1982) *The Reiki Factor: A Guide to Natural Healing, Helping and Wholeness.*

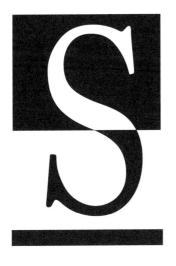

SUICIDE

Suicide can be either individualistic or institutionalized. Individualistic suicide is motivated by personal factors such as revenge, quarrels, depression, grief, or shame. Institutionalized suicide is approved of or perhaps required by the social group. Well-known examples include *hara-kiri*, *tsumebara* (enforced *hara-kiri*), *kamikaze*, and *raidon* in Japan and *suttee* (widow sacrifice or suicide) in India. While Westerners view kamikaze and raidon as suicide, the pilots (airplane and submarine) did not believe they were committing suicide; rather they saw themselves as killing enemy soldiers and believed that their own souls were immortal.

Hara-kiri, when required, is a form of a particular type of suicide known as judicial suicide. Judicial suicide is a type of capital punishment in that a person who is found guilty of a capital crime is forced to kill him- or herself as punishment. Judicial suicide is quite rare, with instances reported in only about 8 percent of cultures. It is found only in complex societies with a strong centralized government headed by a powerful monarch or chief who can force the accused person to commit suicide. Pre-modern Japan fits this model as do the Ashanti in Africa and the Trobriand Islanders and Tikopia in Oceania, all of which have judicial suicide. In Japan, the method was through ritual disembowelment with a ceremonial sword, while Trobrianders jumped from a coconut palm tree and Tikopians paddled out to sea to drown themselves.

Because people often attempt to conceal suicides for personal or religious reasons and because they are hesitant to talk about such matters with outsiders, information on the frequency of suicide is notably unreliable. It is impossible to measure how many societies have suicide and how many do not. And, it is equally difficult to measure the frequency of suicide in a given culture. For example, in a survey of 186 cultures, information about suicide frequency could be obtained for only 47 percent of the cultures, with 4 percent having much suicide, 13 percent a moderate level, and 30 percent very little. The difficulty in counting suicides reliably is indicated by comparing these percentages to those obtained in another survey of 35 societies in which suicide was considered frequent in 35 percent, moderate in 37 percent, and rare in 28 percent of the cultures.

In addition, the meanings and explanations that cultures assign to suicide also vary widely. In some cultures, suicide is a form of conflict resolution mechanism used in settling or airing a grievance. For example, among the Central Thai, relatives might attempt suicide or actually commit suicide in order to let another relative know they are unhappy with their behavior. In this context suicide also serves to assign public responsibility to the person who did them wrong. In other cultures, suicide is a form of punishment. Among the Tikopia of the Pacific, a person likely to be found guilty of committing a serious offense is expected to kill him- or herself. Men usually do this by sailing off alone in a canoe while women are more likely to drown themselves by wading out into the ocean. In either case, "the shark gets his prey." In still other cultures, suicide is seen as a form of aggression directed at the victim by someone else in the community. For example, the Tlingit of Northwest North America believed that all suicides had a cause and when the person who caused the suicide through sorcery was identified his or her relatives were required to compensate the victim's family. Finally, there are some cultures where suicide has no meaning at all. An example are the Aymara of Peru and Bolivia, who cannot comprehend why someone would take his or her

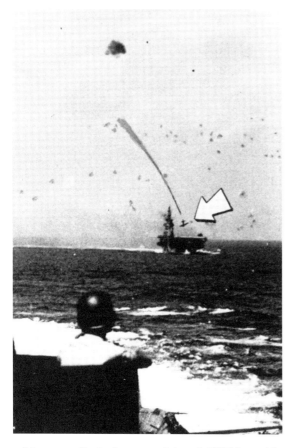

A Japanese pilot is about to crash into the USS Intrepid *during World War II. Westerners thought of the pilots, called kamikazes, as suicide bombers, while the pilots considered themselves heroes on their way to immortality.*

own life. Thus, when told about suicides in other cultures, they can accept that such behavior takes place but cannot understand why it does.

Cultures also vary in the degree to which they consider suicide to be a wrong—a crime or a sin—or to be acceptable. In American culture, suicide is generally disapproved of and surviving relatives prefer not to discuss it. However, the routine acquittals of Dr. Jack Kervorkian in cases where he has admitted assisting terminally ill patients in killing themselves suggests that Americans do accept suicide in certain circumstances. The Ganda of Uganda have a similar view but they worry that the ghost of the suicide victim will cause harm to others. Thus, they quickly remove the body, as with the case of a man who hung himself from a tree in which they cut down the tree and carted the body and tree off to a distant spot in the forest where the ghost could do them no harm. Unlike Americans and Gandans, who usually disapprove of suicide, in many cultures people differentiate among different types of suicide and classify some as wrong and others as acceptable. Among the Ashanti of West Africa, suicide is treated as a capital crime except in special circumstances, when it is considered honorable. Honorable suicides include killing oneself in war to prevent capture, to accompany a master or mistress to the hereafter, or to remove personal dishonor. Otherwise, the Ashanti believe that a person who commits suicide does so to avoid trial and punishment for committing a crime. But the individual does not escape a trial and punishment, as the corpse is tried, found guilty, and beheaded. The beheading prevents the spirit of the deceased from harming the living. It is this fear among the survivors that makes them consider suicide a capital offense.

Both sociocultural and psychological explanations have been used to explain individualistic suicide cross-culturally. Many sociocultural explanations are based on French sociologist Emile Durkheim's research in the 1800s, which suggested that suicide was more likely to occur in social groups that were loosely organized and whose members felt alienated. While this formulation might hold for the modern world or nineteenth-century Europe, in non-Western societies it seems that those who kill themselves are people who feel isolated within a closely knit society.

Psychological explanations stress individual motives, especially feelings of anger and the need to get revenge, even if that revenge is achieved through turning one's anger on oneself. Cultural anthropologist Raoul Naroll sought to combine the sociological and psychological explanations into a single explanation that he called the thwarting disorientation theory of suicide—"thwarting disorientation situations in which a victim blames a person for the victim's loss of social ties, tend to cause suicide." In a sample of 58 cultures, these situations seem to be the cause, with suicide found more often in cultures where couples do not have free choice in selecting a spouse, divorce for men is easy, wives are often beaten, witches are feared, men get drunk and fight, homicide is common, and the group is often at war with other groups. All of these are situations that might break one's social ties to others or to the community. In addition to thwarting disorientation situations, revenge also plays a role. For example, in rural Taiwan, when a woman marries she leaves her childhood home and moves into her husband's childhood home. There she is forced to compete with her mother-in-law and submit to her wishes. The highest suicide rate for Taiwanese women occurs when they are in their early twenties—the time period in which they marry. A young woman may drink poison, throw herself beneath a train, or leap from a bridge. She is motivated partly by a need to escape a difficult social situation and also by revenge, for it is believed that the ghosts of those who commit suicide will not give up until they bring tragedy to those responsible.

Shame also plays a role in suicide for revenge. Among the Lusi-Kaliai people of Papua New Guinea, women who are beaten by their husbands for what they believe are unfair reasons feel terrible shame and powerlessness and seek revenge by killing themselves. The same situation may apply in contemporary North America where the most frequent event preceding suicide by women is beating by their husbands.

While it may often result from broken social ties, suicide, or at least failed attempts at suicide, can also help restore or create ties. Among the !Kung of Botswana, for example, an unhappy young wife might express her feelings by threatening to kill herself. This brings her unhappiness to the attention of other women who rally to offer support.

Cole, John T. (1969) *The Human Soul in the Aymara Culture of Pumasara: An Ethnographic Study in the Light of George Herbert Mead and Martin Buber.*

Counts, Dorothy Ayers, Judith K. Brown, and Jacquelyn C. Campbell, eds. (1992) *Sanctions and Sanctuary: Cultural Perspectives on the Beating of Wives.*

Ember, Carol R., and Melvin Ember. (1992) "Warfare, Aggression, and Resource Problems: Cross-Cultural Codes." *Behavior Science Research* 26: 169–226.

Firth, Raymond. (1949) "Authority and Public Opinion in Tikopia." In *Social Structure: Studies Presented to A. R. Radcliffe-Brown*, edited by Meyer Fortes, 168–188.

Jones, Livingston F. (1914) *A Study of the Tlinghets of Alaska.*

Masamura, Wilfred T. (1977) "Social Integration and Suicide: A Test of Durkheim's Theory." *Behavior Science Research* 12: 251–269.

Naroll, Raoul. (1969) "Cultural Determinants and the Concept of the Sick Society." In *Changing Perspectives in Mental Illness*, edited by Stanley C. Plog and Robert B. Edgerton, 128–155.

Otterbein, Keith F. (1986) *The Ultimate Coercive Sanction: A Cross-Cultural Study of Capital Punishment.*

Rattray, R. S. (1929) *Ashanti Law and Constitution.*

Roscoe, John. (1911) *The Baganda: An Account of Their Native Customs and Beliefs.*

Sharp, Richard L., and Lucien M. Hanks. (1978) *Bang Chan: Social History of a Rural Community in Thailand.*

Shostak, Marjorie. (1981) *Nisa: The Life and Words of a !Kung Woman.*

Smith, David H., and Linda Hackathorn. (1982) "Some Social and Psychological Factors Related to Suicide in Primitive Societies: A Cross-Cultural Comparative Study." *Suicide and Life-Threatening Behavior* 12: 195–211.

Wolf, Margery. (1972) *Women and the Family in Rural Taiwan.*

harmed. For example, the Central Thai believe strongly in the potential harm that might be caused by ghosts. But, the majority of people in rural villages say that they personally have not been harmed by ghosts.

NATURAL EXPLANATIONS

Natural explanations are scientific explanations in the sense that through experimentation or observational studies, one can demonstrate that these naturally occurring factors do cause illness. From the perspective of scientific medicine, there are seven categories of natural explanations for illness:

1. Nutrition, in that too much or too little of a specific substance will cause illness. For example, too little vitamin C causes beriberi while too much fat in the diet causes heart disease in some people.
2. Chemicals that poison or irritate the body or body organs and systems and cause acute or chronic illness. For example, allergies to various plants or foods cause sneezing, runny nose, and other symptoms of physical dysfunction in some people. Similarly, regular exposure to asbestos fibers or coal dust causes lung diseases.
3. Normal physiological changes that may produce illness. For example, a small number of women develop diabetes during pregnancy, and bone deterioration follows menopause for many women.
4. Genetic factors that either cause illness directly or indirectly. Genetic factors are linked indirectly to alcoholism as well as directly to some diseases such as Tay-Sachs disease. It is believed that genetic factors play a significant role in many forms of cancer and heart disease.
5. Emotional stress, including that resulting from daily life and that resulting from

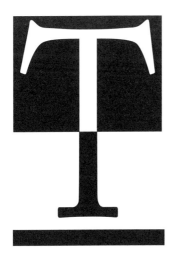

THEORIES OF ILLNESS

Explanations for illness and death across cultures cite either natural causes or supernatural causes. Illness is used here to mean not just disease but also physical injury. While natural causes such as infection, accident, or stress are usually cited in modern societies, which rely primarily on Western medicine for health care, most non-Western cultures in the past and to some extent today attribute illness and death to supernatural causes. And in nearly all cultures (137 out of 139 cultures in one survey), at least some types of illness are attributed to the actions of supernatural forces. This belief is found in all regions of the world and is especially strong in cultures in East Asia and the Mediterranean region. Another survey indicates that in 53 percent of traditional non-Western cultures, all or most illness is attributed to supernatural forces, including witchcraft and sorcery. Of course, while a specific culture may be characterized as having a firm belief in the harmful potential of spirits, this does not mean that all people in the culture share the belief nor that they believe that they will be

undue worry, anger, and unhappiness, plays a part in many physical complaints such as headaches, heartburn, and back pain as well as major disorders such as hypertension.

6. Physical stress caused by overexertion, starvation, and exposure to extreme heat or cold is a major cause of illness.

7. Invading living organisms, including viruses, fungi, bacteria, and parasites, are the cause of numerous diseases and conditions and much scientific research has been devoted to developing natural or chemical agents that will prevent these organisms from causing disease or will halt the progress of the disease.

While these are the explanations cited for illness in scientific medicine, other medical systems such as homeopathy, Ayurvedic medicine, and Chinese medicine also cite "natural causes." However, one major causal agent in these systems is the loss of balance within the human mind-body system, a factor ignored in scientific medicine. Similarly, chiropractic looks to a loss of balance in the "natural alignment" of the nervous system as a major cause of illness.

SUPERNATURAL EXPLANATIONS

Supernatural explanations of illness attribute illness not to the actions of humans or to natural forces such as germs or accidents but to the supernatural world. They fall into three general categories: (1) mystical causation, (2) animistic causation, and (3) magical causation.

Mystical causation describes theories of illness in which the illness is attributed to some impersonal force acting in response to the victim's behavior, including fate, ominous sensations, contagion, and mystical retribution. In mystical explanations no supernatural being directly causes the illness. Fate, ominous sensations

(dreams, sights, sounds that cause illness), and contagion are quite rare across cultures as explanations. In only a minority of cultures are they cited at all, and then only rarely. Examples include the use of judicial ordeals among the Ganda of Uganda in which fate can cause death, certain visions experienced by Pawnee men that cause emotional problems, and contact with ghosts that can cause illness, poverty and other miseries for rural Taiwanese. Mystical retribution, where disease results when someone violates a serious taboo or behaves in an immoral way, is more common and is a major or important explanation for illness in 21 percent of cultures. For example, in Central Thailand, Muslims are thought to be especially susceptible to diseases caused by the water ghost because they wash in ponds or canals after defecation and urination as required by Islam. This angers the water ghost because the water is no longer clean. Buddhists are not subject to such treatment as they wipe but do not wash. For the Sinhalese of Sri Lanka, illness or even supernatural punishment might result from the transgression of sexual mores, particularly if a man has intercourse with a woman who is a relative. And the Mbuti of Central Africa attribute some illnesses or even death to violations of taboos involving the totemic animal of the individual's group. For example, if the totem is a chimpanzee, the individual may not kill it, eat it, eat from a container that held its flesh, or even eat berries, the chimp's favorite food. To avoid violating the taboos and becoming ill, the Mbuti will avoid chimps and hide or flee from them in the forest.

While contagion through contact with a ritually polluting object or person is not a major explanation for illness in general in any culture, it is an important explanation for some illnesses in some cultures. In all cultures there are customary beliefs that allow people to distinguish among objects, places, events, and people that are considered to be unclean and those that are considered to be clean. Some of these beliefs and the rules of behavior based on them are, of course, utilitarian, as they mark unclean items such as a polluted well or spoiled food that might be physically harmful. However, in all cultures people also categorize phenomena as ritually pure or polluting. The idea that certain items are ritually unclean is always accompanied by the notions of pollution and contagion. That is, a person who comes into contact with the item can him- or herself become ritually polluted. These beliefs are accompanied by religious and other behavioral requirements that serve to minimize contact with ritually polluting objects, places, events, and people. As contact with these items is believed to cause illness, misfortune, or even death, there is much reason for following the proper behavior required to avoid contact with them. Across cultures there is enormous variety in the nature and number of items thought to be polluting. In addition, an item might be polluting temporarily or permanently or at certain times but not at others. For example, in many cultures, menstruating women are thought to be polluting to men and their contact with men while they are menstruating is banned or restricted. At all other times, however, they are not thought to be polluting and contact with men is allowed.

A core element of the belief system of Rom Gypsies throughout the world is the notion of *marime*, a complex concept that, depending on the context, means defilement, impurity, shamefulness, pollution, and rejection. Marime is used by Gypsies to order their physical and social worlds, manage male-female relations, maintain distance from outsiders, and maintain order within the group. Unlike the caste system in Hindu India, marime is not linked to the formal religious system, as most Gypsies have traditionally adhered to Roman Catholicism, some follow Eastern Orthodoxy or Islam, and in the last decade significant numbers have been drawn to Pentecostal Christianity. Within the family and the local group, marime focuses on the human body. The parts of the upper half, especially the head and mouth, are considered to be ritually pure while those of the lower half, especially the female genitalia, menstrual blood, and anything associated with birth, are considered polluting or marime. Much ritual activity is devoted to keeping the two spheres separate. The hands, which move between and thereby cross the boundary between the clean upper and marime lower body, are frequently washed, always before cooking or handling religious objects. Items that come into contact with the different body regions are kept clean and stored separately. Newborn infants and the mother—because of involvement with the female genitalia—are considered especially marime and are isolated for days or even weeks before allowed normal contact with men. As regards relations with non-Gypsies, these are restricted to economic matters only, as all non-Gypsies are considered to be marime and the source of disease. Gypsies feel comfortable and safe only at home in the company of other Gypsies. Violation of marime rules is a major source of community disruption and violators are subject to a trial that may result in temporary or permanent isolation or expulsion from the community, both for the violator and his family.

For Gypsies and people in many societies the female genitalia, menstrual blood, and birth are considered polluting for men. While in the majority of societies some restrictions are placed on menstruating women to keep them apart from men, in Gypsy communities the restrictions on male-female contact are far more pervasive. It is marime to touch women's undergarments, to sit on a toilet seat used by a woman, to see the genitalia of a woman who is not one's wife, to engage in sexual intercourse while the woman is menstruating, to engage in oral sex, to touch any objects associated with birth, and for a woman to sit on a man's lap. A Gypsy man goes to considerable lengths to avoid these sources of marime—he might sleep in a bed separate from his wife while she is menstruating, prefer that birth takes place in a hospital, never live on the first floor to avoid women being above him on the second floor, avoid having a woman step over him or his possessions, and ride only in the front seat of cars while women ride only in the rear seat.

Animistic causation refers to the notion of illness as being caused by a supernatural being such as a spirit, or ghost, and is of two types, soul loss and spirit aggression.

In many cultures people believe that the soul is capable of leaving and then returning to the body while the individual is still physically alive. Such travel may be voluntary or involuntary and good or bad for the individual. For the Tarahumara it is voluntary and good, as the soul leaves the body at night when the person sleeps to watch over him, protect his herds, and warn of coyotes. While outside the body, the soul may also act just like a human—singing, dancing, and getting drunk. As in other cultures where the soul leaves voluntarily, it is important that the soul return, or the person will die. The Aymara of Peru are particularly concerned about children accidentally losing their souls. Since children's souls are weak, they are not firmly attached and may be knocked loose when a child falls or is frightened. The soul remains where it fell and must be brought back into the body, usually by the child's mother who waves and yells at it. If it is not brought back, the child is susceptible to possession by evil spirits and might fall ill and die. In about 20 percent of cultures people believe that losing their soul temporarily causes illness. In another 10 percent of cultures, people believe that sorcerers can cause a person to become ill or to die by causing his or her soul to leave the body. Believing that soul loss causes illness seems to be related to the association of soul loss with death, as in most cultures the soul leaves the body when a person dies. Restoring the soul usually requires the expertise of a healer.

Among the Tenino of Oregon, for example, some healers are able to identify the absence of a person's soul as the cause of depression that follows the death of a close relative or friend. The soul of the survivor has departed in order to follow the soul of the deceased to the afterworld. To bring the soul back, the healer dispatches a ghost to the afterworld to bring back the soul, which is then returned to the body and the person's mood lifts.

Spirit aggression is a major supernatural explanation for illness and death across cultures. It is the primary causal factor in 42 percent of cultures and an important cause in another 21 percent of cultures. In many cultures, spirits who cause disease are minor ones (sometimes they are spirits whose main activity is causing disease), in other cultures disease comes from ancestors unhappy with their descendants, and in yet other cultures illness is the work of ghosts, again unhappy with those left behind. In only a small minority of cultures do major spirits or gods concern themselves with the health of individuals.

Spirit aggression as an explanation is part of a more general cultural belief pattern in which supernaturals are defined as either benevolent or generally harmful. For example, the Dani of New Guinea devote considerable ritual activity to pleasing the ghosts of deceased ancestors who lurk about the villages looking to cause disease, bad luck, and illness. The goal of Dani rituals is to drive the ghosts into the forest where they can do little damage. Similarly, the Sara of southern Chad believe in a creator god no longer active in human affairs, and bush spirits and spirits of the dead, both of which are active and potentially harmful. Much of their annual cycle of ceremonies is devoted to pleasing these two categories of spirits in order to maintain or restore order to the natural and social worlds of the Sara. Typical of societies where supernaturals are seen as mainly benevolent are the Tahitians who believe in a hierarchy of supernaturals composed of a high god, superior gods, and ancestor spirits. All are believed to be either potentially malevolent or benevolent, although benevolence is the usual result so long as they are contacted through appropriate ceremonies—the more important the supernatural, the more elaborate the ceremony. In other societies, the nature of supernaturals may be more complex and humans may play a major role in determining their relations with supernaturals. For example, the Mardudjara aboriginals of Australia believe in both benevolent and malevolent spirits but it is humans, under the watch of the spirits, who determine their own fate. Spirits associated with the creation of the Mardudjara and their environment are seen as mainly benevolent and wish humans well, but spirits in distant places are hostile and the Mardudjara prefer to avoid them by staying near home. Whether a culture's customary beliefs about supernaturals is that they are benevolent versus malevolent is closely tied to child rearing practices. In cultures where children are accepted, indulged, and nurtured, supernaturals are usually seen as benevolent. In cultures where children are rejected, severely punished, or ignored, supernaturals are usually seen as malevolent and also as capricious. For example, in the Bahamas, the parents who most frequently beat their children are the ones who are most afraid of supernatural spirits. Thus, people around the world seem to believe that their gods and spirits will treat them as they treat their children.

Magical causation attributes illness and often death to the actions of humans who use magical means to cause others to fall ill or die. These include the evil eye, sorcery, and witchcraft, all three of which are fairly common across cultures as explanations for illness.

Witchcraft is about jealousy, envy, anger, and getting even. In many cultures it is a way that people cause misfortune to happen to others. The Azande of Africa say that if "his condition is bad"

witchcraft is present. Azande witchcraft beliefs are typical of many cultures in the range of misfortune that is attributed to witches:

> A man's ground-nuts [peanuts] are blighted. What does he say? He says, "It is witchcraft. Witchcraft has spoilt my ground-nuts." A man's wife falls ill. What does he say? He says, "Witchcraft has injured my wife." A man is told by the poison oracle that his journey is inauspicious. What does he say? He says, "Witchcraft has spoilt my journey." A man has a nightmare. What does he say? He says, "I have been bewitched in a dream." (Evans-Pritchard 1937: 100)

A witch (a witch is a female, a male witch is called a warlock) is someone who can cause harm to an individual, a family, or even an entire community by simply wishing the harm to take place. A witch is inherently evil and has direct access to the supernatural world and through this supernatural access can cause harm to another person.

The attribution of at least some misfortune to witchcraft is found in 58 percent of societies. Cultures like the Garo in India, where no one "gives a moment's thought to being himself endangered by witchcraft" are in the minority around the world. In cultures with a belief in witchcraft, this belief always involves witchcraft attribution, as people believe it to be a cause of at least some illnesses, accidents, deaths, and other misfortunes. In some cultures witchcraft might not just cause specific misfortunes to befall someone, but may lead to a more general state of harm. The Tlingit of Alaska, for example, say, "You're not yourself when that witch spirit comes on you. You don't even know what you're doing. (de Laguna 1972: 733) Witchcraft is not distributed evenly among the cultures of the world; it occurs far more commonly in societies bordering the Mediterranean Sea, in sub-Saharan Africa, and in communities in the New World formed by descendants of immigrants from the Mediterranean region. It has been suggested that witchcraft beliefs began in Mesopotamia, as beliefs in the evil eye and protective formulae were present among the Babylonians at least as early as 1750 B.C. Witchcraft beliefs were also fairly common in traditional Native American cultures, although unusual elsewhere in the world and virtually absent in East Asia.

In cultures with beliefs in witchcraft attribution, there are often means to protect oneself from witches and to reverse the misfortune they have caused. In many cultures people use protective devices to prevent witch attacks from ever occurring. The Toradja of Indonesia use charms worn on clothing or attached to cradles or placed in cavities in their teeth. The Wolof of Senegal wear amulets and repeat prayers from the Koran in the belief that witches fear God. Iroquois False Face Societies hold pubic rituals to remove disease, storms, witches, and bad luck from the village. In addition, the Iroquois believe that the best way to protect oneself is to behave in an inauspicious manner so as to avoid making anyone jealous. The Tzeltal of Mexico seek to prevent witch attacks by confining their relationships mainly to compadres who are not likely to feel envious.

Short of prevention, in some cultures people watch for signs that help them detect the presence of a witch. The Tlingit know a witch is present by the sound of her footsteps, which sound like cracking ice, while the Toradja believe a witch is present when the tengko bird calls at night instead of day, when a dog repeatedly shows its teeth, or a cat meows at odd times.

Despite efforts to prevent witches from attacking or to detect and avoid them, witches are often successful in causing misfortune. When this happens, the only alternative is to take action to undo the misfortune, which in most cultures and most situations requires the skill and knowledge of a ritual specialist who is often called a shaman, medicine man, witch doctor, sorcerer, or curer. Sometimes the specialist is a general practitioner who deals with all supernatural mat-

ters, not just witchcraft; in other cases he or she might be a witchcraft specialist. As a last resort in some cultures, witches are killed. The Iroquois, for example, would kill only witches who caused great damage or were beyond rehabilitation. When a witch is killed, the concern is that he or she be completely destroyed—the rationale for burning witches or for the Tzeltal practice of hacking the body into dozens of pieces.

Many of the essential features of witchcraft as it exists in contemporary societies are displayed by small-town Mexican-Americans in rural southern Texas. Bewitchment is the most serious of diseases and a matter the people are reluctant to discuss with outsiders. A belief in witchcraft is strongest among lower-class and lower–middle-class adults and generally dismissed as unimportant or ridiculed by those in the upper class and children. Believers fear both male and female witches (*brujos/brujas*), with female witches more common. Witches can fly and often take the form of an animal, usually a cat or an owl. The signs that one has been bewitched include a chronic illness, mental illness, insomnia, and misfortune that soon follow good fortune. Although many are suspected, a witch is rarely identified and accusations are made only after a person dies or leaves town. A person who is a witch can act directly while a nonwitch will hire a witch to place a hex. Witches act out of envy (this is why misfortune after good fortune is attributed to witchcraft), sexual jealousy, and to revenge a real or perceived offense. The hex can be removed by identifying the witch and getting her to remove it, or more often by retaining a specialist to reverse the hex, or by destroying an object thought to cause the hex such as a dead toad or bat.

Although some experts treat sorcery and witchcraft as equivalents, they are different phenomena, and in cultures where both occur the people distinguish between them. Sorcery requires the use of a sorcerer, who, through his or her knowledge of formulae and rituals, can direct supernatural power. Sorcerers, unlike witches, cannot innately cause supernatural forces to affect the lives of the living, as sorcery relies on the use of magical power. For the Ojibwa sorcerer of Canada, that power comes from the plants he uses and from the evil spirits whose assistance he has learned to summon, and whom the Ojibwa believe are only too ready to assist him. The Ojibwa believe that these evil spirits seek to reverse the normal course of events and thus the sorcerer must move in ways opposite the normal. When he digs up a plant to make a potion he must first circle it in a counterclockwise direction and when he calls the spirits by invoking the four directions, he must call east, north, west, and south instead of east, south, west, and north, the normal travel route of the sun. Ojibwa sorcerers have a considerable arsenal of techniques at their disposal, including:

(1) Sketch his victim's image on the ground and place his medicine over the place where he wishes him to feel pain. His victim is stricken immediately.

(2) Carve a wooden image of his victim and tie it by a thread to a poplar tree. The man will die when the thread breaks and the image falls to the ground.

(3) Scratch him with a poisonous spine, *bagamuyak*, imported from the south. Only sorcerers who use these spines know the antidote.

(4) Sprinkle medicine in his victim's food, on his clothes, or on the ground where he walks.

(5) Mix with evil medicine clippings of his victim's fingernails or hair, shreds of fur from his clothing, or charcoal from his campfire. The Indians, therefore, carry away with them a dead coal wrapped in leaves or bark when they break camp, to retain any soul of the fire in their possession; they preserve the souls of old clothing that they give away by keeping a scrap of its wool or hide; and they burn all clippings of their nails or hair.

(6) "Shoot something into his victim's body. To do this he chews with the stick or bone he selects for his missile a leaf of the plant called *zobiginigan* . . . and shoots the two substances together from his mouth in the direction of the enemy. The leaf acts like gunpowder, propelling the stick or stone over the intervening miles until it penetrates the man's body. A *kusabindugeyu* [seer] may extract it and shoot it back at the sorcerer; but unless it penetrates the marrow of his bones he escapes unharmed. Should it penetrate the marrow, however, the sorcerer becomes crippled for life." (Jenness 1935: 85)

Beyond how direct their access is to supernatural power, sorcery and witchcraft differ in other important ways. First, they are found mostly in different cultures. In a survey of 137 cultures, in 47 percent people believed that sorcery was an important cause of illness, in 14 percent people believed that witchcraft was an important cause, in 4 percent people believed that both were important, and in 35 percent people did not believe that either was important. Second, they are found in cultures in different parts of the world. Beliefs in witchcraft as a source of illness predominate in cultures near the Mediterranean Sea, while sorcery beliefs predominate in the New World, in Native American cultures in North and South America. Nearly 50 percent of cultures that attribute illness to sorcery are in the New World. Third, they are found in different types of cultures. Beliefs about sorcery as a cause of illness are found mostly in relatively simple cultures—those with no indigenous writing system, small communities, and an economy based on foraging or horticulture. Witchcraft attribution, on the other hand, is found more often in more complex cultures with larger settlements and agriculture. Fourth, unlike witchcraft, sorcery can be used by anyone. A person can become a sorcerer by learning the spells, formulae, and incantations or can hire a known sorcerer. This suggests that sorcery is more likely to flourish in cultures where people have relatively equal access to the supernatural world. This is more typical of relatively simple cultures where there is less social inequality in all spheres of life. Fifth, witchcraft causes only harm while sorcery can be used to cause harm, to cure, or to benefit others in various ways. Thus, a witch might cause someone to fall ill or die because witches are intrinsically evil but to cause harm a sorcerer must do so intentionally. While attention is often called to harm caused by sorcery, it seems that sorcerers in most cultures also use their skills to do good as well as evil. Some of most sorcerers' work centers on treating, not causing, illness. This is especially true in cultures where sorcery is believed to be a major cause of illness, as sorcery is also the major way to cure illness. Sorcerers who cure are usually called medicine men or shamans.

Sorcery is found primarily in cultures that rely on coordinate control to maintain social order and that do not have agencies of superordinate control. Coordinate control means that conflict is resolved through the direct action of the persons involved such as through retaliation, apology, or avoidance. Superordinate control means that social order is maintained through the actions of culturally recognized authorities such as a council, a chief, or courts. Sorcery acts as a coordinate control in that it causes individuals to pause before causing harm to others for fear that the other person will retaliate by using sorcery to cause them to become ill, have an accident, or even die.

An example of the fear that the threat of sorcery causes is provided by the Toba of Argentina, where sorcery is practiced both in the rural and urban communities. The Toba believe that a sorcerer can cause death through the use of contagious magic, which involves the ritual treatment of physical objects or items associated with the victim—for example, sweat on pieces of clothing, urine, hair, or a cigarette butt. The object is mixed with other objects of magical importance and then burned or buried, causing the victim to become ill and eventually (commonly within a month) die. Death is usually inevitable, although the victim can undo the magic by finding a shaman who can "see" the person causing the victim to fall ill. Additionally, a person dying from sorcery can get revenge by identifying the person causing his death just before he dies; he then dies knowing that his death will be avenged.

The evil eye is the belief that a person can cause harm to another person or their property by simply looking at that person or his or her property. This harm may come in the form of sickness, an accident, or destruction of property such as breaking a valuable pot, burning a house, or killing livestock or crops. A survey of 186 cultures indicates that the belief is present in 36 percent of cultures, although not all people in these cultures believe in the evil eye and believers vary in the intensity of their beliefs. The geographical distribution of the belief is striking. Virtually every culture in India, the Near East, the Middle East, North Africa, East Africa, and Europe has or had an evil eye belief. It also occurs in much of Mexico and a similar belief of "bad air" is found in the Philippines. In regions bordering these areas it occurs only sporadically, and elsewhere in the world it is essentially nonexistent. In North America, the belief is found only among members of immigrant groups from the Old World; there was no such belief among Native Americans. This distribution pattern has led some experts to suggest that the belief began in the Middle East or India and spread to other cultures from there. Others suggest that it may have developed independently in a number of places, although the presence of believers in Mexico and the Philippines is most likely due to the Spanish and Catholic influence on the native cultures of those regions. Wherever it began, the belief goes back at least 5,000 years and was incorporated into the three major world religions that developed in the Middle East—Judaism, Christianity, and Islam—although among many followers of these religions today it is considered a superstition.

Wherever people believe in the evil eye, it is almost always linked with envy. People who are wealthy or good-looking are often the targets, and the destruction of valuable possessions is a widespread result of "casting the evil eye." Cross-culturally and throughout history, the evil eye belief is found mainly in cultures that produce social and physical goods that can be envied. Thus, it is likely that the evil eye belief emerged following the development of agriculture and settled communities about 7,000 years ago. In these communities, wealth distinctions became obvious and people could well envy the pottery, weaving, metal goods, money, cattle, pigs, and sheep of others. Wealth distinctions were accompanied by status distinctions, meaning that there were also categories of people—royalty, upper classes, high castes, chiefs—who could be envied. Another characteristic of evil eye cultures is a strong belief in a high god active in human affairs. This belief, of course, is a central element of Judaism, Christianity, and Islam.

In a survey of evil eye beliefs and practices in twelve nations, anthropologist Clarence Maloney identifies eight general features of the belief:

1. Power emanates from the eye and strikes a person or object
2. The object is something of value
3. The destruction or harm occurs quickly without notice
4. The one casting the evil eye may or may not know that they have the power
5. The victim may or may not know who cast the evil eye

6. The belief is used to explain illness, accidents, and other misfortunes
7. It can be prevented or cured
8. Envy is involved

Many of these features of the evil eye, and especially the link to envy, are found in the evil eye beliefs of the Kandyan Sinhalese of Sri Lanka. The Sinhalese believe in three related phenomena—evil eye, evil mouth, and evil thought—all of which are believed to be motivated by envy. Harm results from a projection of this feeling of envy onto the person who possesses what the jealous person desires. While the caster of the evil eye may do so without awareness, he or she can be identified by a "greedy stare" or in the case of the evil mouth, the making of admiring remarks. Harm resulting from the evil eye includes the destruction of crops and livestock, a reduction in the quality of milk or palm sap, and skin rashes and other maladies. Evil eye accusations are commonly made, but never directly at the accused; often the suspect is an elderly person, a category of person not allowed to be the object of direct expressions of aggression. The Sinhalese take numerous measures to protect themselves from the evil eye, such as keeping food out of the sight of strangers and placing protective signs, objects, and building screens around construction sites.

Within the context of this general pattern suggested by the Sinhalese experience, there is much variation in beliefs and practices associated with the evil eye in cultures around the world. There is even considerable variation within cultures from family to family and individual to individual, especially in regard to measures one must take to prevent the power of the evil from affecting oneself or to reverse its effects. As regards the source of the power, common beliefs are that it comes directly from the evil eye caster, from a certain category of people (the elderly, women, Jews), from a god or supernatural force, from the personal ritual impurity of the caster, from the Devil, or from an evil eye deity. In some cultures it is thought to be always present and always possible, in others it may also be always present and possible, but its consequences are not as serious.

In some cultures anyone is thought capable of casting the evil eye, in others only certain categories of people such as those in low castes, strangers, outsiders, religious officials, witches, babies (also a frequent target), and even animals. Similarly, in many cultures, certain categories of people are more often the target, especially the wealthy and handsome, the dominant group in the community, women, babies, and the weak. Fruits and vegetables, livestock, crops, houses, and all sorts of material objects are frequent targets.

Given the widespread belief that the evil eye can strike anytime an individual admires something about you or something you possess, it is not surprising that thousands of preventative measures are taken to ward off its effects. Incantations are sung, chanted, recited, and spoken to ward off the evil. Amulets in the form of thousands of varieties of charms, necklaces, crosses, pins, and ribbon are worn on the body or attached to clothing. Often, the object must be a certain color. For example, Muslims believe that the color blue is most protective, while Jews and Christians prefer red. Formulae in the form of ritualized sayings and actions may also be used. And, precautions are taken to avoid an evil eye caster. For example, food is prepared in private, one eats in private, one always walks behind someone suspected of being a caster, and a child is called by the name of the opposite sex to confuse the supernatural force behind the evil eye. Cures also include a wide array of incantations, amulets, and rituals. They also may require the intervention of a professional curer such as a sorcerer, exorcist, or priest.

See also ALTERNATIVE AND COMPLEMENTARY MEDICINE; BIOMEDICINE; CULTURE-BOUND SYNDROMES; DEATH; HEALERS; MIND/BODY HEALING.

Ames, David W. (1959) "Belief in 'Witches' among the Rural Wolof of the Gambia." *Africa* 24: 263–273.

Baity, Philip C. (1975) *Religion in a Chinese Town.*

Burling, Robbins. (1963) *Rengsanggari: Family and Kinship in a Garo Village.*

de Laguna, Frederica. (1972) *Under Mount Saint Elias: The History and Culture of the Yakutat Tlingit.*

Downs, Richard E. (1956) *The Religion of the Bare'e-Speaking Toradja of Central Celebes.*

Dundes, Alan, ed. (1981) *The Evil Eye; A Folklore Casebook.*

Evans-Pritchard, Edward E. (1937) *Witchcraft, Oracles and Magic among the Azande.*

Ferndon, Edwin N. (1981) *Early Tahiti as the Explorers Saw It.*

Heider, Karl G. (1990) *Grand Valley Dani: Peaceful Warriors.* 2d. ed.

Hunt, Muriel E. V. (1958) *The Dynamics of the Domestic Group in Tzeltal Villages: A Contrastive Comparison.*

Jenness, Diamond. (1935) *The Ojibwa Indians of Parry Island: Their Social and Religious Life.*

Justinger, Judith M. (1978) *Reaction to Change: A Holocultural Test of Some Theories of Religious Movements.*

Levinson, David, and Martin J. Malone. (1980) *Toward Explaining Human Culture.*

Lumholtz, Carl. (1902) *Unknown Mexico: A Record of Five Years' Exploration of the West-*

ern Sierra Madre; in the Tierra Caliente of Tepic and Jalisco; among the Tarascos of Michoacan.

MacDougall, Robert D. (1971) *Domestic Architecture among the Kandyan Sinhalese.*

Mair, Lucy. (1969) *Witchcraft.*

Maloney, Clarence, ed. (1976) *The Evil Eye.*

Marwick, Max, ed. (1970) *Witchcraft and Sorcery.*

Mascie-Taylor, C. G. N. (1993) *The Anthropology of Disease.*

Masden, William, and Andre Guerrero. (1973) *Mexican-Americans of South Texas.*

Miller, Carol. (1975) "American Rom and the Ideology of Defilement." In *Gypsies, Tinkers, and Other Travelers*, edited by Franham Redhfisch, 41–54.

Miller, Elmer. (1980) *Harmony and Dissonance in Argentine Toba Society.*

Murdock, George P. (1980) *Theories of Illness.*

Naroll, Raoul, Gary L. Michik, and Frada Naroll. (1976) *Worldwide Theory Testing.*

Nash, June. (1970) *In the Eyes of the Ancestors: Belief and Behavior in Maya Community.*

Otterbein, Charlotte S., and Keith F. Otterbein. (1973) "Believers and Beaters: A Case Study of Supernatural Beliefs and Child Rearing in the Bahama Islands." *American Anthropologist* 75: 1670–1681.

Putnam, Patrick. (1948) "The Pygmies of the Ituri Forest." In *A Reader in General Anthropology*, edited by Carlton S. Coon, 322–342.

Reyna, Stephen P. (1995) "Sara." In *Encyclopedia of World Cultures. Volume 9. Africa and the Middle East*, edited by John Middleton and Amal Rassam, 304–307.

Rohner, Ronald P. (1975) *They Love Me, They Love Me Not.*

Roscoe, John. (1911) *The Baganda: An Account of Their Native Customs and Beliefs.*

Swanson, Guy E. (1968) *The Birth of the Gods.*

Textor, Robert B. (1973) *Roster of the Gods: An Ethnography of the Supernatural in a Thai Village.*

Tonkinson, Robert. (1978) *The Mardudjara Aborigines: Living the Dream in Australia's Desert.*

Tschopik, Harry, Jr. (1951) *The Aymara of the Chucuito, Peru: 1. Magic.* Anthropological Papers of the American Museum of Natural History 44: 133–308.

Wallace, Anthony F. C. (1972) *The Death and Rebirth of the Seneca.*

Weltfish, Gene. (1965) *The Lost Universe: With a Closing Chapter on the Universe Regained.*

Whiting, John W. M. (1967) "Sorcery, Sin and the Superego: A Cross-Cultural Study of Some Mechanisms of Social Control." In *Cross-Cultural Approaches*, edited by Clelland S. Ford, 147–168.

Yalman, Nur. (1971) *Under the Bo Tree: Studies in Caste, Kinship, and Marriage in the Interior of Ceylon.*

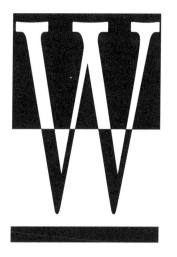

wife beating, and mutual violence. In this scheme, wife beating is defined as physical aggression by a husband against his wife that is considered acceptable by some members of the culture. Wife battering is a pattern of aggression by husbands against wives often accompanied by nonviolent forms of coercion that some people in the culture consider to be abusive. Wife beating/husband beating is the situation where both occur in a given society, with husband beating often a defensive act on the part of the wife. Mutual violence is a situation characteristic of very few cultures, where both husband and wife beating occur, usually independently of each other or with considerable violence. Although this four-type conceptualization has not been explored systematically, it is important to consider because each type may have different causes.

Wife beating is the most common type of family violence found around the world. A survey of 90 cultures indicates that at least some wives are beaten by their husbands in 84.5 percent of societies, a percentage that is consistent with findings of other cross-cultural surveys. Wife beating takes place in most if not all households in 19 percent of cultures, in a majority but not nearly all in 30 percent, in a minority of households in 35.5 percent, and in only a few households or none in 15.5 percent. Additionally, beatings serious enough to permanently injure, scar, or kill a wife occur in 47 percent of cultures.

TYPES OF WIFE BEATING

For a phenomenon so widespread, it is not surprising that wife beating takes a number of different forms. Cross-culturally, societies can be categorized as one of four different types, based on the type of wife beating found there—sexual jealousy, punitive, at will, alcohol-related. In sexual jealousy wife beating cultures, wives are beaten for actual adultery or suspected adultery but are generally not beaten for any other reason. Such cultures constitute 22 percent of

WIFE BEATING

Wife beating is the physical assault of a woman by her husband and includes pushing, shoving, slapping, hitting, hitting with an object, burning, cutting, and shooting. This definition of wife beating can be expanded to include not just husbands and wives but any couple involved in an ongoing, intimate relationship, whether or not they are recognized by society as married. This definition of wife beating encompasses only physical aggression and not other types of nonphysical aggression, such as verbal assault, threats, and ridicule. Cross-culturally, these nonphysical forms of aggression in marriage have been little studied, mainly because they are difficult for outsiders to observe. Wife beating is a major health issue, as such beatings often cause serious physical injury and are part of a pattern of abuse that inflicts emotional distress as well. In many societies, wife beating is a cause of suicide in women.

Some social scientists suggest that wife beating is one of four types of physical violence between spouses found around the world. The three other forms are wife battering, husband beating/

societies with wife beating. In these cultures women experience the most severe beatings and also little or no effort by others in the community to control or prevent the beatings. Sexual jealousy beating societies include a number of Native American groups in North and South America, prior to the reservation period. Here, as in other sexual jealousy beating cultures, men were expected, and even encouraged, to beat wives who had or were suspected of having sexual relations with other men. These beatings were often brutal and the wives might be killed or, among some Plains Indian cultures, facially disfigured, so as to be unattractive to other men. Sometimes—but not always—the wife's lover was also beaten and killed. An example of this pattern is found with the Arapaho:

> Occasionally a suspicious man calmly sent his wife away, either to her paramour or to her home. More often he became angry and jealous. Usually he whipped her, and cut off the tip of her nose or her braids, or both. According to Kroeber (1902, p. 13), he also slashed her cheeks. This treatment of an unfaithful wife was conventional and neither her parents nor the tribe did anything about it. (Hilger 1952: 212)

Punitive beating cultures are ones where men are permitted to beat their wives for reasons that are condoned by others in the community. Usually the reason has to do with the wife's failure or perceived failure to perform her wifely duties or treat her husband correctly. Twenty percent of cultures fall in this category. Beatings in these cultures tend to be less severe and others in the community will intervene if the violence occurs too often or is too severe. The Trukese of Oceania are one example of a culture where beatings for cause are customary:

> Wife beating is quite common but appropriate only if there is good "reason." When

a woman violates the proscriptions on "haughty behavior" or is disobedient, her husband may beat her with no fear of interference from her relatives. However, if a husband beats his wife too frequently, or if the beatings are too severe, the woman's relatives will "pity her" and will cause a separation. (Swartz 1958: 472)

At-will beating cultures are ones where men can and do beat their wives for any reason they deem appropriate. Thus, unlike the first two types, there are no cultural proscriptions governing wife-beating behavior; instead, group norms permit the husband to decide how often and for what reasons to beat his wife. However, others in the community may intervene if beatings occur too often or if they are disruptive to community life. At-will beating cultures constitute 51 percent of cultures with wife beating. Rural Serbs of the early twentieth century displayed many of the typical features of this pattern:

> The peasants consider, and so do their wives, that this is the husband's right as head of the family. If a woman does anything wrong and the husband does not give her a good beating, she begins to despise him, counts him a weakling and strives to assume his place in the home. . . . In the opinion of the village, the husband is the absolute master in the home, who must see that there is order in the home, who has the right to punish the members of the family if they do anything very wrong. (St. Erlich 1966: 270)

In about 8 percent of cultures with wife beating, beatings take place almost exclusively when the husband is drunk, not uncommonly following a public drinking feast that might also include drunken brawling among men. In these cultures, the beatings are highly stylized with the husband apologizing and swearing never to beat the wife again the morning after, the wife forgiving him and excusing his behavior, and the pattern repeating again in the near future.

Since wife beating became a matter of social concern some twenty years ago, numerous social, cultural, economic, political, and psychological explanations have been suggested and tested. It now seems clear that both cross-culturally and in individual cultures, the basic explanation is that wife beating is a means men use to maintain control over women. Both the beatings themselves and the threat of future beatings enable husbands to control the behavior of their wives. Societies where husbands beat their wives regularly are mostly ones where men are able to obtain more wealth than women and where the husband controls the family income. In these cultures men rather than women inherit family property and wealth, men control the fruits of family labor, and men own the family home. Additionally, it is more difficult for women to obtain a divorce and men are the ultimate authority in family decisions. In cultures where women have economic freedom—and especially freedom to control the income produced through their own work—wife beating is unusual, probably because men are no longer in control of their wives and because women have the economic resources that enable them to leave if beaten. A second factor that also encourages wife beating is a cultural pattern that favors the use of physical violence to settle disputes. Thus, wife beating occurs most often in cultures where women are economically unequal and where men and women settle disputes by fighting.

Around the world a variety of interventions are used to prevent a beating from taking place, to end one in progress, or to prevent it from reoccurring. These include:

1. Immediate intervention by a relative, neighbor, or mediator
2. Wife sheltered by a relative or neighbor
3. Public censure of the husband
4. Wife divorces husband
5. Two or more of the above

Interventions occur in nearly all societies, although they are used more often and are most effective in cultures that already have little wife beating. In cultures with much beating the norms that allow or encourage beatings also tend to inhibit the use of interventions.

See also GENITAL MUTILATION; SUICIDE.

Counts, Dorothy Ayers, Judith K. Brown, and Jacquelyn C. Campbell, eds. (1992) *Sanctions and Sanctuary: Cultural Perspectives on the Beating of Wives.*

Daly, Martin, and Margo Wilson. (1988) *Homicide.*

Gelles, Richard J., and Claire P. Cornell. (1983) *International Perspectives on Family Violence.*

Hilger, M. Inez. (1952) *Arapaho Child Life and Its Cultural Background.*

Levinson, David. (1989) *Family Violence in Cross-Cultural Perspective.*

St. Erlich, Vera. (1966) *Family in Transition: A Study of 300 Yugoslav Villages.*

Swartz, M. J. (1958) "Sexuality and Aggression on Romonum, Truk." *American Anthropologist* 60: 467–486.

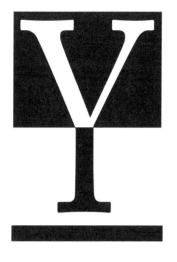

experienced this state and can pass it on to others through teaching. The meditative postures, or asanas, and breathing techniques, or pranayama, are the most common aspects of yoga taught in the West.

Knowledge of yoga first came to the United States through publication of yogic and Hindu texts in the late 1800s. Hindu philosophy became popular among the American Transcendentalist movement in New England at that time. In 1893 Swami Vivekananda, the first guru (or "beloved teacher") came to the United States and attended the World Parliament of Religions in Chicago. He stayed and taught the major branches of yoga. He was followed in the early decades of the twentieth century by a number of yogis who taught the yoga asanas to interested Americans. Indira Devi, a Latvian-born woman, became immersed in yogic philosophy and popularized yoga in Hollywood during the 1950s. Her book, *Yoga for Americans*, was published in 1959.

The asanas are said to bring physical, mental, and spiritual health to those who master the postures and practice them regularly. There are over 200 postures, many of them named after animals and aspects of nature. There are standing, sitting, and prone (laying down) postures. Some require feats of balance and seemingly unnatural twisting, but most can be done, with practice, by any healthy person.

A standing asana—the Tree, for example—requires a person to balance on one leg, while the opposite foot is brought up along the standing leg and placed near the groin. The arms are raised above the head with hands together in a prayerlike fashion. The pose is held for a short time. The Tree is also a balancing posture. Balance poses seek to bring the inner world into balance by causing the person to focus so completely on balancing the body that the mind is clear and a center of peace can be experienced.

A sitting pose, the Lotus, has a person sit upright with legs stretched out in front. Each

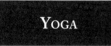

Yoga, a Sanskrit word that means "to unite," is an Indian philosophical system within the religion of Hinduism. Its precepts were set down between 200 and 300 B.C. by Patanjali in the Yoga Sutras. The Yoga Sutras set forth eight steps to attain union with the "ultimate reality," or true self. The steps are: ethics (*yama*), rules of personal conduct (*niyama)*, meditative postures (*asanas*), breathing techniques (*pranayama*), control of the senses (*pratyahara*), concentration (*dharana*), meditation (*dhyana*), and union (*samadhi*).

Samadhi is the culmination of the other seven steps and represents an experience of oneness with the universe. Even though one may "taste" this experience at any time in one's life, it is believed that continued practice of the principles of yoga can lead to more regular experiences of Samadhi.

The experience of Samadhi has been described as an awareness of connection with all of life, a feeling of intense energy, fullness, and bliss. A yogi (male) or yogini (female) is someone who, through his or her mastery of yoga practice, has

foot is then brought into the opposite thigh near the groin area, in a crossed-leg pose. This position is often used in meditation and can be held for long periods of time.

The Cobra, a supine pose, mimics the actions of a snake about to strike. One lies on his or her stomach with the palms of the hands placed on either side of the shoulders. Slowly the head is raised, then the neck, and upper back, using strength in the body. When the back is fully raised, it is supported by the hands. The position is held for a short time.

With practice, yoga students begin to experience an internal flow of energy or well-being while holding the postures. When a session is over, teachers may give several minutes of relaxation for the integration of this energy throughout the body. Teachers of yoga claim that it assists in overcoming physical ailments, "steadies the emotions, and encourages a caring concern for others . . . [and] gives hope." (Mehta, Mehta, and Mehta 1990: 8) Those who practice the asanas as part of the entire yogic system, usually with a master, are expected to develop the other parts of the eightfold system as well. Many in the West who are not Hindus practice the postures for physical health, stress reduction, and relaxation.

Also adapted in the West, and often practiced before relaxation, is pranayama, the special breathing exercises. *Prana* means "life force," and it is believed that regulating the breathing provides another channel to Samadhi. The biologic basis to this is that all of the cells of the body require oxygen, and it is essential to the functioning of the internal organs. The goal of pranayama is the expansion of the breathing capacity.

While sitting in the lotus or a similar crossed-leg position, practitioners focus on the breath. They may inhale in a particular way, holding one nostril closed, then opening it for the exhale. This is called the alternate breath. Use of the throat in the *ujaya* breathing imitates the sounds of ocean waves. One stands up for the cleansing breath, during which the lips are pursed on the exhale for a forceful expulsion of the breath. Again, practitioners experience a sense of wholeness and peace from the practice.

Indian philosophy does not equate the mind with the spirit. Spirit is considered to be unchangeable and related to soul, whereas mind is believed to constantly change. Mind is equated with body as part of the external world—which must be brought in line with the inner spirit in order to reach Samadhi. The purpose of the external world is to provide experiences that help an individual gain spiritual wisdom.

Yoga philosophy teaches that the practice of yoga will strengthen one for the inevitable painful experiences in life. It teaches that while life contains many painful experiences, one can overcome them by learning the peace and serenity of Samadhi. The Hindu concept of conquering "attachment" is an important principle. When one compares the mind, part of the external world, to the true self, the ego is born. From the ego springs a learning toward pleasure and away from pain. But pain and pleasure are transient, so obtaining the habits of steadiness and nonattachment to pain and pleasure is part of the path to true knowledge. Yoga teaches one to obtain a centeredness in the midst of the fluctuations of the mind.

One of the earliest references to yoga in Indian culture is the 3,000-year-old *Ahorbydhyna Samhit*. It describes the idea of union of the true self with the highest self. The Yoga Sutras came 1,000 years later, but it is considered the most authoritative work and is divided into four chapters: Samadhi, practice, accomplishments, and spiritual liberation. There are 196 different aphorisms, or sutras. Because of the detailed descriptions, Hindus think of yoga as a science, including precise technical descriptions of anatomy and benefits to the body as well as showing the path to liberation.

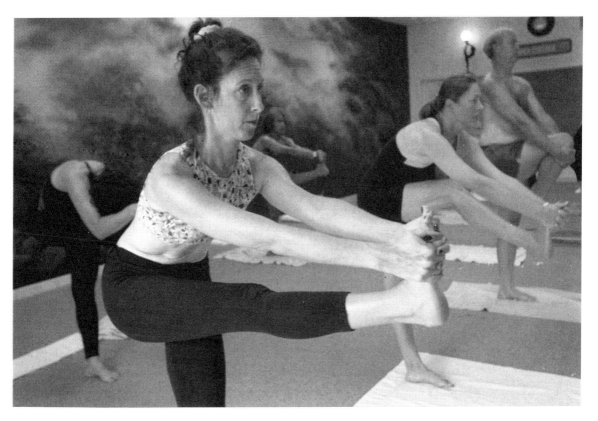

Concentration and stretching precedes a yoga class in Florida in 1995. Originally developed as a Hindu philosophy and practice in India, it has now attracted a following around the world as a complement to scientific medicine.

Many of the asanas are said to have benefits for particular organs. The plough, for example, is done with the shoulders supporting the body and the legs reaching over the head. It increases flexibility in the spine, but also is said to have positive effects on the thyroid, the liver, and the spleen.

Yoga is mentioned in the classical Indian texts of the *Mahabharata*—a long Indian historic epic—and the 18-chapter scriptural portion of the *Bhagavad Gita*. In the *Mahabharata*, the protagonists stop and use yoga and meditation before making decisions.

Hindu concepts of reincarnation (the idea that we have lived before and will be reborn into a new body after death) and polytheism (multiple gods and goddesses) have an impact on the philosophy of yoga. Patanjali wrote that there were two ways of attaining Samadhi: the way of technique and the way of nature. One may practice the asanas and become a yogi, or one may be a god or a superbeing and simply acquire it naturally. It is believed that Samadhi may come spontaneously to a person who studied yoga in a previous life.

In Samadhi, or Nirvana, the self becomes free of the mind in a state where there is no mental conditioning or intellectual structure to interfere with the rapture of one's original being. Intellect is no longer needed and withdraws. Spirit remains. One is said to live no longer within the framework of time, but in "the eternal present."

Yogis often separated themselves from normal human activity and even today many live an ascetic lifestyle. Yoga was once only practiced by men. They were/are often chaste, and, if married, engage in sexual intercourse to conceive children only, then preach a continuation of a chaste lifestyle.

A number of yogic practices seek to find a common internal biological rhythm with the movement of the celestial bodies—especially the sun and moon. The word *hatha* combines the words for sun and moon in Sanskrit. This idea of "cosmicization" is believed to be a stage in the process of liberation. Beyond this great experience of unity is the withdrawal and separation from the cosmos—and the achievement of complete autonomy. In this state there is knowledge of unity and bliss. It can be compared to a return to the state of grace in Christian theology—of the life of Adam and Eve in the garden before they met the serpent. But unlike Adam and Eve, a yogi in this state is *conscious* of his or her freedom.

TYPES OF YOGA

There are a number of different types of yoga, as well as different styles of teaching the asanas. Some styles were created in India and some were created as yoga practice moved out of India into different cultures. China and Japan, for example, have their own particular brands of yoga.

Hatha yoga is a vigorous type of yoga that teaches that there is dormant divine power (kundalini) in the base of the spine, which is released through the asanas and other special practices (including pranayama). It stresses flexibility. Other types of yoga are Iyengar, Kripalu, Ashtanga, Kundalini, and Shwandanda.

The focus of Iyengar yoga is the mastery of the physical body. One seeks to do the postures with perfect alignment and precision. It can be a very demanding form and was developed in In-

dia by B. K. S. Iyengar. Kripalu yoga, popularized in the United States by Yogi Amrit Desai at the Kripalu Center in Massachusetts, has a "softer" approach, which encourages the practitioner to witness the inner world. The first stage of Kripalu is to master the asanas as much as possible without forcing the body. The second is to focus on the feelings and sensations that occur when the form is taken. Finally there is a point where the practitioner surrenders and the body continues the form as the feelings dissolve.

In Ashtanga yoga, a particularly energizing and systematic form of yoga, students repeat one series of asanas with continuous breathing until the poses are mastered. Students work toward higher levels of complexity. The series goes up the spine one vertebra at a time and stimulates the internal organs. There is no break or relaxation between asanas; one pose simply flows into the next, using the breath as a bridge from one to the next.

Kundalini yoga, introduced to the United States by Yogi Bhajan in the 1970s, stresses the release of the kundalini energy. But it is also called the yoga of awareness and seeks to strengthen the inner aims of the spirit. The kundalini is believed to be the energy of the highest potential or motivating evolutionary force. Shwandanda yoga is a very intense aerobic yoga popular in India.

Still other types of yoga do not focus on the physical form of the asanas. Mantra yoga requires the repetition of a particular sound until perfection is attained. The syllable "aum," or "Om," said to include the sound of all the vowels combined and believed to be a sacred sound, is one such mantra. A practitioner often sits in the lotus position or other crossed-leg pose, while quietly repeating the mantra. A mantra is often assigned to the student by his guru. Maharashi Mahesh Yogi brought mantra yoga to the West.

Laya yoga combines breathing, mantra, and rhythm to attain freedom from desire and absorption in bliss. Raja yoga is mastery of the mind and senses. Naad yoga explores the effect of sound vibration on one's state of being. Bahkti yoga is the yoga of devotion to a particular Hindu god or goddess. Karma yoga is the yoga of selfless service, and Yana yoga is the yoga of study and the development of the mind. Kriya yoga is a cleansing yoga.

Tantric yoga is the yoga of sexuality and includes the practice of regulating sexual energy. New England teacher Nancy Simonson, one of the first yoga practitioners to teach in Massachusetts, says that it is not surprising that there are so many kinds of yoga. "Yoga means union," she says. "The art of awareness in peeling an apple can be yoga."

See also HOLISTIC HEALTH AND HEALING; MIND/BODY HEALING.

Dasgupta, Surendranath. (1924) *Yoga as Philosophy and Religion*.

Devi, Indira. (1959) *Yoga for Americans*.

Eliade, Mircea. (1969) *Yoga: Immortality and Freedom*.

Mehta, Silva, Mira Mehta, and Shyam Mehta. (1990) *Yoga, the Iyengar Way*.

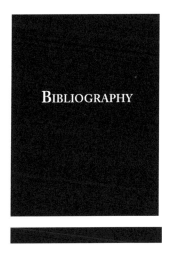

BIBLIOGRAPHY

Abbink, Jon. (1993) "Famine, Gold and Guns: The Suri of Southwestern Ethiopia, 1985–1991." *Disasters* 17: 218–225.

Ackman, Lonnelle. (1977) *Nature's Healing Arts: From Folk Medicine to Modern Drugs.*

Adriani, N., and Albert C. Kruyt. (1951) *The Bare'e-Speaking Toradja of Central Celebes (the East Toradja).* Translated from the Dutch by Jenni K. Moulton.

Ahern, Emily M. (1975) "Sacred and Secular Medicine in a Taiwan Village: A Study of Cosmological Disorders." In *Medicine in Chinese Cultures: Comparative Studies of Health Care in Chinese and Other Societies*, edited by Arthur Kleinman et al., 91–113.

Albert, Steven M., and Maria G. Cattell. (1994) *Old Age in Global Perspective.*

Ames, David W. (1959) "Belief in 'Witches' among the Rural Wolof of the Gambia." *Africa* 24: 263–273.

Andersen, Johannes C. (1995) *Myths and Legends of the Polynesians.* First published in 1928.

Anderson, David, Dale Buegel, and Dennis Chernin. (1978) *Homeopathic Remedies for Physicians, Laymen and Therapists.*

Aptekar, Lewis. (1994) *Environmental Disasters in Global Perspective.*

Arguelles, Jose. (1992) *Mandala.*

Armelagos, George J., Kathleen C. Barnes, and James Lin. (1996) "Disease in Human Evolution: The Re-Emergence of Infectious Disease in the Third Epidemiological Transition." *Anthro Notes* 18: 1–7.

Atkinson, Jane M. (1992) "Shamanisms Today." *Annual Review of Anthropology* 21: 307–330.

Avery, Jeanne. (1982) *The Rising Sign: Your Astrological Mask.*

Babor, Thomas. (1986) *Alcohol: Customs and Rituals.*

Baginski, Bodo J., and Shalila Sharamon. (1988) *Reiki Universal Life Energy: Self-Treatment and the Home Professional Practice.*

Baity, Philip C. (1975) *Religion in a Chinese Town.*

Balch, James F., and Phyllis A. Balch. (1990) *Prescription for Nutritional Healing.*

Balzer, Marjorie M., ed. (1990) *Shamanism: Soviet Studies of Traditional Religion in Siberia and Central Asia.*

Barrett, Robert J., and Rodney H. Lucas. (1994) "Hot and Cold in Transformation: Is Iban Medicine Humoral?" *Social Science Medicine* 38: 383–393.

Barton, Roy F. (1922) *Ifugao Economics.*

———. (1946) *The Religion of the Ifugao.*

Bastien, Joseph. (1989) "Differences between Kallaway-Andean and Greek-European Humoral Theory." *Social Science Medicine* 28: 45–51.

Becker, Robert O. (1990) *Cross Currents: The Perils of Electropollution, the Promise of Electromedicine.*

Belshaw, Cyril S. (1951) "Social Consequences of the Mount Lamington Eruption." *Oceania* 21: 241–252.

Benet, Sula. (1974) *Abkhasians: The Long-Living People of the Caucasus.*

Blong, R. J., and D. A. Radford. (1993) "Deaths in Natural Hazards in the Solomon Islands." *Disasters* 17: 1–11.

Bogin, Barry. (1991) "The Evolution of Human Nutrition." In *The Anthropology of Medicine,* edited by Lola Romanucci-Ross et al., 158–195.

Bohannan, Paul, and Laura Bohannan. (1958) *Three Source Notebooks on Tiv Ethnography.*

———. (1969) *A Source Notebook on Tiv Religion in 5 Volumes.*

Bolinder, Gustaf. (1925) *The Indians of the Tropical Snow-Capped Mountains: Investigations in Northernmost South America.* Translated from the German by Frieda Schutze.

Bollig, Laurentius. (1927) *The Inhabitants of the Truk Islands.* Translated from the German.

Bott, Victor. (1982) *Anthroposophical Medicine: An Extension of the Art of Healing.*

Bouroncle-Carreon, Alfonso. (1964) "Contribucion al Estudio de los Aymaras." *America Indigenista* 24: 129–169, 233–269.

Boyd, Hamish. (1981) *Introduction to Homeopathic Medicine.*

Brennan, Barbara A. (1993) *Light Emerging: The Journey of Personal Healing.*

Brennan, Barbara Ann. (1988) *Hands of Light: A Guide to Healing through the Human Energy Field.*

Brower, Barbara A. (1987) *Livestock and Landscape: The Sherpa Pastoral System in Sagarmatha (Mt. Everest) National Park, Nepal.*

Brown, Fran. (1992) *Living Reiki—Takata's Teachings.*

Bryant, Alfred T. (1966) *Zulu Medicine and Medicine-Men.*

Burling, Robbins. (1963) *Rengsanggari: Family and Kinship in a Garo Village.*

Burton-Bradley, B. G. (1985) "The Amok Syndrome in Papua and New Guinea." In *The Culture-Bound Syndromes: Folk Illnesses of Psychiatric and Anthropological Interest,* edited by Ronald C. Simons and Charles C. Hughes, 237–249.

Button, John. (1988) *A Dictionary of Green Ideas.*

Carreiro, Mary. (1987) *The Psychology of Spiritual Growth, A Gentle Winds Book.*

Carrington, Patricia. (1977) *Freedom in Meditation.*

Centers for Disease Control and Prevention. (1991) "The HIV/AIDS Epidemic: The First Ten Years." *Morbidity and Mortality Weekly Report* 40: 357–369.

A Century of Christian Science Healing. (1966).

Champion, Jean R. (1963) *A Study in Cultural Persistence: The Tarahumaras of Northern Mexico.*

Chernin, Kim. (1985) *The Hungry Self: Women, Eating and Identity.*

Child, Alice B., and Irvin L. Child. (1993) *Religion and Magic in the Life of Traditional Peoples.*

Chopra, Deepak. (1989) *Quantum Healing: Exploring the Frontiers of Mind/Body Medicine.*

———. (1991) *Perfect Health: The Complete Mind/Body Guide.*

Christensen, James B. (1952) *Double Descent among the Fanti.*

Christian Science: A Sourcebook of Contemporary Materials. (1990).

Christian Science Board of Directors. (1991) *Humanity's Quest for Health. Christian Science Sentinel* (Special Issue).

Christian Science Publishing Society. *The Christian Science Sentinel* (weekly).

Cohen, Ronald. (1966) *The Kanuri of Bornu.*

Colbin, Annemarie. (1986) *Food and Healing.*

Cole, John T. (1969) *The Human Soul in the Aymara Culture of Pumasara: An Ethnographic Study in the Light of George Herbert Mead and Martin Buber.*

Collinge, William. (1996) *The American Holistic Health Association's Complete Guide to Alternative Medicine.*

Conzemius, Eduard. (1932) *Ethnographical Survey of the Miskito and Sumu Indians of Honduras and Nicaragua.*

Counts, Dorothy, and David Counts. (1985) *Aging and Its Transformations: Moving toward Death in the Pacific.*

Counts, Dorothy Ayers, Judith K. Brown, and Jacquelyn C. Campbell, eds. (1992) *Sanctions and Sanctuary: Cultural Perspectives on the Beating of Wives.*

Culshaw, W. J. (1949) *Tribal Heritage: A Study of the Santals.*

Cummings, Stephen, and Dana Ullman. (1984) *Everybody's Guide to Homeopathic Medicines: Taking Care of Yourself and Your Family with Safe and Effective Remedies.*

Currier, Richard L. (1966) "The Hot-Cold Syndrome and Symbolic Balance in Mexican and Spanish-American Folk Medicine." *Ethnology* 5: 251–263.

Daly, Martin, and Margo Wilson. (1988) *Homicide.*

Dasgupta, Surendranath. (1924) *Yoga as Philosophy and Religion.*

Davis, Adelle. (1954) *Let's Eat Right to Keep Fit.*

Davis, Patricia. (1995) *Aromatherapy A–Z.*

de Laguna, Frederica. (1972) *Under Mount Saint Elias: The History and Culture of the Yakutat Tlingit.*

Densmore, Frances. (1929) *Chippewa Customs.*

Desai, Meghnad. (1988) "The Economics of Famine." In *Famine*, edited by G. Ainsworth Harrison, 107–138.

Deshen, Shlomo. (1992) *Blind People: The Private and Public Life of Sightless Israelis.*

Devi, Indira. (1959) *Yoga for Americans.*

DeWaal, M. (1980) *Medicinal Herbs in the Bible.*

Diamond, Norma. (1969) *K'un Shen: A Taiwan Village.*

Dirks, Robert. (1993) "Starvation and Famine: Cross-Cultural Codes and Some Hypothesis Tests." *Cross-Cultural Research* 27: 28–69.

Doorkendoo, Efua. (1995) *Cutting the Rose: Female Genital Mutilation, the Practise and Its Prevention.*

Dorsey, George A. (1940) *Notes on Skidi Pawnee Society.*

Dossey, Larry. (1993) *Healing Words: The Power of Prayer and the Practice of Medicine.*

Downs, Richard E. (1956) *The Religion of the Bare'e-Speaking Toradja of Central Celebes.*

D'Souza, Frances. (1988) "Famine: Social Security and an Analyses of Vulnerability." In *Famine*, edited by G. Ainsworth Harrison, 1–56.

Ducey, Paul R. (1956) *Cultural Continuity and Population Change on the Isle of Skye.*

Dundes, Alan, ed. (1981) *The Evil Eye; A Folklore Casebook.*

Dunkin, Amy. (1995) " 'Complementary' Medicine: Is It Good for What Ails You?" *Business Week* (November 27): 134.

East, Ruppert, ed. (1939) *Akiga's Story: The Tiv Tribe as Seen by One of Its Members.*

Eaton, S. B., and M. Konner. (1985) "Paleolithic Nutrition." *New England Journal of Medicine* 312: 283–189.

Eddy, Mary Baker. (1875) *Science and Health with Key to the Scriptures.*

Eisenberg, D. M., et al. (1993) "Unconventional Medicine in the United States: Prevalence, Costs, and Patterns of Use." *New England Journal of Medicine* 328: 246–252.

Eliade, Mircea. (1964) *Shamanism: Archaic Techniques of Ecstacy.*

———. (1969) *Yoga: Immortality and Freedom.*

Eliade, Mircea, ed. (1990) *The Encyclopedia of Religion.*

Elliot, C. (1969) *Japanese Buddhism.*

Ember, Carol R., and Melvin Ember. (1992) "Warfare, Aggression, and Resource Problems: Cross-Cultural Codes." *Behavior Science Research* 26: 169–226.

Emboden, William A., Jr. (1972) *Narcotic Plants.*

Etkin, Nina L. (1990) "Ethnopharmacology: Biological and Behavioral Perspectives in the Study of Indigenous Medicines." In *Medical Anthropology: A Handbook of Theory and Method*, edited by Thomas M. Johnson and Carolyn F. Sargent, 149–158.

Evans, Michael, and Iain Rodger. (1992) *Anthroposophical Medicine: Healing for Body, Mind and Spirit.*

Evans-Pritchard, Edward E. (1937) *Witchcraft, Oracles and Magic among the Azande.*

Ferndon, Edwin N. (1981) *Early Tahiti as the Explorers Saw It.*

Finerman, Ruthbeth. (1989) "The Forgotten Healers: Women as Family Healers in an Andean Indian Community." In *Women as Healers: Cross-Cultural Perspectives*, edited by Carol S. McClain, 24–41.

———. (1989) "Tracing Home-Based Health Care Change in an Andean Indian Community." *Medical Anthropology Quarterly* 3: 162–174.

Firth, Raymond. (1949) "Authority and Public Opinion in Tikopia." In *Social Structure: Studies Presented to A. R. Radcliffe-Brown*, edited by Meyer Fortes, 168–188.

Forrest, Steven. (1984) *The Inner Sky: The Dynamic New Astrology for Everyone.*

Foulkes, Edward F. (1972) *The Arctic Hysterias.*

Frayser, Suzanne. (1985) *Varieties of Sexual Experience.*

Gallin, Bernard. (1966) *Hsin Hsing, Taiwan: A Chinese Village in Change.*

Garb, Paula. (1987) *Where the Old Are Young: Long Life in the Soviet Caucasus.*

Garrett, Laurie. (1994) *The Coming Plague: Newly Emerging Diseases in a World out of Balance.*

Geertz, Hildred. (1968) "Latah in Java: A Theoretical Paradox." *Indonesia* 5: 93–104.

Gelles, Richard J., and Claire P. Cornell. (1983) *International Perspectives on Family Violence.*

Gennep, Arnold Van. (1960) *The Rites of Passage.* Originally published 1909.

Gladwin, Thomas, and Seymour B. Sarason. (1953) *Truk: Man in Paradise.*

Glascock, Anthony P. (1984) "Decrepitude and Death-Hastening: The Nature of Old Age in Third World Societies." *Studies in Third World Societies* 22: 43–67.

Glascock, Anthony P., and Richard A. Wagner. (1986) *HRAF Research Series in Quantitative Cross-Cultural Data. Vol. II: Life Cycle Data.*

Godwin, Austin. (1872) "On the Stone Monuments of the Khasi Hill Tribes, and on Some of the Peculiar Rites and Customs of the People." *Journal of the Anthropological Institute of Great Britain and Ireland* 1: 122–143.

Good, Mary-Jo Del Vecchio, et al., eds. (1992) *Pain as Human Experience: An Anthropological Perspective.*

Gottlieb, Bill, ed. (1995) *New Choices in Natural Healing.*

Gottschalk, Stephen. (1990) "Christian Science." In *Christian Science: A Sourcebook of Contemporary Materials.*

Gould-Martin, Emily. (1983) *Women Asking Women: An Ethnography of Health Care in Rural Taiwan.*

Granzberg, Gary. (1973) "Twin Infanticide—A Cross-Cultural Test of a Materialistic Explanation." *Ethos* 4: 405–412.

Gregerson, Edgar. (1982) *Sexual Practices: The Story of Human Sexuality.*

Groce, Nora. (1990) *Everyone Here Spoke Sign Language: Hereditary Deafness on Martha's Vineyard.*

Gusinde, Martin. (1931) *The Fireland Indians. Vol. 1. The Selk'nam: On the Life and Thought of a Hunting People of the Great Island of Tierra del Fuego.* Translated from the German by Frieda Schutze.

Haberly, Helen. (1990) *Reiki—Hawayo Takata's Story.*

Hamlyn, E. C. (1979) *The Healing Art of Homeopathy: The Organon of Samuel Hahnemann.*

Hanneman, Holger. (1995) *Magnet Therapy: Rebalancing Your Body's Energy Flow for Self-Healing.*

Hansen, Art. (1994) "The Illusion of Local Sustainability and Self-Sufficiency: Famine in a Border Area of Northwestern Zambia." *Human Organization* 53: 11–20.

Harner, Michael. (1982) *The Way of the Shaman: A Guide to Power and Healing.*

Harrell, Clyde S. (1981) "Growing Old in Rural Taiwan." In *Other Ways of Growing Old: Anthropological Perspectives,* edited by Pamela T. Amos and Stevan Harrell, 193–210, 259–260.

Harrison, G. Ainsworth, ed. (1988) *Famine.*

Hastings, James, ed. (1908–1926) *Encyclopedia of Religion and Ethics.*

Hausfater, G., and S. Blaffer Hardy, eds. (1984) *Infanticide: Comparative and Evolutionary Perspectives.*

Hay, Louise. (1984) *You Can Heal Your Life.*

Heath, Dwight B., ed. (1995) *International Handbook on Alcohol and Culture.*

Heider, Karl G. (1990) *Grand Valley Dani: Peaceful Warriors.* 2d. ed.

Hilger, M. Inez. (1939) *A Social Study of One Hundred Fifty Chippewa Indian Families of the White Earth Reservation of Minnesota.*

———. (1952) *Arapaho Child Life and Its Cultural Background.*

Hill, Ann, ed. (1979) *A Visual Encyclopedia of Unconventional Medicine: A Health Manual for the Whole Person.*

Homer-Dixon, Thomas F. (1994) "Environmental Scarcities and Violent Conflict: Evidence from Cases." *International Security* 19: 5–40.

Hosken, Fran. (1982) *The Hosken Report; Genital and Sexual Mutilation of Females.*

Howell, Signe. (1984) *Society and Cosmos: Chewong of Peninsular Malaya.*

Hsu, Francis. (1943) *Magic and Science in Western Yunan: The Problem of Introducing Scientific Medicine in a Rustic Community.*

Hulke, Malcolm, ed. (1979) *The Encyclopedia of Alternative Medicine and Self-Help.*

Hultkranz, Åke. (1992) *Shamanic Healing and Ritual Drama: Health and Medicine in Native North American Religious Traditions.*

Human Relations Area Files. (1964) *Food Habits Survey.*

Hunt, Muriel E. V. (1958) *The Dynamics of the Domestic Group in Tzeltal Villages: A Contrastive Comparison.*

Hunter, William W. (1879) *Statistical Account of the District of the Garo Hills.*

———. (1897a) *Statistical Account of Assam. Vol. 2.*

———. (1897b) *Statistical Account of the Khasi and Jantia Hills.*

Ingersoll, Jasper C. (1969) *The Priest and the Path: An Analysis of the Priest Role in a Central Thai Village.*

Jankowiak, William, and Dan Bradburd. (1996) "Using Drug Foods to Capture and Enhance Labor Performance: A Cross-Cultural Perspective." *Current Anthropology* 37: 717–720.

Jenness, Diamond. (1922) *Report of the Canadian Arctic Expedition, 1913–1918, Vol. XII, Part A.*

———. (1935) *The Ojibwa Indians of Parry Island: Their Social and Religious Life.*

Jochelson, Waldemar. (1933) *The Yakut.* Anthropological Papers of the American Museum of Natural History, vol. 33 (2): 33–335.

Johnson, Thomas M., and Carolyn F. Sargent, eds. (1990) *Medical Anthropology: A Handbook of Theory and Method.*

Jones, Livingston F. (1914) *A Study of the Tlinghets of Alaska.*

Jones, Marc Edmund. (1972) *Astrology: How and Why It Works.*

Jordan, Mary Kate. Personal communication.

Justinger, Judith M. (1978) *Reaction to Change: A Holocultural Test of Some Theories of Religious Movements.*

Kanami, Beena. (1991) "Taking Care of Mankind's Needs." *Humanity's Quest for Health. Christian Science Sentinel* (Special Issue).

Kastner, Mark, and Hugh Burroughs. (1993) *Alternative Healing: The Complete A–Z Guide to over 160 Different Therapies.*

Kaufman, Martin. (1971) *Homeopathy in America: The Rise and Fall of a Medical Heresy.*

Keen, David. (1994) "In Africa, Planned Suffering." *The New York Times* (August 15): A15.

Kemp, Phyllis. (1935) *Healing Ritual: Studies in the Technique and Tradition of the Southern Slavs.*

Kendall, Laurel. (1985) *Shamans, Housewives, and Other Restless Spirits: Women in Korean Ritual Life.*

Kennedy, John G. (1963) "Tesguino: The Role of Beer in Tarahumara Culture." *American Anthropologist* 65: 620–640.

Kiev, Ari (1972) *Transcultural Psychiatry.*

Kleinman, Arthur. (1978) *Culture and Healing in Asian Societies.*

Kleinman, Arthur, et al., eds. (1975) *Medicine in Chinese Cultures: Comparative Studies of Health Care in Chinese and Other Societies.*

Knaster, Mirka. (1996) *Discovering the Body's Wisdom.*

Knez, Eugene I. (1960) *Sam Jong Dong: A South Korean Village.*

Krauss, Friedrich S. (1888) *Yakut Shamanism.*

Krieger, Dolores. (1995) *Therapeutic Touch.*

LaBarre, Weston. (1948) *The Aymara Indians of the Lake Titicaca Plateau, Bolivia.*

Langer, William L. (1974) "Infanticide: A Historical Survey." *History of Childhood Quarterly: The Journal of Psychohistory* 1: 353–365.

Langone, John. (1982) *Chiropractors: A Consumers Guide.*

Lappé, Francis Moore. (1970) *Diet for a Small Planet.*

Larson, David E., ed. (1996) *Mayo Clinic Family Health Book.*

Leroi-Gourhan, Andre. (1953) *French Somaliland.* Translated from the French by Bernard Scholl.

Lesser, Alexander. (1933) *The Pawnee Ghost Dance Hand Game.*

Leventhal, Howard, and Linda Patrick-Miller. (1993) "Emotion and Illness: The Mind Is in the Body." In *Handbook of Emotions,* edited by Michael Lewis and Jeanette M. Haviland, 365–379.

Levine, Barbara. (1991) *Your Body Believes Every Word You Say: The Language of the Body/Mind Connection.*

Levinson, David. (1989) *Family Violence in Cross-Cultural Perspective.*

Levinson, David, and Karen Christensen. (1996) *The Global Village Companion: An A–Z Guide to Understanding Current World Affairs.*

Levinson, David, and Martin J. Malone. (1980) *Toward Explaining Human Culture.*

Leviton, Richard. (1988) *Anthroposophical Medicine Today.*

Lewis, Bernard. (1995) *The Middle East: A Brief History of the Last 2,000 Years.*

Lewis, Oscar. (1973) *The Effects of White Contact on Blackfoot Culture with Special Reference to the Role of the Fur Trade.*

Lofthus, Myrna. (1980) *A Spiritual Approach to Astrology.*

Logan, Michael. (1977) "Humoral Medicine in Guatemala and Peasant Acceptance of Modern Medicine." In *Culture, Disease and Healing,* edited by David Landay, 487–495.

Lumholtz, Carl. (1902) *Unknown Mexico: A Record of Five Years' Exploration of the Western Sierra Madre; in the Tierra Caliente of Tepic and Jalisco; among the Tarascos of Michoacan.*

McClain, Carol S., ed. (1989) *Women as Healers: Cross-Cultural Perspectives.*

McClintock, Walter. (1968) *The Old North Trail; or Life, Legends and Religion of the Blackfeet Indians.*

McCoy, Elin, and Frederick Walker. (1976) *Coffee and Tea.* 3d ed., revised.

MacDougall, Robert D. (1971) *Domestic Architecture among the Kandyan Sinhalese.*

McElroy, Ann, and Patricia K. Townsend. (1989) *Medical Anthropology in Ecological Perspective.*

McFee, Malcolm. (1971) *Modern Blackfeet: Contrasting Patterns of Differential Acculturation.*

McGilvery, Carole, and Jimi Reed. (1994) *Essential Aromatherapy.*

McLean, Scilla, and Stella Efua Graham, eds. (1983) *Female Circumcision, Excision, and Infibulation: The Facts and Proposals for Change.*

MacNeil, William H. (1976) *Plagues and People.*

Magner, Lois N. (1992) *A History of Medicine.*

Maharishi Mahesh Yogi. (1968) *Science of Being and Art of Living.*

Maine, Margo. (1991) *Father Hunger: Fathers, Daughters, and Food.*

Mair, Lucy. (1969) *Witchcraft.*

Mairesse, Michelle. (1981) *Health Secrets of Medicinal Herbs.*

Malinowski, Bronislaw. (1929) *The Sexual Life of Savages in Northwestern Melanesia.*

Maloney, Clarence, ed. (1976) *The Evil Eye.*

Marano, Lou. (1985) "Windigo Psychosis: The Anatomy of an Emic-Etic Confusion." In *The Culture-Bound Syndromes: Folk Illnesses of Psychiatric and Anthropological Interest,* edited by Ronald C. Simons and Charles C. Hughes, 411–448.

Marshall, Mac. (1979) "Natural and Unnatural Disaster in the Mortlock Islands of Micronesia." *Human Organization* 38: 265–272.

Marshall, Mac, ed. (1979) *Beliefs, Behaviors & Alcoholic Beverages: A Cross-Cultural Survey.*

Marwick, Max, ed. (1970) *Witchcraft and Sorcery.*

Masamura, Wilfred T. (1977) "Social Integration and Suicide: A Test of Durkheim's Theory." *Behavior Science Research* 12: 251–269.

Mascie-Taylor, C. G. N. (1993) *The Anthropology of Disease.*

Masden, William, and Andre Guerrero. (1973) *Mexican-Americans of South Texas.*

Maxwell, Robert J., and Philip Silverman. (1989) "Gerontocide." In *The Contents of Culture: Constants and Variants: Studies in Honor of John M. Roberts*, edited by Ralph Bolton, 511–523.

Mehta, Silva, Mira Mehta, and Shyam Mehta. (1990) *Yoga, the Iyengar Way.*

Messegue, Maurice. (1973) *Of Men and Plants.*

Messing, Simon. (1957) *The Highland Plateau Amhara of Ethiopia.*

Micozi, Marc S. (1996) "The Need to Teach Alternative Medicine." *The Chronicle of Higher Education* (August 16): 48.

Miller, Carol. (1975) "American Rom and the Ideology of Defilement." In *Gypsies, Tinkers, and Other Travelers*, edited by Franham Redhfisch, 41–54.

Miller, Elmer. (1980) *Harmony and Dissonance in Argentine Toba Society.*

Minturn, Leigh, and Jerry Stashak. (1982) "Infanticide as a Terminal Abortion Procedure." *Behavior Science Research* 17: 70–90.

Moerman, Daniel. (1986) *Medicinal Plants of Native America.* 2 vols.

Montgomery, Ruth. (1973) *Born to Heal.*

Morehouse, Geoffrey. (1972) *Calcutta.*

Moyers, Bill. (1993) *Healing and the Mind.*

Mukherjea, Charulal. (1962) *The Santals.*

Murdock, George P. (1980) *Theories of Illness.*

Murphy, Robert. (1987) *The Body Silent.*

Murray, Michael, and Joseph Pizzorno. (1991) *Encyclopedia of Natural Medicine.*

Mushtaque, A., et al. (1993) "The Bangladesh Cyclone of 1991: Why So Many People Died." *Disasters* 17: 291–304.

Naroll, Raoul. (1969) "Cultural Determinants and the Concept of the Sick Society." In *Changing Perspectives in Mental Illness*, edited by Stanley C. Plog and Robert B. Edgerton, 128–155.

Naroll, Raoul, Gary L. Michik, and Frada Naroll. (1976) *Worldwide Theory Testing.*

Nash, June. (1970) *In the Eyes of the Ancestors: Belief and Behavior in Maya Community.*

Ness, Robert C. (1985) "The Old Hag Phenomenon as Sleep Paralysis: A Biocultural Interpretation." In *The Culture-Bound Syndromes: Folk Illnesses of Psychiatric and Anthropological Interest*, edited by Ronald C. Simons and Charles C. Hughes, 123–146.

Nichter, Mark. (1992) *Anthropological Approaches to Ethnomedicine.*

Norman, Laura. (1988) *Feet First: A Guide to Foot Reflexology.*

O'Connor, Bonnie B. (1995) *Healing Traditions: Alternative Medicine and the Health Professions.*

Olsen, Kristin G. (1989) *The Encyclopedia of Alternative Health Care.*

Otterbein, Charlotte S., and Keith F. Otterbein. (1973) "Believers and Beaters: A Case Study of Supernatural Beliefs and Child Rearing in the Bahama Islands." *American Anthropologist* 75: 1670–1681.

Otterbein, Keith F. (1986) *The Ultimate Coercive Sanction: A Cross-Cultural Study of Capital Punishment.*

Palau-Marti, Monserrat. (1957) *The Dogon.* Translated from the French by Frieda Schutze.

Panoff, Françoise. (1970) "Maenge Remedies and Conceptions of Disease." *Ethnology* 9: 68–84.

Panos, Maesimund B., and Jane Heimlick. (1980) *Homeopathic Medicine at Home: Natural Remedies for Everyday Ailments and Minor Injuries.*

Paulme, Denise. (1940) *Social Organization of the Dogon of French Sudan.* Translated from the French by Frieda Schutze.

Payer, Lynn. (1988) *Medicine and Culture.*

Peel, Robert. (1971) *The Biography of Mary Baker Eddy, Vol. II, The Years of Trial.*

Prevention Magazine Health Books. (1989) *Hands-On Healing: Massage Remedies for Hundreds of Health Problems.*

Putnam, Patrick. (1948) "The Pygmies of the Ituri Forest." In *A Reader in General Anthropology*, edited by Carlton S. Coon, 322–342.

Quain, Buell. (1948) *Fijian Village.*

Questions and Answers on Christian Science. (1974).

Rattray, Robert S. (1916) *Ashanti Proverbs.*

———. (1927) *Religion and Art in Ashanti.*

———. (1929) *Ashanti Law and Constitution.*

Ray, Barbara Weber. (1982) *The Reiki Factor: A Guide to Natural Healing, Helping and Wholeness.*

Reichel-Dolmatoff, Gerardo. (1951) *The Kogi: A Tribe of the Sierra Nevada de Santa Marta, Colombia.* Vol. 2. Translated from the Spanish by Sydney Muirden.

Reyna, Stephen P. (1995) "Sara." In *Encyclopedia of World Cultures. Volume 9. Africa and the Middle East*, edited by John Middleton and Amal Rassam, 304–307.

Reynolds, Holly B. (1978) *To Keep the Tali Strong: Women's Rituals in Tamilnad, India.*

Richards, Audrey I. (1939) *Land, Labour, and Diet in Northern Rhodesia: An Economic Study of the Bemba Tribe.*

Risse, Gunther, ed. (1973) *Modern China and Traditional Chinese Medicine.*

Rivers, W. H. R. (1914) *The History of Melanesian Society.*

Rivers, William H. R., ed. (1926) *Psychology and Ethnology.*

Rohner, Ronald P. (1975) *They Love Me, They Love Me Not.*

Roizman, Bernard, and James M. Hughes. (1995) *Infectious Disease in an Age of Change.*

Roscoe, John. (1911) *The Baganda: An Account of Their Native Customs and Beliefs.*

Rose, Barry. (1992) *The Family Health Guide to Homeopathy.*

Rosenblatt, Paul C., R. Patricia Walsh, and Douglas A. Jackson. (1976) *Grief and Mourning in Cross-Cultural Perspective.*

Rosenow, Hill Gates. (1970) *Prosperity Settlement: The Politics of Paipai in Taipei, Taiwan.*

Roth, H. Ling, ed. (1892) *The Natives of Borneo.*

Rousseau, R. (1933) *Senegal in Former Times: Study on Cayor, Notebooks of Yoro Dyao.* Translated from the French by Ariane Brunel.

Rubel, Arthur J. (1964) "The Epidemiology of a Folk Illness: Susto in Hispanic America." *Ethnology* 3: 268–283.

Rubenstein, R., ed. (1990) *Anthropology and Aging: Comprehensive Reviews.*

Sahlins, Marshall D. (1958) *Social Stratification in Polynesia.*

St. Erlich, Vera. (1966) *Family in Transition: A Study of 300 Yugoslav Villages.*

Santillo, Humbart. (1984) *Natural Healing with Herbs.*

Savage-Landor, A. Henry. (1895) *Corea or Chosen: The Land of the Morning Calm.*

Schaden, Egon. (1962) *Fundamental Aspects of Guarani Culture.* Translated from the Portuguese by Lars-Peter Lewinsohn.

Schlagen, Kurt H., D.C. Personal communication.

Seaman, Gary W. (1983) *Temple Organization in a Chinese Village.*

Seavoy, Ronald E. (1986) *Famine in Peasant Societies.*

Segal, Gerald. (1993) *The World Affairs Companion.*

Selby, John. (1992) *Kundalini Awakening: A Gentle Guide to Chakra Activation and Spiritual Growth.*

Sen, Amartya. (1981) *Poverty and Famines: An Essay on Entitlement and Deprivation.*

Sharp, Richard L., and Lucien M. Hanks. (1978) *Bang Chan: Social History of a Rural Community in Thailand.*

Shostak, Marjorie. (1981) *Nisa: The Life and Words of a !Kung Woman.*

Siegel, Alan, and Phil Young. n.d. *Polarity Therapy: The Power That Heals.*

Simons, Ronald C., and Charles C. Hughes, eds. (1985) *The Culture-Bound Syndromes: Folk Illnesses of Psychiatric and Anthropological Interest.*

Slack, Alison T. (1988) "Female Circumcision: A Critical Appraisal." *Human Rights Quarterly* 10: 437–486.

Slick, Rosemary Gladstar. (n.d.) *Herbs for the Nervous System.*

———. (n.d.) *Herbs for Winter Health.*

Smith, David H., and Linda Hackathorn. (1982) "Some Social and Psychological Factors Related to Suicide in Primitive Societies: A Cross-Cultural Comparative Study." *Suicide and Life-Threatening Behavior* 12: 195–211.

Sokolovsky, Jay, ed. (1990) *Culture, Aging, and Society.*

Spencer, Walter B., and Francis J. Gillen. (1927) *The Arunta: A Study of a Stone Age People.*

Stanfield, Peggy. (1986) *Nutrition and Diet Therapy.*

Stern, Gerald M. (1976) *The Buffalo Creek Disaster: The Story of the Survivors' Unprecedented Lawsuit.*

Stiffarm, Lenore A., and Phil Lane, Jr. (1992) "The Demography of Native North America: A Question of Native American Survival." In *The State of Native America*, edited by M. Annette James, 23–54.

Stillerman, Elaine. (1996) *The Encyclopedia of Bodywork.*

Stoff, Jesse A., and Charles R. Pellegrino. (1988) *Chronic Fatigue Syndrome: The Hidden Epidemic.*

Swanson, Guy E. (1968) *The Birth of the Gods.*

Swartz, M. J. (1958) "Sexuality and Aggression on Romonum, Truk." *American Anthropologist* 60: 467–486.

Tan, Leong T., Margaret Y. C. Tan, and Veith Ilza. (1973) *Acupuncture Therapy: Current Chinese Practice.*

Tappan, Frances M. (1980) *Healing Massage Technique: A Study of Eastern and Western Methods.*

Teicher, Morton. (1960) *Windigo Psychosis.*

Textor, Robert B. (1973) *Roster of the Gods: An Ethnography of the Supernatural in a Thai Village.*

Thakkur, Chandrashekhar (1974) *Ayurveda: The Indian Art and Science of Medicine.*

Theiss, Barbara, and Peter Theiss. (1989) *The Family Herbal.*

Thompson, Laura. (1940) *Southern Lau, Fiji: An Ethnography.*

Tisserand, Robert. (1988) *Aromatherapy: To Heal and Tend the Body.*

Titiev, Mischa. (1971) *Old Oraibi: A Study of the Hopi Indians of Third Mesa.*

Tonkinson, Robert. (1978) *The Mardudjara Aborigines: Living the Dream in Australia's Desert.*

Torry, William I. (1978) "Bureaucracy, Community, and Natural Disasters." *Human Organization* 37: 302–308.

———. (1978) "Natural Disasters, Social Structure and Change in Traditional Societies." *Journal of Asian and African Studies* 13: 167–183.

———. (1979) "Anthropology and Disaster Research." *Disasters* 3: 43–52.

Tschopik, Harry, Jr. (1951) *The Aymara of the Chucuito, Peru: 1. Magic.* Anthropological Papers of the American Museum of Natural History 44: 133–308.

Turnbull, Colin. (1965) *The Mbuti Pygmies: An Ethnographic Survey.*

United Methodist Book of Worship (1992).

University of California at Berkeley. (1991) *The Wellness Encyclopedia.*

Van Esterik, John L. (1978) *Cultural Interpretation of Canonical Paradox: Lay Meditation in a Central Thai Village.*

Wall, Lewis. (1988) *Hausa Medicine: Illness and Well-Being in a West African Culture.*

Wallace, Anthony F. C. (1972) *The Death and Rebirth of the Seneca.*

Watts, Alan. (1957) *The Way of Zen.*

Weil, Andrew. (1983) *Health and Healing: Understanding Conventional and Alternative Medicine.*

Weiss, Gaea, and Shandor Weiss. (1992) *Growing & Using the Healing Herbs.*

Weltfish, Gene. (1965) *The Lost Universe: With a Closing Chapter on the Universe Regained.*

Whiting, John W. M. (1967) "Sorcery, Sin and the Superego: A Cross-Cultural Study of Some Mechanisms of Social Control." In *Cross-Cultural Approaches*, edited by Clelland S. Ford, 147–168.

Williamson, Marianne. (1994) *Illuminata.*

Winkelman, Michael. (1986) "Magico-Religious Practitioner Types and Socioeconomic Conditions." *Behavior Science Research* 20: 17–46.

———. (1990) "Shaman and Other 'Magico-Religious' Healers: A Cross-Cultural Study of Their Origins, Nature, and Social Transformations." *Ethos* 18: 308–352.

Winzeler, Robert L. (1991) "Latah Is Sarawak, with Special Reference to the Iban." In *Female and Male in Borneo: Contributions and Challenges to Gender Studies,* edited by Vinson H. Sutlive, Jr., 317–333.

Wolf, Margery. (1972) *Women and the Family in Rural Taiwan.*

Woodham, Anne. (1994) *HEA Guide to Complementary Medicine and Therapies.*

Yalman, Nur. (1971) *Under the Bo Tree: Studies in Caste, Kinship, and Marriage in the Interior of Ceylon.*

Yamamoto, Shizuko, and Patrick McCarthy. (1993) *Whole Health Shiatsu.*

Yogananda, P. (1946) *Autobiography of a Yogi.*

Young, Allan L. (1971) *Medical Beliefs and Practices of the Begemder Amhara.*

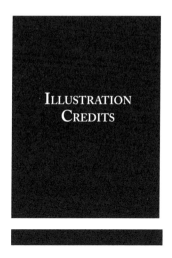

ILLUSTRATION CREDITS

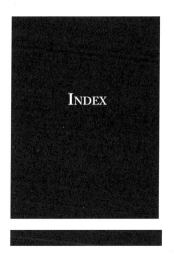

INDEX

.